MW00838137

AMERICAN
MEDICAL
ASSOCIATION

AMA Guides™
to the
Evaluation of Work Ability and Return to Work

Second Edition

James B. Talmage, MD
J Mark Melhorn, MD
Mark H. Hyman, MD

American Medical Association
Chicago, Illinois

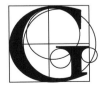

Executive Vice President, Chief Executive Officer: Michael D. Maves, MD, MBA
Chief Operating Officer: Bernard L. Hengesbaugh
Senior Vice President, Publishing and Business Services: Robert A. Musacchio, PhD
Vice President, Business Operations: Vanessa Hayden
Vice President, AMA Publications and Clinical Solutions: Mary Lou White
Manager, Book and Product Development and Production: Nancy Baker
Senior Developmental Editor: Michael Ryder
Production Specialist: Meghan Anderson
Director, Sales Marketing & Strategic Relationships: Joann Skiba
Director of Sales, Business Products: Mark Daniels
Manager, Marketing and Strategic Planning: Erin Kalitowski
Marketing Manager: Lauren Jones

Copyright 2011 by the American Medical Association. All rights reserved.
Printed in the United States of America

No part of this publication may be reproduced, stored in a retrieval system, or transmitted, in any form or
by any means electronic, mechanical, photocopying, recording, or otherwise, without the prior written
permission of the publisher.

Internet address: www.ama-assn.org

The American Medical Association ("AMA") and its authors and editors have consulted sources believed
to be knowledgeable in their fields. However, neither the AMA nor its authors or editors warrant that the
information is in every respect accurate and/or complete. The AMA, its authors, and editors assume no
responsibility for use of the information contained in this publication. Neither the AMA, its authors or editors shall be responsible for, and expressly disclaims liability for, damages of any kind arising out of the use
of, reference to, or reliance on, the content of this publication. This publication is for informational purposes
only. The AMA does not provide medical, legal, financial or other professional advice and readers are
encouraged to consult a professional advisor for such advice.

The contents of this publication represent the views of the author[s] and should not be construed to be the
views or policy of the AMA, or of the institution with which the author[s] may be affiliated, unless this is
clearly specified.

Additional copies of this book may be ordered by calling 800 621-8335 or from the secure AMA Web site
at www.amastore.com. Refer to product number OP324011.

Library of Congress Cataloging-in-Publication Data

AMA guides to the evaluation of work ability and return to work / [edited by] James B. Talmage, J. Mark
Melhorn, Mark H. Hyman. — 2nd ed.
   p. ; cm.
   Guides to the evaluation of work ability and return to work
   Rev. ed. of: A physician's guide to return to work / editors, James B. Talmage, J. Mark Melhorn. c2005.
   Includes bibliographical references and index.
   Summary: "This book will help the reader think through helping patients with return-to-work decisions
when persisting symptoms and problems from illness or injury make work difficult"—Provided by publisher.

ISBN 978-1-60359-530-8

   1. Work capacity evaluation—United States. 2. Disability evaluation--United States. 3. Vocational
rehabilitation—United States. 4. Workers' compensation—United States. 5. Work—Psychological aspects.
6. Convalescence—Psychological aspects. I. Talmage, James B. II. Melhorn, J. Mark. III. Hyman, Mark H.
IV. American Medical Association. V. Title: Guides to the evaluation of work ability and return to work.
   [DNLM: 1. Rehabilitation—psychology. 2. Convalescence—psychology. 3. Disability Evaluation.
4. Employment—psychology. WB 320]
   RC963.4.P48 2011
   616.07'5—dc22   2011010018

22 23 24 / PG-MG / 9 8 7 6 5 4

BP05:08/22

Dedication

This book is dedicated to my parents, George and Helen Talmage, who taught me the importance of a strong work ethic, and to my wife, Jill, and daughter, Heidi, who love me despite it.

Jim Talmage

This book is dedicated to my patients who taught me the benefits and value of work and to my family who have enriched my life while allowing me the opportunity to share this knowledge with others.

J. Mark Melhorn

This book is dedicated to my two families—the one at home and the one at work: Sheryl, Ari, Micah, Jesse, Noah, Joan, Susan, Erika, Pam, and Gabriella.

Mark Hyman

Acknowledgments

For help in the creation of this book I would like to thank Richard A. Hoffmeister, MD, and Sam T. Barnes, MD, who taught me how to think "like an orthopedist"; John LoCasio, MD, who first introduced me to the concepts of risk, capacity, and tolerance; and my patients over the past 39 years, who taught me about the human experiences of life and work.

James B. Talmage

For help in the creation of this book I would like to thank Henry O. Marsh, MD, and Herbert H. Stark, MD, who contributed to my development as an occupational orthopaedic hand surgeon; Peggy Gardner, PhD, who nurtured my interest in researching the prevention of work-related musculoskeletal pain; the medical librarians at Via Christi Regional Medical and Wesley Medical Center, who continue to obtain references for me; and my office staff at The Hand Center, who help to communicate the message to my patients about the benefits of staying at work and early return to work.

J. Mark Melhorn

We would like to thank Michael Ryder, Senior Development Editor at AMA Press, and Meghan Anderson, Production Specialist, at AMA Press, who assisted us in the production of this book. We would like to acknowledge, for the use of their materials, ACOEM Guidelines, the Reed Group and MDG, and Official Disability Guidelines.

James B. Talmage, J. Mark Melhorn, Mark H. Hyman

Contributors

Karen (Edinger) Belkić, MD, PhD
Adjunct Professor of Preventive Medicine Physician Specialist in
Internal Medicine

Department of Oncology-Pathology
Karolinska Institute, Stockholm, Sweden

School of Community and Global Health
Claremont Graduate University, Claremont, California

Institute for Health Promotion & Disease Prevention Research University of
Southern California School of Medicine, Los Angeles, California

Gina Bruns, MA
American University
Washington, DC

David J. DePaolo, JD, MBA
CEO, President
WorkCompCentral
Camarillo, CA

Dwight K Dowda, MB, BS, MPH
Consultant Occupational Physician
Sydney—Australia

Marjorie Eskay-Auerbach, MD, JD
SpineCare & Forensic Medicine, PLLC
Tucson, AZ

Michael Feuerstein, PhD, MPH
Professor
Departments of Medical and Clinical Psychology and Preventive Medicine
and Biometrics Uniformed Services University of the Health Sciences
Bethesda MD

Elizabeth Genovese MD MBA (posthumous)

Douglas P. Gross, PhD, BScPT
Associate Professor, Department of Physical Therapy
University of Alberta
Edmonton, Alberta

Kurt T. Hegmann MD, MPH
Department of Family & Preventive Medicine
University of Utah
Salt Lake City, UT

Philip Harber, MD, MPH
Professor Emeritus, UCLA
Former Chief, Division of Occupational and Environmental Medicine

Jawali Jaranilla, MD, MPH
Internal Medicine-Hospitalist
HealthPartners Medical Group & Clinics

Les Kertay, PhD
AVP and Medical Director, Lincoln Financial Group

Edwin H. Klimek, MD
Private practice (neurology), St. Catherines

Cynthia W. Ko, MD, MS
Associate Professor
Department of Medicine/Division of Gastroenterology
University of Washington.

Thomas E. Kottke, MD, MSPH
Consulting Cardiologist, HealthPartners Medical Group
Medical Director for Evidence-Based Health, HealthPartners
Senior Clinical Investigator, HealthPartners Research Foundation

Randall Lea, MD
Center of Orthopedic Care and Evaluative Medicine
Baton Rouge, Louisiana

Clement Leech, MD
Chief Medical Advisor
Department of Social Protection
Government of Ireland

David Linklater, MD, MBA
Medical Manager
WCB Alberta

Douglas Martin, MD
Director
St. Luke's Occupational Health Service
Sioux City, SD

Michael P. Porter, MD
Associate Professor, Urology Section,
VA Puget Sound Health Care System, Seattle, WA
Department of Urology, University of Washington, Seattle WA

James R. Rainville, MD
Physical Medicine & Rehabilitation
New England Baptist Hospital
Boston, MA

Michiel F. Reneman, PhD, PT
Department of Rehabilitation Medicine, Center for Rehabilitation,
University Medical Center Groningen
University of Groningen

Shirley M. Seaman, PA-C
The Hand Center
Wichita, KS

David Silver, MD
Associate Clinical Professor of Medicine, UCLA School of Medicine
Former Clinical Chief of Rheumatology, Cedars Sinai Medical Center

Stuart Silverman, MD
Medical Director, Bone Center of Excellence
Cedars-Sinai Medical Center
Clinical Professor of Medicine, David Geffen UCLA School of Medicine

Joel Steinberg, MD
Assistant Clinical Professor of Medicine and of Psychiatry, Case Western
Reserve Univ. School of Medicine
Willoughby, OH

Jong Uk Won, MD, Dr.PH
Dept. of Preventive Medicine, Yonsei Univ. College of Medicine
Institute for Occupational Health

Anjel Vahratian, PhD, MPH
Assistant Professor
Department of Obstetrics and Gynecology
The University of Michigan at Ann Arbor

Christopher J. Welty, MD
Department of Urology, University of Washington, Seattle WA

Table of Contents

Reviewers

Bruce Gruberman, MD
Huntington, West Virginia

LuAnn Haley, JD
Tucson, Arizona

Richard T. Katz, MD
St. Louis, Missouri

Henry Jules Roth, MD
Denver, Colorado

E. Randolph Soo Hoo, MD, MPH, FACOEM
Tucson, Arizona

David B. Torrey, AB, JD
Pittsburgh, Pennsylvania

Preface to the Second Edition

The Second Edition of *AMA Guides*™ *to the Evaluation of Work Ability and Return to Work* is supported by an incremental increase in evidence-based science regarding return to work. Since the first edition, many individuals have provided suggestions and materials that have been incorporated into this new edition. The editors encourage future communications and suggestions.

The editors wish to thank the chapter authors and the many individuals who have contributed to this edition. This book is dedicated to their day-to-day efforts to improve the quality of life for injured patients.

Preface to the First Edition

Work. For most individuals, work is part of what gives life meaning and purpose, as well as what provides the income for life's necessities—food, shelter, clothing, and medical care. *A Physician's Guide to Return to Work* is designed to help employees (ill and injured workers), employers, administrative staff, legal and legislative bodies, and healthcare providers understand the importance of staying at work or appropriate early return to work.

A Physician's Guide to Return to Work approaches return-to-work issues from the healthcare provider's point of view, because the healthcare provider is often looked to by the other parties for guidance. Science is the standard to which the healthcare provider looks for answers. This book is based on the science but also provides insight into the art of medicine as it applies to the dilemmas encountered when patients ask, "Can I work despite my [*fill in the blank*]?"

An etymological analysis of several of the languages of Europe reveals that *work* means "worry, trouble, and/or toil." The French word, *travailler,* was derived from the Latin, *tripotium,* or "feared instrument of torture."[1] Yet, work for man is necessary (see Chapter 1). If the reader is a believer in the theory of evolution, man has evolved while working over eons. Work is part of the environment to which man has adapted. Taking work away from man is thus like placing penguins at the equator. If the reader is a creationist, man was created to work, or perhaps work was created for man by a benevolent God.[2,3] Thus, either way, man has been intertwined with work since the beginning of time.

The editors and authors of this text have the firm belief, supported by science and consensus, that work is good for man,[1] and that it is the physician's role to encourage work and return to work, as part of treatment.[4–7]

Many brief work absences occur due to minor illness or minor injury. On a daily basis physicians deal with requests for work-absence certification for such events. According to Canadian Medical Association policy, absences for five or fewer days should not need physician certification of disability, and such certification is inappropriate retrospectively (the physician must have attended to the patient for the illness or have satisfactory knowledge of such illness).[8]

This book is not about minor, brief illness or injury. This is a text dedicated to the problem of long-term medical certification of disability by physicians. Despite the fact that work in developed nations is getting progressively easier due to automation, ergonomics, and labor legislation, and despite the disappearance of diseases such as polio and improvements in medical care, the rate of medical disability certification in working-age adults is increasing dramatically, and faster than the population is increasing.[9,10] This book is about how physicians can help patients by thinking through the issues of "risk," "capacity," and "tolerance" when return-to-work decision making occurs in the context of persistent problems from illness or injury.

Disability can be viewed in many ways. These include at least a biomedical model, a biopsychosocial model, and a naturalistic sociolegal model.[11] Less than severe illness or injury with alleged disability conforms much better to the biopsychosocial model than to the biomedical model. However, employers, disability insurers, and the United States Social Security Administration all utilize a biomedical model for disability assessment, assuming that impairment or pathology equates to work capacity and risk. Thus far Hadler[12] has been the clearest voice calling for logic and compassion to change the current Western way of thinking about disability. Until Western society changes the "system," physicians caring for patients will be forced to use the biomedical model. As such, this book uses the biomedical model to think through return-to-work issues based on this current general acceptance of the biomedical model.

Return to work is not a subject about which physicians have received extensive training in their medical educations. Patients, employers, and disability insurers believe physicians have the necessary knowledge and experience to scientifically answer disability certification questions. The employers and insurers who have developed forms for physician documentation of disability certification may not realize that few physicians have had any formal training in such certification. There are organizations teaching these principles at physician Continuing Medical Education (CME) meetings.

The authors of the chapters in this book are all practicing physicians (except Chapter 8, which was written by lawyers) who face these issues on a frequent basis. Many are involved in teaching disability evaluation to physicians in CME conferences. Some chapter authors think and write with a "workers' compensation mindset," while others think and write with a "long term disability insurance mindset." While the term they use for the patient may differ (either *injured worker*, *patient*, or *disability applicant*), the approach they advocate is consistent.

A Physician's Guide to Return to Work is a text, and not a systematic review. On many disability certification issues, there is little pertinent scientific literature. Wherever possible, the authors have included and cited relevant medical literature.

This book does not cover all body systems. Each chapter on a body system discusses only a few common problems to teach the thought process of assessing risk, capacity, and tolerance. Examples of consensus-defined disability durations are included. There are more extensive texts on appropriate disability durations for individual illnesses and injuries.[13–15] Of the three most commonly used texts, the editors[*] chose to include data from *The Medical Disability Advisor*, based on the fact that the MDA includes data from physician-coded *International Classification of Diseases, Ninth Revision, Clinical Modification* (ICD-9-CM) diagnoses, and based on the need to keep this text brief. For help with the many conditions not discussed in this text, the reader is referred to these three excellent texts.[13–15]

A Physician's Guide to Return to Work attempts to describe a methodology for physicians to use to think through return-to-work issues based on risk, capacity, and tolerance. Relevant scientific literature, consensus documents, and "common sense" are the tools available. This text is meant to be read "cover to cover," as the material in the later chapters assumes the reader has read the beginning chapters.

Every patient is unique, and must be evaluated by a physician intimately familiar with that patient's condition and co-morbidities. Medicine is both an art and a science. There is no guarantee that an individual will not be re-injured or sustain a new injury if he or she chooses to return to work with, or despite, physician recommendations.

In the final analysis, return-to-work decisions are always those of the patient and his or her employer. The physician's role is merely one of advisor. The advice for a particular patient must come from the physician who knows intimately the unique aspects of the patient's illness or injury, co-morbidities, and personality.

In light of ongoing research and changes in clinical experience and in governmental regulations, readers are encouraged to confirm the information contained herein with additional sources.

---

[*]James B. Talmage, MD, was a paid contributor to *The Medical Disability Advisor*, 3rd and 4th editions and is currently on the Advisory Board of the Official Disability Guidelines (ODG). J. Mark Melhorn, MD, is on the Advisory Board of the ODG, and will be involved in future editions of *The Medical Disability Advisor*. Neither was involved in the *American College of Occupational and Environmental Medicine's Occupational Medicine Practice Guidelines, 2nd Edition*.

References

1. Nordin M. 2000 International society for the study of the lumbar spine presidential address: back to work—some reflections. *Spine*. 2001;26:851–856.

2. Genesis 2:15.

3. Genesis 3:17.

4. Canadian Medical Association. *CMA Policy: The Physician's Role in Helping Patients Return to Work After an Illness or Injury (Update 2000)*. Available at: www.cma.ca/multimedia/staticContent/HTML/N0/l2/where_we_stand/return_to_work.pdf. Accessed May 21, 2004.

5. American College of Occupational and Environmental Medicine. *ACOEM Consensus Opinion Statement: The Attending Physician's Role in Helping Patients Return to Work after an Illness or Injury*. Available at: www.acoem.org/guidelines/pdf/Return-to-Work-04-02.pdf. Accessed May 21, 2004.

6. American Academy of Orthopaedic Surgeons. *AAOS Position Statement: Early Return to Work Programs*. Available at: www.aaos.org/wordhtml/papers/position/1150.htm. Accessed May 21, 2004.

7. American Medical Association. *Report 12 of the Council on Scientfic Affairs (A-04) Full Text*. Available at: www.ama-assn.org/ama/pub/article/print/2036-8668.html. Accessed May 24, 2004.

8. Canadian Medical Association. *CMA Policy: Certificate of Disability*. Available at: www.cma.ca/index.cfm/ci_id/3212/la_id/1.htm. Accessed May 24, 2004.

9. Waddell G, Aylward M, Sawney P. *Back Pain, Incapacity for Work and Social Security Benefits: An International Literature Review and Analysis*. London, England: The Royal Society of Medicine Press, Ltd; 2002.

10. Leopold RS. *A Year in the Life of a Million American Workers*. New York, NY: Metropolitan Life Insurance Company; 2003.

11. Halligan PW, Bass C, Oakley DA. Willful deception as illness behavior. In: Halligan PW, Bass C, Oakley DA. *Malingering and Illness Deception*. New York, NY: Oxford University Press, Inc; 2003.

12. Hadler NM. *Occupational Musculoskeletal Disorders*. 2nd Ed. Philadelphia, Pa: Lippincott, Williams, & Wilkins; 1999.

13. Reed P. *The Medical Disability Advisor: Workplace Guidelines for Disability Duration*. 5th ed. Westminster, Colo: Reed Group, Ltd; 2005.

14. Denniston P, ed. *Official Disability Guidelines*. 9th ed. Encinitas, Calif: Work Loss Data Institute; 2004.

15. Glass L, ed. *American College of Occupational and Environmental Medicine: Occupational Medicine Practice Guidelines*. 2nd ed. Beverly Farms, Mass; 2004.

Why Staying at Work or Returning to Work Is in the Patient's Best Interest

**James B. Talmage, MD, J. Mark Melhorn, MD
and Mark Hyman, MD**

No other technique for the conduct of life attaches the individual so firmly to reality as laying emphasis on work; for his work at least gives him a secure place in a portion of reality, in the human community.

—Sigmund Freud[1]

An unemployed existence is a worse negation of life than death itself. Because to live means to have something definite to do—a mission to fulfill—and in the measure in which we avoid setting our life to something, we make it empty. … Human life, by its very nature, has to be dedicated to something.

—Josè Ortega y Gasset[1]

Without work all life goes rotten.

—Albert Camus[1]

Work is not man's punishment. It is his reward and his strength and his pleasure.

—George Sand[2]

Philosophers and psychiatrists have grasped the central importance of work to human existence. This book will help the reader think through helping patients with return-to-work decisions when persisting symptoms and problems from illness or injury make work difficult. This chapter is devoted to why physicians should encourage early and ultimate return to work whenever possible. Simply stated: it is usually in the patient's best interest to remain in the workforce.

There are serious injuries and illnesses that clearly leave patients unable to engage in any meaningful work activity. In these circumstances, the severity of the impairments is objectively obvious, and Western society has provided the protection of a "social security disability" safety net. The chapters that deal with specific body systems refer to the US Social Security Administration's criteria for such severe and disabling conditions. Other developed countries typically have similar criteria in somewhat similar systems. This type of social support system is typically absent in third world countries.

This book focuses on the less obvious and less severe illness and injury situations in which many patients with similar problems work, and yet some patients consult with physicians seeking medical information to support a disability application. In these cases the disability is not obvious, and patients, employers, and disability insurers may request information from treating physicians and from "second opinion" physicians or independent medical examiners. In cases in which there is neither obvious severe disability nor obvious major pathology (and thus returning to work is clearly indicated), what weight should be given to the benefits of patients returning to work?

US Social Security Administration data from 2008 show that from 1978 to 2006 the US population increased by 35%, yet the number of Americans on government funded disability increased by 236%.[3] These "disabled" Americans were not primarily those dying of cancer or awaiting heart transplants, but rather were primarily middle-aged folks with common health conditions. Most of these were individuals with musculoskeletal disorders. Thus the majority of this disability would seem to be preventable.

Consensus Statements

In the introduction to this book, the consensus statements of the Canadian Medical Association,[4] the American College of Occupational and Environmental Medicine,[5] and the American Academy of Orthopaedic Surgeons[6] were introduced. All three documents strongly recommend that physicians return patients to their usual work roles as soon as possible.

Prolonged absence from one's normal roles, including absence from the workplace, is detrimental to a person's mental, physical, and social well-being. Physicians should therefore encourage a patient's return to function and work as soon as possible after an illness or injury.[4]

> ... medically related withdrawal from normal social roles, including work, is destabilizing and may be detrimental to a patient's mental, physical, and social well-being; maintaining or returning a patient to all possible relevant life activities as soon as is safely possible has many beneficial psychosocial and physical effects ...[5]

The American Academy of Orthopaedic Surgeons and the American Association of Orthopaedic Surgeons (AAOS) support safe, early return-to-work programs that help injured workers improve their performance, regain functionality, and enhance their quality of life. ... As patient advocates, physicians realize that early return to work results in many benefits for the injured worker, including the prevention of deconditioning and the psychological sequels of prolonged time off work.[6]

At its summer 2004 meeting, the American Medical Association (AMA) adopted its version of this policy statement:

> The AMA encourages physicians everywhere to advise their patients to return to work at the earliest date compatible with health and safety and recognizes that physicians can, through their care, facilitate patients' return to work.[7]

A similar statement was published by the United Kingdom Department of Work and Pensions:

> As a certifying doctor you will need to consider and manage your patient's expectations in relation to their ability to continue working. In summary, you should always bear in mind that a patient may not be well served in the longer term by medical advice to refrain from work, if more appropriate clinical management would allow them to stay in work or return to work.[8]

Physicians are familiar with prescribing medications for patients. If a physician looked up a drug in the Physician's Desk Reference[9] and found a "black box" warning required by the Food and Drug Administration (FDA) like this one:

> **Warning:** This drug is detrimental to your patient's mental, physical, and social well-being.

would physicians prescribe that medication?

Physicians should have the same mind-set when filling out return-to-work forms as when about to prescribe a medication with the above black box warning.

What is the science behind the consensus statements by these organizations? Is it really true that being out of work is hazardous to one's health?

A Review of the Literature

A 1995 review from Canada of 46 original articles concluded that, on an epidemiologic basis, unemployment has a strong positive association with many adverse health outcomes.[10] Despite a reduction in mortality from motor vehicle accidents, unemployment was positively associated with increased overall mortality and with mortality from cardiovascular disease and suicide. Workers laid off because of factory closure have more symptoms and objectively validated illnesses and are more likely to take medication and be hospitalized.

A 1996 review concluded that unemployment is pathogenic, with increased mortality and decreased physical and mental health.[11] The most common documented disorders were emotional and cardiopulmonary disease. A 1998 review from Australia concluded that unemployment itself is detrimental to health and that it is associated with increasing mortality rates, causes physical and mental illness, and results in a greater use of health services.[12]

Three large studies add to the certainty of these conclusions. Nylen and Floderus[13] reported in 2001 from the Swedish Twin Registry data on all-cause mortality in 9500 women and 11132 men followed from 1973 to 1996. Unemployment was associated with a relative risk of mortality of 1.98 (95% confidence interval [CI] 1.16–3.38) for women and of 1.43 (95% CI 0.91–2.25) for men, even when controlled for potential social, behavioral, work, and health-related confounders.

Quaade et al.[14] reported in 2002 on the effect of early retirement. Some retire early because they are ill with serious disease(s), but what is the subsequent health status of those who are financially able to retire early while apparently healthy? This study utilized the Danish population-based register of individuals born between 1926 and 1936 who were evaluated from 1986 to 1996. Those who continued to work had the lowest mortality. Those who were retired because of disease or injury disability had the highest mortality. Those who were well, but were able to choose an "early" retirement, had an intermediate mortality rate, consistent with an adverse effect on health of retirement itself.

In 2003, Gerdtham and Johannesson[15] described the mortality experience of 30000 Swedes followed for 10 to 17 years, concluding that unemployment increased the risk of death by nearly 50% (from 5.36% to 7.83%).

There are also reviews showing the effects of unemployment on specific diseases such as cancer and heart disease.[16–18] A study of 24,036 Swedes with complete employment records from biennial national Swedish Work Environment Surveys from 1989 to 1999 confirmed that unemployment due to employer downsizing was associated with health risks.[19]

A similar study found increased rates of cardiovascular disease in Americans who became unemployed when their company relocated to a foreign country.[18]

A study of employees of Shell Oil in Texas[20] and of Greeks[21] found similar increases in mortality among the unemployed. In the Greek study, a 5-year delay in retirement was associated with a 10% decrease in mortality (95% CI = 4 to 15).

A review of 5 Swedish studies had the same conclusion:

> Subjects with a disability pension had increased mortality rates as compared with non-retired subjects, only modestly affected by adjustments for psycho-socio-economic factors, underlying disease, etcetera. It is unlikely that these factors were the causes of the unfavorable outcome. Other factors must be at work. [Unemployment itself is a toxin.][22]

Barth and Roth[23] published a review of some of the pertinent articles on the mental health effects of unemployment.

Waddell and Burton have published a 257-page systematic review of studies on the effects of unemployment on health and concluded that work meets important personal goals (material well-being, psychosocial needs, identity, etc) and that there is strong evidence that unemployment is harmful to health (higher mortality, poorer physical and mental health, increased health care utilization). There is also strong evidence that re-employment leads to improved self-esteem, physical health, and mental health.

Thus, there is sound science indicating that unemployment is hazardous to a patient's physical, mental, and social well-being. As patient advocates, physicians therefore should strongly urge patients to return to work or to stay at work and should decline to certify disability unless it is obvious. Ethically, in these cases, beneficence trumps autonomy.

References

1. Peter LJ. Peter's Quotations: Ideas for Our Time. New York, NY: Bantam Books; 1977.

2. http://www.finestquotes.com/select_quote-category-Work-page-1.htm. Accessed January 15, 2011.

3. http://www.socialsecurity.gov/policy/docs/statcomps/ssi_asr/2008/. Accessed October 21, 2010.

4. Canadian Medical Association. CMA policy: the physician's role in helping patients return to work after an illness or injury (Update 2000). Available at: www.cma.ca/multimedia/staticContent/HTML/N0/l2/where_we_stand/return_to_work.pdf. Accessed May 21, 2004.

5. American College of Occupational and Environmental Medicine. ACOEM policies & position statements: the personal physician's role in helping patients with medical conditions stay at work or return to work. (2008) Available at: http://www.acoem.org/guidelines.aspx?id=5460. Accessed 10/21/2010.

6. American Academy of Orthopaedic Surgeons. AAOS position statement: early return to work programs. Available at: www.aaos.org/wordhtml/papers/position/1150.htm. Accessed May 21, 2004.

7. American Medical Association. Report 12 of the council on scientific affairs (A-04) full text: physician's guidelines for return to work after injury or illness. Available at: www.ama-assn.org/ama/pub/article/print/2036-8668.html. Accessed June 24, 2004.

8. Medical evidence for Statutory Sick Pay. Statutory Maternity Pay and Social Security Incapacity Benefit purposes. A Guide for Registered Medical Practitioners. http://www.dwp.gov.uk/medical/medicalib204/ib204-june04/ib204.pdf. Accessed January 15, 2011.

9. Physician's Desk Reference. 58th ed. Montvale, NJ: Medical Economics Co, Inc; 2004.

10. Jin RL, Shah CP, Svoboda TJ. The impact of unemployment on health: a review of the evidence. *CMAJ*. 1995;153:529–540.

11. Shortt SE. Is unemployment pathogenic? A review of current concepts with lessons for policy planners. *Int J Health Serv*. 1996;26:569–589.

12. Mathers CD, Schofield DJ. The health consequences of unemployment: the evidence. *Med J Aust*. 1998;168:178–182.

13. Nylen L, Floderus B. Mortality among women and men relative to unemployment, part time work, overtime work, and extra work: a study based on data from the Swedish Twin Registry. *Occup Environ Med*. 2001;58:52–57.

14. Quaade T, Enghlom G, Johansen AM, et al. Mortality in relation to early retirement: a population-based study. *Scand J Public Health*. 2002;30:216–222.

15. Gerdtham UG, Johannesson M. A note on the effect of unemployment on mortality. *J Health Econ*. 2003;22:505–518.

16. Lynge EI. Unemployment and cancer: a literature review. In: Kogavinas M, Oearce N, Boffetta P, eds. Social Inequalities and Cancer. Lyon, France: International Agency for Research on Cancer; 1997. IARC Scientific Publications No. 138.

Chapter 1

17. Brenner MH. Heart disease mortality and economic changes; including unemployment; in Western Germany 1951–1989. *Acta Physiol Scand Suppl.* 1997;640:149–152.

18. Gallo WT, Bradley EH, Falba TA, et al. Involuntary job loss as a risk factor for subsequent myocardial infarction and stroke: findings from the Health and Retirement Survey. *Am J Indust Med.* 2004;45:408–416.

19. Westerlund H, Ferrie J, Hagbert J, et al. Workplace expansion, long-term sickness, absence, and hospital admission. *Lancet.* 2004;363:1193–1197.

20. S P Tsai et al. Age at retirement and long term survival of an individual industrial population: prospective cohort study. *British Medical Journal.* 2005;331:995–997.

21. C Bamia, et al. Age at retirement and mortality in a general population sample. *Am J Epidem.* 2008;167(5):561–569.

22. Wallman et al. The prognosis for individuals on disability retirement: an 18-year mortality follow-up study of 6887 men and women sampled from the general population. *BMC Public Health* 2006;6:103. doi:10.1186/1471-2458-6-103.

23. Barth RJ, Roth VS. Health benefits of returning to work: review of the literature. *Occup Environ Med Rep.* 2003;17:13–17.

24. http://www.workingforhealth.gov.uk/documents/is-work-good-for-you.pdf. Accessed October 21, 2010.

Chapter 2

How to Think About Work Ability and Work Restrictions: Risk, Capacity, and Tolerance

James B. Talmage, MD, J. Mark Melhorn, MD and Mark Hyman, MD

> "It is the working man who is the happy man. It is the idle man who is the miserable man."

> "The Constitution only gives people the right to *persue* happiness. You have to catch it yourself."

> Benjamin Franklin, quoted in the *Nashville Tennessean*, Section D, page 1, January 15, 2011

Chapter 1 reviewed the consensus documents and scientific literature indicating that it is generally in the patient's best interest to remain at work or return to work. For worker illness, physicians are usually asked for medical information and work status certification. Physicians cooperate with these tasks by completing forms describing what patients can or cannot do at work. While physicians are well trained in diagnosis and treatment, most have received little or no training in how to evaluate their patient's work ability. Whenever asked about a patient's work ability, physicians should think through the issues by considering three terms: *risk, capacity*, and *tolerance*.

Risk

Risk refers to the chance of harm to the patient, co-workers, or to the general public, if the patient engages in specific work activities. One familiar example is the Department of Transportation's medical certification processes requiring examining physicians to disqualify individuals with uncontrolled seizure disorders from working as aircraft pilots and as commercial motor vehicle drivers. When patients should *not* attempt certain work activities because of known risk, this is clearly the basis for physician-imposed "work restrictions." A *work restriction* is something a patient can do, but should not do, as opposed to a *work limitation*, which is defined later in this chapter (under "capacity") as something the patient cannot physically do. The terms *work restriction* and *work limitation* are frequently seen on work status certification forms.

Unfortunately, there is little scientific literature on the real-world observed risks of working despite known medical conditions. Ideally, this would be the type of information on which to base work restrictions. Where generally accepted sound scientific evidence exists, there should logically be universal agreement among physicians about the issue in question. Sometimes, there are consensus documents that are helpful in assigning work restrictions based on risk. One example is the American College of Cardiology guidelines for physicians in approving participation in competitive sports.[1] While this is a consensus document, and thus not scientifically proven, following these guidelines is our best approach to achieve consistency among physicians. In the chapters in this book that deal with specific organ systems (Chapters 11–23), each author discusses the existing scientific studies on the risk of working as they relate to that organ system.

If a patient or examinee is applying for work, the US physician performing the pre-placement medical examination for the employer must remember that the Americans with Disabilities Act of 1990 permits the employer to deny the tentatively offered employment *only if*, on the basis of objective information, the work activities of the "essential job functions" pose a substantial risk of significant harm to self or others that is imminent. Under this law, these criteria would be the basis for physician-imposed work restrictions that would disqualify an applicant from working. Jurisdictions in other countries may have similar laws or rules.

Substantial harm means an objectively verifiable worsening in the patient's condition, and not merely an increase in previously present symptoms, like pain or fatigue. This US law says that individuals may choose to work despite pain or fatigue. While physicians in pre-placement examinations generally remember and adhere to the maxim that "if there is not objective evidence of substantial risk of significant harm, the patient may choose whether or not to work despite symptoms," many times the obverse of this principle is forgotten when physicians are asked by patients to certify work disability based on subjective symptoms (tolerance) without evidence of risk of harm. If seeking work despite symptoms is the patient's decision (and not the physician's decision) when the patient is a willing job applicant, logically *the decision is still the patient's* when the patient is requesting disability certification.

There are recurring situations in which physicians have historically restricted patients on the basis of medically plausible risk assessment. Examples include heavy overhead lifting after shoulder rotator cuff repair and heavy lifting, carrying, and jumping in the presence of combined knee anterior and medial instability. In these cases, it is plausible to argue that recurrent cuff rupture or progressive knee osteoarthritis may occur, despite the lack of prospective human studies to prove real, quantifiable risks. Until studies disprove these risks, they will be "generally accepted" and noted by consensus groups.

For decades, spine surgeons placed permanent lifting and other activity restrictions on patients who had good results after a first-operation lumbar diskectomy. Recently, studies have shown that those with good results can return quickly to full work with no increase in the incidence of disk re-rupture.[2,3]

Capacity

Capacity refers to concepts such as strength, flexibility, and endurance. These are measurable with a fair degree of scientific precision. Actually, "capacity" indicates that the individual is already maximally trained and fully acclimated to the job or activity in question. Thus, an athlete trained and ready to run a marathon and a worker accustomed to a heavy construction labor job may function at near "capacity." This current level of fitness can be quantified.

Physicians most often deal with an individual's *current ability*. Current ability can increase with exercise and activity, or it can decrease with inactivity. The aphorism "use it or lose it" summarizes the concept that the cardiopulmonary and musculoskeletal systems are affected by activity level. Current ability may increase up to capacity with exercise. This exercise may be rehabilitative exercise, recreational exercise, or even progressively more difficult work activity. Current ability may decrease with inactivity (deconditioning), and the effects of a sedentary lifestyle on exercise ability are well known.

The individual with a rotator cuff tear in the shoulder who can not raise his arm high enough to reach the overhead controls of a factory press is an example of lack of capacity. Another is the individual with heart disease who can exercise only to 4 METs (metabolic equivalents) on a treadmill before she reaches her maximal predicted heart rate, and who thus cannot return to a job that requires frequent 6 MET exertion. While physicians *impose* work restrictions (proscribe certain activities), physicians *describe* work limitations (what the patient is not physically able to do).

There are situations in which a patient lacks the "current ability" for specific work activities. If lifting 100 pounds is required, a significant percentage of the population will not have this ability. However, many, but not all, can acquire this ability with an exercise training program. Physicians are often asked to certify whether a patient has the "current ability" to perform certain work tasks (or perhaps the misnomer "capacity" appears on the form). Sometimes it is objectively obvious whether or not the patient has the ability in question. Many times the physician has no objective way to decide whether the patient does or does not have the current ability to do a task. This is the scenario in which a functional capacity evaluation (FCE) test is frequently ordered. (Chapter 6 reviews the reliability and validity of this testing in detail.) The term *functional capacity evaluation* is a misnomer in that it tells the physician whether or not, on the day of testing, the patient was or was not willing to demonstrate the "current ability" to do a job or job tasks. Unless the individual is already trained to maximal ability, it does not measure capacity. It usually reflects tolerance for symptoms, and not necessarily current ability.

If there are no scientific data on risk, and if it is not objectively obvious that the patient lacks the current ability to do certain job tasks, then whether he or she will work is usually a question of tolerance.

Tolerance

Background

Tolerance is a psychophysiologic concept. It is the ability to tolerate sustained work or activity at a given level. Symptoms such as pain and/or fatigue are what limit the ability to do the task(s) in question. The patient may have the ability to do a certain task (no work limitation) but not the ability to do it comfortably. Thus, tolerance is not scientifically measurable or verifiable. Tolerance is frequently less than either capacity or current ability.

Tolerance is dependent on the rewards available for doing the activity in question. Tolerance is exemplified when an individual chooses, because of pain, not to work for minimum wage at a job he dislikes, but, when offered a much more physically demanding job at three or four times minimum wage, he happily works and endures (tolerates) even greater pain. This confirms that tolerance is not scientifically measurable and explains why different physicians seeing the same individual will often find it difficult to agree on issues relating to tolerance.

When a patient describes his or her activity tolerances, a physician may feel that this should be the basis for physician-imposed activity restrictions. However, on a medical certification form, the term *work restrictions* means what the patient should *not* do on the basis of risk of harm to self or others. Symptoms do not harm, so "work restrictions" are not appropriate if based only on symptoms. The term *work limitations* describes what current abilities the patient lacks or tasks he or she is unable to perform. In this example (patient-described activity tolerance), work limitations are not appropriate. This patient clearly can perform the activity but chooses not to (tolerance) because he dislikes the symptoms associated with the activity.

If multiple physicians see the same patient in a contested work ability/disability case, the physicians are likely to agree on questions of risk and capacity. Serious "risk of harm" situations are rare and easily analyzed with common sense. Most often there is no scientific study that can clearly be generalized to the specific patient's work risk questions.

When multiple physicians provide widely ranging opinions on work tolerance but wrongly present the information as *work ability* (capacity) or *work restrictions* (risk), the physicians appear to patients, employers, insurers, judges, and juries to be either unscientific, biased, or "paid for." This obviously reflects poorly on medicine as a profession. Yet, many times, two equally well-qualified and honest physicians will testify in contested cases to exactly opposite conclusions about whether a given patient can do a specific job. The physicians will have agreed on diagnosis and treatment, because those are scientific subjects, and yet will have disagreed on work ability based on the patient's self-described interest in working despite symptoms.

Again, tolerance is not a scientifically verifiable concept. When two physicians offer strongly held but contradictory testimony on work ability in which both claim to be scientific ("reasonable medical probability"), not recognizing that they are arguing about the nonscientific concept of tolerance, they confuse the legal system and potentially diminish the medical profession.

When objective pathology is dramatic, physicians generally agree that working despite pain or fatigue the patient considers to be intolerable is not reasonable, and thus physicians generally agree that this patient has believable "problems" based on tolerance, but this is not a situation for work restrictions or work limitations. For example, if severe osteoarthritis of the hip is present radiographically, and the patient describes severe pain when attempting work that requires prolonged heavy lifting and carrying (proving that he has the current ability to do this task), a work problem is "believable," and physicians agree on the pathology and the problem it causes. In this example, the patient would meet the criteria for total hip replacement surgery on the basis of believable pain and radiographic severe hip arthritis. This patient may also meet the Social Security Administration (SSA) "listing" of an impairment severe enough to qualify for social security disability.[4]

When there is no objective pathology, or mild pathology, but symptoms that are clearly out of proportion to the physical examination and test results, most physicians agree that working despite symptoms poses no major risk, and the patient is free to work if he or she wishes. Thus, a patient with no objective findings who alleges intolerable pain when attempting to lift a postage stamp would clearly have an issue of tolerance, and not an issue of risk or current ability. Most physicians would certify that this patient can work. In this case the tolerance is not believable. There are conditions, such as fibromyalgia, in which there are significant symptoms but no objective findings, in which some physicians (inappropriately) impose severe activity "restrictions" solely on the basis of tolerance. (See Chapter 19 for more information about working with functional syndromes.)

Models

Almost all Western societies use a "biomedical model" to determine disability. This is a model in which objective medical fact is all that is considered and "severe objective impairment equals disability." A "biopsychosocial model" is much better at explaining disability in problematic cases (who will choose to work despite symptoms).[5] Thus, third parties (employers, disability insurers, etc) inquire of physicians about "work restrictions" (based on risk) and "work limitations" (based on capacity) expecting scientific answers based on the biomedical model of severe impairment-based disability. When some physicians answer these questions using the patient's symptom tolerance as a basis for the opinion under the biopsychosocial model and inappropriately state answers as "work restrictions," physicians appear to be biased, unscientific, or influenced by financial considerations.

Physicians may believe strongly about the biopsychosocial model for disability, and they may believe that employers and insurers who ask about disability in terms of the biomedical model are asking the wrong question. However, "there is no right answer to the wrong question."[6] As long as Western society asks questions phrased in the biomedical model of disability, physicians will be expected to answer using the biomedical model.

There is a continuum from no objective pathology to severe objective pathology. Where in this continuum physicians should logically accept a patient's report of intolerable symptoms and advise the patient to pursue a different job or even to pursue disability status based only on tolerance can not be answered scientifically. In contested disability cases the scenario frequently is similar to the following:

> Dr A: "I usually declare patients like Joe fit to work despite his symptoms. They usually remain at work in this type job and do fine, so I must be correct."

> Dr B: "I usually declare patients like Joe to require work limitations. They usually cannot tolerate staying at work in this type job, so I must be correct."

Both physicians are honest, well trained, and experienced, yet they have diametrically opposed answers to the question, "Can Joe do this job?" This is because there is no scientific answer to the question, and both physicians are answering on the basis of either anecdotal experience with similar patients or personal bias. When these two physicians fill out forms, write reports, and testify under oath with these contradictory answers to what seems to be a simple question, they again give the appearance to patients, employers, insurers, judges, and juries of being either unscientific, biased, or "paid for."

Faced with this predicament, physicians have 4 choices:

1. "Play secretary" and write down on return-to-work forms what work activities the patient is willing to do.

2. Try to assess tolerance.

3. Guess (Gestalt).

4. Abstain, and leave the tolerance decision to the patient.

Tolerance Choice #1, "Play Secretary"

The "playing secretary" scenario often looks like this:

1. The patient brings a form to the doctor asking about work ability (capacity) and work restrictions (risk). The first question on the form is "How much can this individual lift?"

2. The doctor asks the patient, "How much can you lift?"

3. The patient says, "Ten pounds."

4. The doctor writes in "ten pounds" and signs the form.

This scenario demonstrates how many physicians actually fill out work ability/work guidelines forms.[7] In this scenario the physician merely asks the patient what activity he or she can tolerate and functions as a secretary taking dictation. If looked at logically, the patient could actually fill out the form himself without the aid, or expense, of a physician.

Tolerance Choice #2, Try to Assess Tolerance

Functional capacity evaluation (FCE) is an attempt to assess tolerance, although, as is discussed in Chapter 6, it is far from a perfect tool. It lacks proven reliability and validity.[8–12] In the only published study in which an FCE was performed on patients with back pain and the FCE result was then ignored, when patients were sent back to full duty even though the FCE frequently said that the patients were not capable of full duty, ignoring the FCE findings improved the treatment results.[13]

FCEs are really a "tolerance test" and not a "capacity test." Because the therapists who administer these exams don't want to be successfully sued for injuring a patient during testing, before the actual testing starts, the therapist has an "informed consent" session with the examinee and instructs the examinee not to do anything during testing that would injure the examinee (not "knowingly be reinjured"). Thus the examinee is instructed to stop functioning during testing if significant pain suggests to the examinee the possibility of re-injury.

Tolerance Choice #3, Guess (Gestalt)

Faced with this dilemma, many physicians guess using Gestalt. In this system the "educated guess" cannot be scientifically described but seems to be: "Based on my anecdotal experience, patients like this usually do, or usually do not, function at this level of work with this medical problem." Two physicians will have had different anecdotal experiences, and they will have different biases, which explains why two seemingly equally well-trained and qualified physicians will agree on diagnosis and treatment but have diametrically opposed opinions on work ability/ guidelines. This is like Aesop's fable of the blind men examining the elephant, in which each physician has a different anecdotal experience (piece of the elephant) and different biases (blindfolds), leading to different conclusions about the nature of elephants—or of patients' work abilities.

Tolerance Choice #4, Abstain

Because pain cannot be measured, how does a physician assess a patient's tolerance for work? Can any two physicians come to the same conclusion?

Plato taught that the ideal form of government was the "Philosopher King."[14] If Plato appointed you (the reader) Philosopher King, would you want to tell an individual that as king you have decided that on a 0 to 10 visual analog pain scale:

- At work your average pain will be a _____.

- Your minimum pain at work will be _____.

- Your peak pain at work will be a _____, lasting for _____ minutes.

- You will get only _____ hours of sleep because of your pain.

- On Mondays your pain will be only a _____, but by Fridays it will be a _____.

- On the weekend if you rest your pain will decrease to a _____, but not until you've been out of work for _____ hours.

If physicians will never be able to agree on what activity a given patient should be able to tolerate in terms of symptoms like pain and fatigue, it is best that physicians not pretend there is a medical answer to this question. Recalling the discussion in Chapter 1, that remaining at work has clear health benefit for the individual and thus is in his or her long-term best interest, the best answer a physician can give to such a patient may be the following:

You do not appear to meet the Social Security Administration's criteria for total disability. Thus, in our society, there is some job you're expected to be able to do. Because there is no medical evidence that you are at high risk of significant harm by working, I cannot certify that you're disabled for this job. There is no basis for work restrictions based on risk. I realize that you have pain (or fatigue, etc), but you have the ability to do many things despite your pain. Whether the rewards of working are sufficient for you to choose to remain at work, or whether the pain you feel is sufficient for you to choose a different type of work, or not to work at all, is a question only you can answer. I can record on this form what you feel to be your current activity tolerances, but not as "work restrictions" or as "work limitations." These tolerances are not scientific, and they may change in the future.

If this type of statement is included in a medical report or work ability form, it should be on the line for "comments," and the "work guides" should be clearly labeled as based only on patient-described tolerance. The physician should include a disclaimer that medicine is both a science and an art, and that the future is not foreseeable. (See Chapters 4 and 8 for more information about disclaimers and legal considerations in return-to-work decisions.)

Unfortunately, physicians have not done a good job of educating patients, employers, insurers, and judges that there is some science on risk assessment, but that tolerance for symptoms is the usual problem in contested disability cases, and tolerance is *not* scientifically measurable.

How to Evaluate Work Ability: A Seven-Step Process

By using an organized approach, a physician can determine appropriate work guides for an individual. Understanding the principles discussed in this chapter permits such an approach:

1. What is the job in question? Do I have an adequate job description? Do I have information from both the individual and the employer as to what this patient is expected to do at work? If "no," request such information before answering.

2. What is this patient's medical problem? What are the objective signs of pathology? What are the symptoms? Is this permanent or temporary during recovery from injury/surgery? Is this problem improvable with time, or medical treatment, or exercise (which includes work)? If the condition is temporary or improvable, record this fact.

3. Does this patient have severe pathophysiology that appears to meet the Social Security Administration's criteria for total disability? If "yes," tell this fact to the patient and support his or her disability application if he or she chooses to apply for disability. If not, consider risk.

4. Is there significant risk of substantial harm with work activity (not merely an increase in subjective symptoms)? If "yes" on the basis of sound science or a major consensus document, certify that work *restrictions* are appropriate on the basis of risk. If "no," consider current ability.

5. Is this patient actually able to physically do the task in question (not considering symptoms, but ability)? If "no," state the reason as a *limitation* ("lacks shoulder range of motion to reach overhead machine controls"). If "yes," consider tolerance.

6. If the patient has the ability to do the work task, at acceptable risk, and wants to do the job, certify that he or she is medically able.

7. If the patient has the ability to do the work task, at acceptable risk, and does not like doing the job based on tolerance for symptoms like pain and fatigue, is there severe objective pathology present that makes physician agreement on work problems based on tolerance likely? If "yes," certify that work "problems" are present "on the basis of believable symptoms and severe objective pathology," but certify that the patient may work despite the symptoms if he or she wishes. (Note that there will usually not be a line or box on the work ability form for "work problems" but there frequently is a line for "comments.") If "no," and the objective pathology is only mild or moderate, certify that the patient may work at the job in question, but that he or she describes symptoms at a certain level of work activity. This scenario represents a "medically unanswerable question" and should be labeled as such by physicians. The decision whether or not to work despite symptoms is *ultimately the patient's*, and not the physician's.

Summary

Most physicians have not been trained in work ability assessment. Multiple physicians often give contradictory answers to questions of work ability if tolerance (symptoms) is what limits work performance. There is limited science on work risk assessment. There are some consensus documents that give useful information. Significant risk of injury or harm to self or others should justify work restrictions.

Few individuals function at capacity. Current ability can be measured but can increase with activity or decrease with inactivity. If individuals lack the current ability to do a work task, this is a work limitation.

Tolerance for symptoms such as pain and fatigue is what in most cases gives patients work problems. Multiple physicians will not agree on work guidelines based on tolerance unless there is severe objective pathology associated with the symptoms. This level of impairment usually means the individual meets the Social Security Administration's "listing" of conditions severe enough to qualify for total disability and/or the indications for major reconstructive surgery.

If there is no medical answer to when a condition with mild or moderate pathology is significant enough that the individual should choose to pursue a different career or to stop work entirely, physicians should not pretend there is a medical answer, and thus physicians should decline to certify such individuals as disabled or unable to work. This is ultimately the patient's decision. Employers and insurers ask about work restrictions and work limitations, phrasing the questions in the biomedical model in which severe impairment equals disability. Physicians should not try to answer these questions based on tolerance using the biopsychosocial model (despite its superiority at predicting who will choose to work despite symptoms). "There is no right answer to the wrong question." As a patient advocate, the physician should have a discussion with the patient as to why he or she is not eligible for disability certification. Suggested wording for this discussion is offered, and a seven-step process to think through specific work ability questions is recommended.

References

1. Pelliccia A, Zipes DP, Maron BJ. Bethesda Conference #36 and the European Society of Cardiology Consensus Recommendations revisited: a comparison of U.S. and European criteria for eligibility and disqualification of competitive athletes with cardiovascular abnormalities. *JACC*. 2008;52(24):1990–1996.

2. Carragee EJ, Han MY, Yang B, et al. Activity restrictions after posterior discectomy: a prospective study of outcomes in 152 cases with no postoperative restrictions. *Spine*. 1999;24:2346–2351.

3. Carragee EJ, Helms E, O'Sullivan GS. Are postoperative activity restrictions necessary after posterior lumbar discectomy? A prospective study of outcomes in 50 consecutive cases. *Spine*. 1996;21:1893–1897.

4. Disability Evaluation Under Social Security. Baltimore, MD: Social Security Administration; January 2003. SSA publication 64-039.

5. Waddell G. The biopsychosocial model. In: Waddell G, ed. *The Back Pain Revolution*. 2nd ed. London, England: Churchill Livingstone; 2004.

6. Carolyn Acuff, personal communication with the author (JBT).

7. Pransky G, Katz JN, Benjamin K, Himmelstein J; Improving the physician role in evaluating work ability and managing disability: a survey of primary care practioners. *Disabil Rehabil*. 2002;24:867–874.

8. Gouttebarge V, Wind H, Kuijer P, et al. Reliability and validity of Functional Capacity Evaluation methods: a systematic review with reference to Blankenship system, Ergos work simulator, Ergo-Kit, and Isernhagen work system. *Int Arch Occup Environ Health*. 2004;77:527–537

9. Gross DP, Battie MC, Cassidy JD. The prognostic value of functional capacity evaluation in patients with chronic low back pain, part 1: timely return to work. *Spine*. 2004;29:914–919.

10. Gross DP, Battie MC. The prognostic value of functional capacity evaluation in patients with chronic low back pain, part 2: sustained recovery. *Spine*. 2004;29:920–924.

11. Gross DP, Battie MC. Functional capacity evaluation performance does not predict sustained return to work in claimants with chronic back pain. *J Occup Rehabil*. 2005;15:285–94.

12. Gross DP, Batti MC. Does functional capacity evaluation predict recovery in workers compensation claimants with upper extremity disorders? *Occup Environ Med*. 2006;63:404–410.

13. Hall H, McIntosh G, Melles T, Holowachuk B, Wai E. Effect of discharge recommendations on outcome. *Spine*. 1994;19:2033–2037.

Chapter 2

Chapter 3

How to Negotiate Return to Work

J. Mark Melhorn, MD and James R. Rainville, MD

> "I still hurt! How can you even think I can go back to work?"

Disagreements about the ability to work are common between patients with painful musculoskeletal conditions and the physicians responsible for their care, especially as symptoms become more chronic.[1–4] Many times, these disagreements reflect basic differences in the factors that are being considered by each party. Physicians tend to rely heavily on established medical facts, such as clinical findings, work capacity, and risk. (As discussed in Chapter 2, *risk* is the possibility of re-injury or worsening of the medical condition; *capacity* is the physical ability based on the injury and the current medical condition.) On the other hand, patients tend to base their opinions on job related factors, such as anticipated tolerance for the discomfort produced while performing the physical aspects of their jobs.[5] *Tolerance* refers to the decision by the individual to endure symptoms such as pain or fatigue in exchange for the benefits of work (Chapter 2). As tolerance incorporates decision making, it is influenced by psychosocial issues such as previous pain experiences (learned behavior), fear-avoidance beliefs, and economic considerations such as direct and indirect financial gains. Because anticipated tolerance is multifactorial, it can be quite dynamic and can change rapidly in response to modifications of its subcomponents.

It is an inherent role of the physician to address patients' concerns about tolerance for work while presenting the medical facts about risk and capacities that are the basis for medical work recommendations. Often by addressing these concerns, discordance about work expectations is lessened and a successful return to work ensues. (For the remainder of this chapter *return to work* will refer to both stay-at-work and return-to-work options.) Unfortunately, when differences in expectation are great, this process can cause substantial stress on the physician-patient relationship. It is the premise of this chapter that the injured worker can be successfully returned to work and good physician-patient relationship can be preserved if the physician has a clear understanding of the many factors and players that are involved in successful return to work and combines this knowledge with effective negotiation skills during return-to-work discussions.

The Scope of the Problem

Workers' compensations systems exist to offer benefits to employees injured during the course of work, while limiting the liability exposure of employers to claims of injured employees. The four objectives of the workers' compensation system are listed here:

- Provide prompt and reasonable income and medical benefits to injured workers, or income benefits to the dependents of injured workers, regardless of fault.

- Provide a single and exclusive remedy for work-related injuries.

- Reduce court delays, costs, and workloads arising out of personal injury litigation, and eliminate attorney and witness fees.

- Encourage employers to be interested in safety and rehabilitation through appropriate experience-rating mechanisms.

By law, work-related injuries or illnesses are those that require medical treatment (other than first aid), result in lost work time, cause loss of consciousness, lead to restriction of work activities, or mandate a transfer to another job.[6] Of great interest, *injuries*, defined as conditions that occur from specific traumatic events, are decreasing, whereas *illnesses*, defined as conditions that do not occur from specific traumatic events, are increasing.[7] Poorly understood chronic musculoskeletal pain (also labeled *cumulative trauma disorders*, *musculoskeletal disorders*, or *nontraumatic soft-tissue musculoskeletal disorders*) is the fastest growing category within the illness group.[8,9]

Nationally, the magnitude and costs of this issue are staggering. Private industry reports 6.1 million injuries and illnesses per year, with a case rate of 7.1 cases per 100 equivalent full-time workers.[10] Viewed from a different perspective, consider that an estimated 8 million American workers are at home and not working because of illness or injury. The resulting paid disability leave costs employers more than $100 billion per year through sick pay, salary continuation, workers' compensation indemnity benefits, and long-term and short-term disability benefits.[11] In 1997, the nation's costs for work-related injuries and illnesses were estimated at $837 billion.[12] Reducing the total costs has clearly become a priority for the American public and the American business community.

The consumption of time for health care providers is equally staggering. It is estimated that 11% of primary care encounters involve return-to-work discussions.[13,14] Because of the frequency of musculoskeletal complaints, orthopedic surgeons report the highest frequency of encounters dealing with return-to-work cases.[15] In summary, return-to-work discussions consume countless hours of physician time during millions of medical encounters each year.

The Return-to-Work Decision Makers

Chapter 3

Though physicians often assume that their work recommendations are the determining factors for returning injured employees to work, there are actually four groups involved in making return-to-work decisions: the physician, the injured worker, the employer, and the supplementary players (administrators, attorneys, benefit adjudicators, case managers, consultants, insurers, judicial or physician reviewers, rehabilitation managers, unions, and the state-specific workers' compensation system).[16] With so many players involved in the process, communication is often poor, misunderstandings are common, and unnecessary time off work often occurs.[17–20] Unfortunately, when considering physicians' work recommendations after an injury, both the employer and the employee often adapt a negative point of view that focuses on the injured worker's incapacity or limitations rather than on retained ability. This often taints their response to restrictions included in physician's work recommendations. Employers and injured workers should be reminded about the wisdom in the old question, "Is the glass half empty or half full?" and learn to view physicians' work recommendations as defining ability rather than incapacity or limitations.

The advantage to employers is that, by offering work opportunities compatible with medical recommendations, they gain substantial leverage to encourage return to work. Under most jurisdictions, employees receiving workers' compensation salary replacement benefits are required to accept offers for modified work, unless their medical condition precludes travel to and from work, being at work, or being able to perform assigned tasks and duties. If the employee does not comply with a work assignment compatible with medical recommendation, the employer may not legally be required to approve the employee's absence and the linked workers' compensation benefits. (In other words, the employer is able to modify the subcomponent of economic considerations and strongly influence the employees' decision about their ability to tolerate work.) Additionally, the early and appropriate return to work of injured employees means a reduction in the employer's workers' compensation benefits or disability payments and therefore a reduction of the cost of the claim. This may help to control the rise of workers' compensation and health insurance premiums that are based on usage and past claims experiences.

Of course the employer may also take an alternative position by not accommodating medical limitations but requiring that the injured employee be classified as "100%" or "capable of full duty" before allowing a return to work. This is sometimes precipitated when there were employee-employer relations problems before the injury. By refusing to take back the worker with restrictions and/or limitations, the employer temporarily solves its personnel problem by keeping the problem employee off the job site and on workers' compensation. This is invariably a costly mistake as this decision further delays the employee's return to work, forces additional wage replacement, and ultimately increases workers' compensation costs. Beyond this, the unwillingness of employers to accommodate an injured employee's restrictions and/or limitations may impact employer-employee relationships. Additionally, this approach causes employees to also focus on their limitations instead of their abilities and therefore feel much less capable than they really are. It can also send a message to the employee that the employer does not care about him as an individual. This increases the likelihood the injured worker will hire an attorney, which is associated with increased claim cost.[21] Depending on application, this decision may also violate the Americans with Disabilities Act of 1990 for covered disabilities, under which employers are required to make reasonable accommodations that enable employees to perform the essential functions of their jobs.[22] (See Chapter 7 for more information about legal considerations in return-to-work decisions.)

For the employee, taking advantage of work opportunities made available by the physician's recommendations means a restoration of at least partial earnings, benefits, and social esteem or status. It also means that the employee is back in the running for any advancement or lateral job opportunities that may arise. Conversely, prolonged absence from one's normal roles, including absence from the workplace, may be detrimental to a person's mental, physical, and social well-being.[19] In addition, one study has shown that being unemployed results in an increased mortality for men and their families.[23] (See Chapter 1 for more information about the health consequences of being unemployed.)

For all players involved, a return to work, even in a light-duty position or with accommodation, also means the transition from incapacitated patient to productive employee, thus enhancing recovery and reducing disability.[19]

As key players in the return-to-work process, physicians have the decisive opportunity to support a patient's return to function and work after an illness or injury by instituting a successful interaction (negotiation) with the injured workers (patient, employee) about appropriate abilities.[19] Assuming the employer is willing and able to accommodate restrictions and limitations and the supplementary players are supportive, the physician's efforts are usually rewarded with their patients' successful return to work. Unfortunately, many factors ultimately influence the employee's decision to stay at work or return early to work (tolerance) that are out of control of the physician. It is therefore useful to remember that taking advantage of every opportunity to communicate with all members of the four groups listed above increases the physician's ability to influence as many of these factors as possible, increasing the likelihood of the injured employee returning to appropriate work in the shortest period of time.

The Five Steps From Injury to Resolution

Return to work is only one part of a sequence of events that also includes the injury and the restoration of function. The injured worker must move through five steps from injury to resolution in order to allow closure of the workers' compensation claim and to allow the individual to reach maximum medical improvement. These steps are:

1. Establishing a relationship between injury and the workplace

2. Diagnosis and treatment

3. Time off work and return to work

4. Impairment and disability

5. Settlement and resolution

Establishing a Relationship between Injury and the Workplace

The injury or illness is the event that triggers the workers' compensation claim. *Occupational injuries* result from a work-related event or from a single instantaneous exposure in the work environment as defined by the Occupational Safety and Health Administration (OSHA), while *occupational illness* is any abnormal condition or disorder (other than one resulting from an occupational injury) caused by exposure to a factor(s) associated with employment.[6] Injuries are easy to understand. The individual usually has a cut, break, or strain. The relationship to the workplace is often straightforward, with a specific event, a specific injury, and a specific diagnosis. Illnesses, as discussed in this chapter, are limited to musculoskeletal disorders, such as tendinitis, nerve entrapments, and musculoskeletal pain or disorders, which are sometimes called *cumulative trauma disorders (CTDs)*. With the longer onset of symptoms and lack of a specific event, and often the lack of distinct pathology, it is sometimes difficult to demonstrate their relationship to work. Regardless, physicians are often asked to do so. This requires an understanding of the symptoms (what hurts), the signs (the clinical examination), supporting tests (such as nerve conduction studies or X rays), the diagnosis, and the natural disease process underlying the diagnosis (causation). This opinion for causation is often given to a reasonable degree of medical probability (more likely than not, sometimes described as more than 51% of the time), which is a legal, not a medical, definition of probability. Causation is discussed in Chapter 5 or in the companion book *Guides to the Evaluation of Disease and Injury Causation*.

Diagnosis and Treatment

Diagnosis and treatment are the most familiar to the physician. The diagnosis is based on collecting the information from symptoms, signs, and tests that are analyzed for a conclusion. The diagnosis may be easy or difficult, depending on the information available and the physician's experience and skills. Treatment is traditionally based on the diagnosis. For example, a nondisplaced (simple) fractured wrist is treated with a cast because medical outcome studies have demonstrated a reasonable outcome with casting. Treatment protocol or guides have been developed for many diagnoses by professional organizations such as the AAOS Clinical Practice Guidelines (CPG)[24] and ACOEM Practice Guidelines[25] or by commercial products such as the Official Disability Guidelines.[26] When a specific diagnosis is not available, the treatment becomes less specific and often less effective.

Time Off Work and Return to Work

Many consider modified work as the cornerstone in job rehabilitation. A systematic review of the 2345 articles in the scientific literature on return-to-work issues published since 1985 supported the following findings: modified work programs facilitate early return to work for the temporarily and permanently disabled worker; the likelihood of continued employment is increased by twofold by early return to work; individual physical impairments and costs for the employer are often decreased; and the quality of life for the employee is improved with early return to work.[27]

Employers, patients, lawyers, and the courts often assume that time away from work after an illness or injury is necessary. They typically remain unquestioning as long as there is ongoing treatment. However, they often

Chapter 3

neglect to ask the physician whether the patient is safely able to do any productive work. Certainly, some injuries or illnesses will require that the employee be off work. Other injuries or illnesses may allow the employee back to work with restrictions, accommodations, or modifications. Lost work days because of poor or slow communication between the physician and the employer, inadequate information, litigation over benefits, disputes over other matters, lack of cooperation by any party, administrative delays, or lack of desire on the part of the employee reflect inefficiencies in the system and are medically unnecessary.

The cost of unnecessary lost work days is substantial. The national average lost time claim costs more than $19000 in medical and indemnity payments, compared with the average medical-only claim that costs less than $400.[28] Christian[29] surveyed occupational health physicians on their clinical experience regarding medically necessary days off work after injury. The majority said that less than 10% of the employee-patients would require a few days off work. Almost half of the physicians surveyed placed the percentage at 5%. The actual national average is 24%. Using this range of 5% to 10% would suggest that 60% to 80% of the lost work days involve medically unnecessary time off from work.

More than two-thirds of the physicians surveyed gave the following reasons for the medically unnecessary time off work: the treating physician is unwilling to force a reluctant patient back to work (the most common reason cited); the treating physician is not equipped to determine the right restrictions and limitations on work activity; the employer has a policy against light-duty work; the employer cannot find a way to temporarily modify a job; the treating physician feels caught between the employer's and the employee's version of events; the treating physician has been given too little information about the physical demands of the job to issue a work release for the patient; and a conflict exists between the opinions of two physicians.[29]

Often, appropriate return to work can be greatly improved by the physician engaging case managers and ergonomists. Involvement of these professionals has been shown to produce a direct benefit–to–cost savings ratio of 6.8.[30] These professionals can inform the physician of important issues such as performance or job dissatisfaction problems that may enhance the injured employee's resistance to return to work under any circumstance.[31] Additionally, well-informed case managers can educate physicians about state-specific law for workers' compensation benefits, which have a significant effect on the results of medical treatment, return-to-work status, and the cost of medical care.[32] Indeed, evidence suggests that physicians resistance to engage all involved parties and fully commit to return-to-work goals can be a major obstacle for early return to work.[33]

Chapter 3

Understanding Impairment and Disability

Impairment is defined by the American Medical Association's (AMA's) *Guides to the Evaluation of Permanent Impairment 5th Edition (the Guides)* as the loss, loss of use, or derangement of any body part, system, or function,[34] while the *Guides, Sixth,* defines it as a significant deviation, loss, or loss of use of any body structure or body function in an individual with a health condition, disorder, or disease.[35] It is the physician's task to identify and document impairment that results from work-related injuries such as loss of neurological, musculoskeletal, or cognitive function. The physician may also need to determine whether the impairments are permanent and to identify impairments that could lead to sudden or gradual incapacitation, further impairment, injury, transmission of a communicable disease, or other adverse occurrence.

Disability refers to the loss of ability to perform normal human tasks and has been defined in a number of ways to reflect this. The AMA *Guides, Fifth,* defined disability as a decrease in, or the loss or absence of, the capacity of an individual to meet personal, social, or occupational demands, or to meet statutory or regulatory requirements because of an impairment,[34] while the *Guides, Sixth,* defines disability as activity limitations and/or participation restrictions in an individual with a health condition, disorder, or disease.[35] It is these definitions that are most relevant to this current discussion.

Physicians should be aware that other definitions of disability exist. The Americans with Disabilities Act of 1990 uses the term *disability* to represent a concept that is similar to the concept of impairment used in the AMA *Guides.* It is important to note that under the Americans with Disabilities Act, identification of an individual with a "disability" does not depend on the results of a medical evaluation. An individual may be identified as having a disability if there is a record of an impairment that has substantially limited one or more major life activities or, of greater concern, if the individual is regarded as having a disability. *Disability* is also sometimes used to describe the time away from work due to a loss of full physical capacity, whether minor or major, temporary or permanent, as a result of a work-related injury or illness.

Settlement and Resolution

After injury, diagnosis, treatment, and return to work or time off work, the physician is often asked to provide an impairment rating, which is converted to a disability by the legal system to offer a settlement and provide for resolution of the process. The *Guides, Sixth,* defines *impairment rating* as a consensus-derived percentage estimate of loss of activity reflecting severity for a given health condition and the degree of associated limitations in terms of activities of daily living (ADLs). Notice that this definition does not include work activities.

It is useful for physicians to remember that workers' compensation systems represents a compromise for both employers and employees and are designed to be a no-fault and exclusive remedy. The workers and their dependents are not required to prove fault for personal injuries, diseases, or deaths arising out of and in the course of employment. The employer agrees to provide rapid payment to the injured worker for lost wages and medical care costs in exchange for limiting or eliminating the employer's potential liability for said occupational illness, injuries, and death and, thereby, the possibility of large tort verdicts. Although described as a system, each state, each US territory, and the US federal government have state-, territory-, and federal-specific workers' compensation laws and regulations. Although not specifically part of the workers' compensation system, Title XIV of the federal Social Security Disability Program provides benefits to disabled workers younger than 65 years who are expected to be totally disabled for at least 12 months.

Return-to-Work Guides

Chapters 12 to 19 expand on determining capacity, understanding tolerance, and assessing risk for return-to-work guides. This section provides a general overview to assist in understanding how to negotiate return-to-work decisions.

Not surprisingly, return to work is often less dependent on the medical factors surrounding the actual injury than it is about the unique characteristics of an injured employee and his or her employer. Important predictive factors for return to work are outlined in Table 3-1. In general, increasing age,[36,37] female gender,[38] and strong psychosocial issues make return to work more difficult.[39] A treating physician can look for and respond to the "five *D*'s" as described by Brena et al.[40]: dramatization (vague, diffused nonanatomic pain complaints), drugs (misuse of habit-forming pain medications), dysfunction (unwillingness to function in various personal, social, and occupational roles), dependency (passivity, depression, and helplessness), and disability (unwillingness to return to work).

Table 3-1 Predictive Factors for Return to Work

Individual Risk	Job Risk
Age	Job or task demands
Gender	Organizational structure
Biosocial issues	Physical work environment

Predictive factors for the job include task demands, organizational structure, and the physical work environment.[41,42] Job satisfaction is the foremost factor correlating with an early return to work.[43,44] Persons with high levels of discretion are more than two times as likely to be working as those with less autonomy. Those with high demands and little autonomy to deal with them are far less likely to return to work after what should be a temporarily disabling injury. An unpleasant and stressful work environment will greatly reduce the probability of return to work. The individual employer has the greatest opportunity to reduce losses in the workers' compensation system and to return the injured employee to work. A single supportive telephone call from the employer to the injured worker would be a strong force in motivating the patient to return to work, especially if the patient is experiencing depression or has a need for emotional support.

Unfortunately, some employers respond angrily to the injured worker and refuse to file an initial report of injury. As mentioned earlier, occasionally the employer is simply happy to be rid of the injured worker and does as little as possible to promote his or her return to work. Considering the prevalence of psychiatric comorbidity, it is possible to understand that attitude. Depressed, anxious, or substance-abusing people do not make the most desirable and productive employees.

In addition, unions with rigid seniority policies may limit access to the easier jobs. Often, seniority is the only consideration during job bidding, and work limitations cannot be used to override seniority. Similarly, union rules can strictly prohibit a worker from crossing trades and thus limit work options. These policies essentially tie the hands of an employer, making the employer unable to offer many less physically demanding jobs to an injured worker and thereby hampering return-to-work efforts. In many communities, experienced physicians are aware of specific union policies of major employers in their area and work to actively address these issues to facilitate the transitional work. This requires a working partnership among the physician, patient, employer, union, and insurer.

For the physician, the overriding objective is a safe, speedy return to work with the interests of the patient being the primary responsibility. Early recognition of psychosocial issues, and efforts by the physician to keep the focus on rapid return to work based on the medical and not the psychosocial issues, is the most likely strategy to produce a successful outcome. The physician must realize that these psychosocial issues affect the patient's perception of recovery. The physician must try to dissociate the patient's perceptions from true recovery as understood through medical science.

Physicians can make a fair estimate of the time required for healing based on empiric knowledge of specific injuries. This recognition is essential, because it is the power invested in physicians based on their knowledge of medical science that allows them to redirect patients' inappropriate concerns and replace them with valid medical explanations about the role of resuming function in the healing and recovery process.[45]

Medical principles of healing can be matched with available information about specific job tasks to design logical return-to-work recommendations. Job information can be acquired from the employer, the employee, or through the US Department of Labor.[46–49] By combining these elements, safe and reasonable work guides can be provided that will allow the injured employee to return to the appropriate work while using the workplace as an integral part of the therapy program, thus providing for cost-effective rehabilitation. Physicians who treat work-related injuries realize that there is no easy table for developing work guides. The process is slow, time consuming, and often frustrating for both the patient and the physician. The benefits to the employee are significant and worthy of the effort.[50]

Chapter 3

Why Physicians May Feel Uncomfortable Recommending Early Return to Work

Often physicians feel uncomfortable recommending early return to work because of the medical issues surrounding the decision. For example:

- Recommending a patient return to work early is outside the realm of the traditional medical model that focuses on anatomy, physiology, and pathology.

- Each individual and his or her work situation is unique. This makes translation of academic generalities difficult to apply to each individual.

- Standards for defining work capacities for injured workers are limited.

- Often the physician's position on return to work reflects his or her attitudes about pain and function as much as scientific knowledge.[51]

Patient and physician relationship issues may also prevent physicians from recommending early return to work. For example:

- There may be a significant difference between the physician's opinions and those of the patient, the family, the case manager, the employer, the insurer, or even other health care providers.

- The normal partnership between the physician and the patient may be disrupted by this difference.

- If differences in opinions exist, then negotiations must take place. These take time and are emotionally uncomfortable. This time is usually not "codable" or "reimbursable."

Negotiation Strategies for Return to Work

Negotiation is defined as coming to terms; a dialogue, talk, or discussion intended to produce an agreement. *Agreement* is defined as a compatibility of observations. Synonyms include accord, arrangement, concord, correspondence, and understanding.[52] Because the patient and the physician have the same goal—maximum restoration of function with the least pain—reaching an agreement on return to work should be easy. Unfortunately, this patient-physician interaction often results in the patient feeling that the physician is pushing him or her back to work. This perspective is often the result of lack of knowledge of the significance of pain, the benefits of physical activities to the healing process, and therefore a lack of understanding of the benefits of work. As a patient advocate, the physician will need to take more time to transfer knowledge, which will enable the physician to negotiate a successful return to work based on the medical sciences involving pain, musculoskeletal physiology, healing, capacity, and risk while still appreciating the patient's concerns about work tolerance.

Whether physicians realize it or not, they are actually involved with negotiation every time they encounter a patient. So why are physicians not more successful in providing appropriate return-to-work guides?

Negotiations require strategies; strategies require understanding; understanding requires knowledge; acquiring knowledge requires communication; and communication results in understanding. Because many injured workers have little knowledge of the workers' compensation system, it is important for the physician to communicate that he or she is first a patient advocate, and that appropriate early return to work is part of the recovery process and is in the patient's best interests. A general discussion of the four objectives of workers' compensation as listed earlier (providing prompt and reasonable income and benefits, providing a single remedy for work-related injuries, reducing court delays and costs, and encouraging employer interest in safety and rehabilitation) is helpful. The physician should acknowledge that, on occasion, the workers' compensation system does not run smoothly and delays may occur. Patients should be encouraged to communicate these occurrences and their other concerns with appropriate parties. Physicians will work with them to assist in the process, but patients must also take responsibility for their part and actively participate. Together, many of the obstacles to successful return to work can be overcome. This builds a relationship for successful negotiations to occur.

Like other capabilities learned by physicians, negotiation is both a skill and an art form. The key to negotiation is to be firm on the science (healing, capacity, and risk) and soft on the patient (tolerance) while making recommendations that the physician believes are in the patient's best interest for improving recovery and restoring function with the least amount of pain.[53]

A commonsense approach is outlined by the word "success":

*S*et the stage.

*U*ncover the issues.

*C*onfine the issues.

*C*onfirm intent and authority.

*E*valuate the issues.

*S*olve the problem.

*S*atisfaction check.

As with other skills, the more the physician practices, the better his or her ability to negotiate.[54] Studies suggest that the best way to begin learning negotiation skills is by examples.[55,56] The following are several examples of negotiation strategies between the physician and the injured worker.[57]

1. Judging Negotiation	2. Positional Bargaining
The success of negotiation can be judged in several ways. Of greatest importance, negotiations should result in a wise decision that fulfills as many of the goals of all parties as possible. The process of negotiating should be efficient and completed in a reasonable amount of time. At the completion of negotiations, the important relationship between physician and patient should not be damaged.	Positional Bargaining is probably the type of negotiation that most people are familiar with. Each side takes a position, argues over it, and makes concessions to reach a compromise. Results are based on willpower.

Statement/Question	
Physician:	It's time for you to go back to work.
Injured Worker:	I don't think that I am ready yet.
Physician:	How much more time do you think you need?
Injured Worker:	I don't know. I don't seem any better.
Physician:	How about by the end of this month?
Injured Worker:	It seems you're only worried about my work and not my pain. I don't see how I can get better by then.

Positional bargaining can produce an agreement, though not always a wise one. This approach can be inefficient and stressful on the physician-patient relationship, especially if the physician holds his or her ground.[55]

Principled Negotiation is an alternative approach to negotiating that focuses on identifying the basic interests of both parties, explores mutually satisfying options, and establishes fair standards on which to base the negotiations.

The first component of principled negotiation is to separate the *people* from the *problem*, and to go hard on the *problem* and soft on the *people*. For all parties involved with return-to-work negotiations after a work-related illness or injury, the central issues are the implications of work on healing, and of capacities and risk on the ability to perform the various tasks of work. These issues are medical issues that the physician can address with great expertise. Therefore the physician should consciously keep the focus of negotiations on medical issues. It is essential that the physician avoid focusing on the relationship issues. It is undeniable that human emotions are involved in the negotiation process, but the physician should try not to react to these and to instead stay focused on the central medical issues.

The second principle is to identify and focus on mutual *interest* instead of *positions*. The physician can often translate the patient's position into interest (concern about injury, restoring normal lifestyle, financial security, etc). In most situations, patient's and physician's interests are similar. This can be revealed to patients by talking about those interests and explaining how return-to-work recommendations are not contrary, but compatible with, those interests. Discussions of common interest will often reveal *options* for mutual gain.

The third principle includes insisting on using *objective (medical)* criteria during return-to-work negotiations. Physicians' recommendations have the greatest legitimacy when they are based on medical principles and objective in nature. Physicians should remain open to discussions about these medical principles but not respond to pressure to abandon medical principles during negotiations. If they do so, the legitimacy of their recommendations will be seriously undermined.

3. Principled Negotiation

Statement/Question	Approach
Physician: By law I am required to define work capacities that are reasonable for a person with your injury.	Focus on problem, not people
Injured Worker: I don't feel that I am ready to go back to work yet.	Statement of Position
Physician: By law I am required to define work capacities that are reasonable for a person with your injury.	Focus on problem, not people
Injured Worker: I don't feel that I am ready to go back to work yet.	Statement of Position
Physician: By law I am required to define work capacities that are reasonable for a person with your injury.	Focus on problem, not people

Chapter 3

Statement/Question	Approach
Injured Worker: I don't feel that I am ready to go back to work yet.	Statement of Position
Physician: I understand your concern. I too am interested in your full recovery, and we will continue to work toward that goal.	Identify mutual interests
I also know that you must be interested in returning to your job as quickly as you are able.	
From a medical viewpoint, you do not fulfill the necessary criteria for being totally disabled.	Move to medical criteria
Don't you agree that you are able to safely perform many useful activities at this point?	Look for consensus on principles
Injured Worker: Such as what?	Opening to explore options
Physician: Let's first look at hours of work per day. You are still in therapy three times per week and your workplace must accommodate that.	Address mutual medical interests
Injured Worker: I don't feel that I could work a full day!	Statement of position
Physician: At this time there is no medical justification for rest, and these work recommendations must be based on medical criteria.	Move to medical criteria
What is the reason that you feel that you cannot work a full day?	Address concern

Useful Responses to Three Common Attacks

Regardless of our skill as physicians or negotiators, some patients will try to manipulate the negotiations by bringing up nonmedical concerns, threats, or personal attacks. All physicians have experienced the discomfort produced by these encounters. These are some examples of the use of principled negotiations to help manage these negotiations by staying focused on the problem not the people, identifying mutual interests, and keeping the negotiations focus on the medical issues at hand.

Help Me Against My Big, Bad Employer

Injured Worker: You don't know my boss. He won't follow these restrictions.	Focus on a person
Physician: I am sorry to hear that your boss may be unreasonable. You might want to bring this concern to your personnel manager or his boss.	Separate the people from the problem
As your doctor, my recommendations must be based solely on the medical issues related to your injury. …	Move to medical criteria

The Threat

Injured Worker: If I hurt myself, I'll hold you responsible.	Personal threat
Physician: My responsibility is to continue to help you recover from your current injury, and to help you return to your normal lifestyle, including work.	Recast an attack on you as an attack on the problem
It is a fact of life that all of us face a risk of future illness and injury. No one can alter that.	Move to medical criteria
The work recommendations that we have agreed upon today are based on your current situation. If something dramatically changes, please call me, as I am here to help you. Regardless, let's see each other again in a month to see how you're doing.	Reinforce your commitment to the physician-patient relationship

You Are a Incompetent Doctor

Injured Worker: You said I would be fine after the surgery, but I don't feel any better. And now you want to send me back to work!	Personal attack
Physician: It is unfortunate that surgery did not eliminate all your symptoms. This possibility was explained to you before the surgery.	Review of medical fact
I am committed to continue to work with you to improve your symptoms. However, at this time we are legally required to define work capacities that are reasonable for you.	Reinforce your commitment to the physician-patient relationship
Let's review the criteria we use to do this.	Move to medical criteria

Chapter 3

So Why Should Physicians Care About Disability?

Physicians are patient advocates. Reducing unnecessary disabilities days (days away from work) are in their patients' best interest. The specific benefits for the patient have been outlined in other chapters. So why aren't more physicians helping to reduce unnecessary disabilities days? Lack of training, lack of understanding, limited communication skills, or limited time to spend with patients, to name a few. This has often been summed up as less use of the "art of Medicine" and more dependence on the "gizmos of Medicine." Western medicine and the training of physicians have moved toward "Gizmo Idolatry." "Gizmo" is defined by the American Heritage Dictionary as "a mechanical device or part whose name is forgotten or unknown; a gadget."[52] Gizmo Idolatry has a commonsense appeal because so many gizmos make so much sense, in the absence of evidence or even the presence of evidence to the contrary, their value or utility is persuasive prima facie.[58] Furthermore, humans love bells and whistles, so increasing the technological complexity of treatment appears to increase the significance of an illness and the appeal of an intervention. Gizmo utilization can also be used as proof of competence. Unfortunately, little of this is useful in returning a patient back to work where the limiting factor is often tolerance (biopsychosocial issues), which cannot be measured by gizmos. Much has been published on strategies for developing negotiation skills by bridging gaps and achieving compromise,[55,57] but these suggestions must be balanced with the ability to say "No" in a clinical setting in which ethical or safety issues may affect decisions.[59]

Summary

For early return to work to be successful and to reduce unnecessary work disability, a partnership between the patient, the family, the health care provider, the employer, and the insurer is required.[19] Communication and education are key issues. The work guides must be safe and allow for speedy return to work, with the interests of the patient being the primary responsibility. Early return to work has been demonstrated to be in the patient's best interest.[60–76] Examples of these benefits include better self-image,[77] improved ability to cope,[78] improved work survivability,[50] and improved ability to be self-sufficient.[67] These benefits result in a win-win situation for employee and employer.[66,70,79–80]

Conversely, prolonged time away from work makes recovery and return to work progressively less likely.[81] Prevention of disability is challenging. Physicians cannot prove or disprove the existence of pain clinically.

A person complaining of pain may or may not have nociception, suffering, pain behavior, impairment, or disability. When diagnostic evaluation has ruled out treatable nociception, and when impairment has been addressed, targets for intervention include the suffering component (emotional distress), pain behaviors, and disability issues.

The scientific benefits of early return to work will eventually change physicians' opinions and their application of early return-to-work approaches. However, the real question is whether we as physicians can convert the mind-set and motivational level of an injured worker who has comorbidity and overt barriers to behavioral change. Although the focus of this chapter has been on how the physician should approach the patient, change is only possible if motivation abounds. Overcoming this comorbidity is critical in promoting a degree of motivation to change that will allow the injured worker to create long-term behavioral changes and coping strategies to successfully return to society.

Traumatic injuries occur at a rate of 7.1 per 100 equivalent full-time employees in the private business sector at an estimated cost of more than $1.25 trillion;[82] therefore, the need for better management of work-related injuries has clearly become a priority for the American public and the American business community. Work-related injuries require complex decision making and require the physician to draw on an understanding of basic medical and surgical principles, prior experiences, and familiarity with the literature to formulate a reasonable diagnosis, an appropriate treatment plan, and consideration for reasonable return-to-work guides. In today's environment, where outcomes are important and economics matter greatly, the physician is in a unique position to provide better management of work-related injuries. Improved outcomes are possible when the physician treats the whole patient. This whole-patient approach requires an understanding of the factors that contribute to the poorer outcomes, medical treatment plans that include options to address the psychosocial issues, and early return-to-work guides. These inclusive medical treatment plans aid in the patient's recovery and rehabilitation while avoiding many of the pitfalls of the workers' compensation system. This approach requires a team effort on the part of the patient, physician, employer, insurer, and government, but the benefits are significant and well worth the additional effort.

References

1. Lofgren A, Hagberg J, Arrelov B, et al. Frequency and nature of problems associated with sickness certification tasks: a cross-sectional questionnaire study of 5455 physicians. *Scand J Prim Health Care*. 2007;25:178–85.

2. von Knorring M, Sundberg L, Lofgren A, et al. Problems in sickness certification of patients: a qualitative study on views of 26 physicians in Sweden. *Scand J Prim Health Care*. 2008;26:22–8.

3. Kapoor S, Shaw WS, Pransky G, et al. *J Occup Environ Med*. 2006;48: 1173–80.

4. Reiso H, Gulbrandsen P, Brage S. Doctors' prediction of certified sickness absence. *Fam Pract*. 2004;21:192–9.

5. Reiso H, Nygard JF, Frage S, et al. Work ability assessment by patients and their GPs in new episodes of sickness certification. *Fam Pract*. 2000;17:139–44.

6. Bureau of Labor Statistics. *Occupational Injuries and Illnesses: Counts, Rates, and Characteristics, 1994*. Washington, DC: US Department of Labor; 1997.

7. Bureau of Labor Statistics. *Workplace Injuries and Illnesses in 2002*. Washington, DC: US Department of Labor; 2003.

8. Melhorn JM. *Work-Related Injuries to the Upper Extremities*. Topeka, Kan: Kansas Department of Human Resources, Division of Workers Compensation; 2000.

9. Melhorn JM. Work injuries: the history of CTD/RSI in the workplace. In: Melhorn JM, Zeppieri JP, eds. *Workers' Compensation Case Management: A Multidisciplinary Perspective*. Rosemont, Ill: American Academy of Orthopaedic Surgeons; 1999:221–250.

10. Bureau of Labor and Statistics. *Workplace Injuries and Illnesses in 1997*. Washington, DC: US Department of Labor; 1999.

11. Hebert L. Analytical focus reduces anxiety over CTD claims. *Occup Health Safety*. 1993;62:56–62.

12. Brady W, Bass J, Royce M, et al. Defining total corporate health and safety costs: significance and impact. *J Occup Environ Med*. 1997;39:224–231.

13. Englund L, Svardsudd K. Sick-listing habits among general practitioners in a Swedish county. *Scand J Prim Health Care*. 2000;18;81–86.

14. Pransky, G., Katz, J.N., Benjamin, K., et al. Improving the physician role in evaluating work ability and managing disability: a survey of primary care practitioners. *Disabil Rehabil*. 2002;24:867–874.

15. Arrelov, B., Alexanderson, K., Hagberg, J., Lofgren, A., Nilsson, G., Ponzer, S. Dealing with sickness certification - a survey of problems and strategies among general practitioners and orthopaedic surgeons. *BMC Public Health*. 2007;7:273.

16. Zeppieri JP. The physician, the illness, and the workers' compensation system. In: Beaty JH, ed. *Orthopaedic Knowledge Update 6*. Rosemont, Ill: American Academy of Orthopaedic Surgeons; 1999:131–137.

17. Melhorn JM. *Reducing Unnecessary Workplace Disability: Treating More Than the Injury*. Sacramento, Calif: California Industrial Medicine Council; 2003.

18. Melhorn JM. Occupational orthopaedics. *J Bone Joint Surg Am*. 2000;82A:902–904.

19. Melhorn JM. Workers' compensation: avoiding the work-related disability. *J Bone Joint Surg Am*. 2000;82A:1490–1493.

20. Melhorn JM. Treating more than the injury—reducing disability with early return to work. In: Mandell PJ, ed. *Occupational Health at the Dawn of the New Millennium*. Sacramento, Calif: California Orthopaedic Association; 2000:1–15.

Chapter 3

21. Victor RA, Savych B. Factors Influencing Attorney Involvement. *IAIABC Journal 2010*;47(1):13–22.

22. Americans with Disabilities Act, 42 USC 12101 (1991).

23. Wilson SH, Walker GM. Unemployment and health: a review. *Public Health*. 1993;107:153–162.

24. AAOS Clinical Practice Guidelines (CPG) viewable at http://www.aaos.org/research/guidelines/guide.asp.

25. ACOEM Practice Guidelines viewable at http://www.acoem.org/practiceguidelines.aspx.

26. Official Disability Guidelines viewable at http://www.disabilitydurations.com/.

27. Melhorn JM. The benefits of returning the injured worker to work early: a review of the research. *J Workers Comp*. 2000;10:60–75.

28. Macher A. *Annual Statistical Bulletin*. Boca Raton, Fla: National Council on Compensation Insurance Inc; 1998.

29. Christian J. Reducing disability days: healing more than the injury. *J Workers Comp*. 2000;9(2):30–55.

30. Arnetz BB, Sjogren B, Rydehn B, Meisel R. Early workplace intervention for employees with musculoskeletal-related absenteeism: a prospective controlled intervention study. *J Occup Environ Med*. 2003;45:499–506.

31. Abramson JH, Gofin J, Habib J. Work satisfaction and health in the middle-aged and elderly. *J Epidemiol*. 1994;23:98–104.

32. Bednar JM, Baesher-Griffith P, Osterman AL. Workers compensation effect of state law on treatment cost and work status. *Clin Orthop*. 1998;351:74–77.

33. Anema JR, Van Der Giezen AM, Buijs PC, Van Mechelen W. Ineffective disability management by doctors is an obstacle for return-to-work: a cohort study on low back pain patients sicklisted for 3–4 months. *Occup Environ Med*. 2002;59:729–733.

34. American Medical Association. *Guides to the Evaluation of Permanent Impairment*. 5th ed. Chicago, Ill: American Medical Association; 2001.

35. American Medical Association. *Guides to the Evaluation of Permanent Impairment*. 6th ed. Chicago, Ill: American Medical Association; 2009.

36. Melhorn JM. Return to work issues: arm pain. In: Melhorn JM, Strain RE Jr, eds. *Occupational Orthopaedics and Workers' Compensation: A Multidisciplinary Perspective*. Rosemont, Ill: American Academy of Orthopaedic Surgeons; 2002.

37. Melhorn JM. Evidence to support early return to work: how to write appropriate return to work guides. In: *Annual Meeting 2003*. Sacramento, Calif: California Orthopaedic Association; 2002:75–98.

38. Melhorn JM. Upper extremities: return to work issues. In: Melhorn JM, Spengler DM, eds. *5th Annual Occupational Orthopaedics and Workers' Compensation: A Multidisciplinary Perspective*. Rosemont, Ill: American Academy of Orthopaedic Surgeons; 2003:256–285.

39. Melhorn JM. Return to work: the employer's point of view. In: *2003 Safety and Health Conference*. Topeka, Kan: Kansas Department of Human Resources; 2003.

Chapter 3

40. Brena SF, Chapman SL, Stegall PG, Chyatte, SB. Chronic pain states: their relationship to impairment and disability. *Arch Phys Med Rehabil.* 1979;60:387–389.

41. Melhorn JM. Return to work: workplace guides. In: Melhorn JM, Zeppieri JP, eds. *Workers' Compensation Case Management: A Multidisciplinary Perspective*. Rosemont, Ill: American Academy of Orthopaedic Surgeons; 1999:451–458.

42. Melhorn JM. Work restrictions for return to work. In: Zeppieri JP, Spengler DM, eds. *Workers' Compensation Case Management: A Multidisciplinary Perspective*. Rosemont, Ill: American Academy of Orthopaedic Surgeons; 1997:249–266.

43. Bigos SJ, Battie MC, Spengler DM, et al. A longitudinal, prospective study of industrial back injury reporting. *Clin Orthop.* 1992;279:21–34.

44. Fordyce WE, Bigos SJ, Battie MC, Fisher LD. MMPI Scale 3 as a predictor of back injury report: what does it tell us? *Clin J Pain.* 1992;8:222–226.

45. Melhorn JM. The advantages of early return to work. *IAIABC J.* 2003;41:128–147.

46. American College of Occupational and Environmental Medicine. *ACOEM's Eight Best Ideas for Workers' Compensation Reform*. In: *American College of Occupational and Environmental Medicine Conference*. Chicago, Ill: American College of Occupational and Environmental Medicine. 1997;4.

47. Colledge AL, Johns RE Jr, Thomas MH. Functional ability assessment: guidelines for the workplace. *J Occup Environ Med.* 1999;41:172–180.

48. Equal Employment Opportunity Commission. *Job Advertising and Pre-Employment Inquiries Under the Age Discrimination in Employment Act*. Washington, DC: Equal Employment Opportunity Commission; 1989.

49. Equal Employment Opportunity Commission. Equal Employment Opportunity Commission issues final enforcement guidance on preemployment disability-related questions and medical examinations under the Americans With Disabilities Act. *Equal Employment Opportunity Commission News*. 1995;95:1–5.

50. Melhorn JM. CTD injuries: an outcome study for work survivability. *J Workers Comp.* 1996;5:18–30.

51. Rainville J, Carlson N, Polatin P, Gatchel RJ, Indahl A. Exploration of physicians' recommendations for activities in chronic back pain. *Spine.* 2000;25: 2210–2220.

52. *The American Heritage Dictionary of the English Language, Fourth Edition*, 2006. Online at dictionary.reference.com.

53. Melhorn JM. Negotiating return to work: strategies to deal with the dreaded moment. In: Melhorn JM, Barr JS Jr, eds. *Occupational Orthopaedics and Workers' Compensation: A Multidisciplinary Perspective*. Rosemont, Ill: American Academy of Orthopaedic Surgeons; 2001.

54. Di Guida AW. Negotiating a successful return to work program. *AAOHN J.* 1995;43:101–106.

55. Fisher R, Ury W. *Getting to Yes: Negotiating Agreement Without Giving In*. New York, NY: Penguin Books; 1981.

56. Linney BJ. The successful physician negotiator. *Physician Exec.* 1999;25:62–65.

57. Melhorn JM. Getting to yes: negotiating successful return to work. In: Melhorn JM, Spengler DM, eds. *Occupational Orthopaedics and Workers' Compensation: A Multidisciplinary Perspective.* Rosemont, Ill: American Academy of Orthopaedic Surgeons; 2003:517–534.

58. Leff B and Finucane TE. Gizmo idolatry. *JAMA.* 2008;299(15):1830–1832.

59. Paterniti DA, Fancher TL, Cipri CS, Timmermans S, Heritage J, and Kravitz RL. Getting to "no": strategies primary care physicians use to deny patient requests. *Arch Intern Med.* 2010;170(4):381–388.

60. Cook AC, Birkholz S, King EF, Szabo RM. Early mobilization following carpal tunnel release: a prospective randomized study. *J Hand Surg.* 1995;20B:228–230.

61. Melhorn JM, Wilkinson LK. *CTD Solutions for the 90's: A Comprehensive Guide to Managing CTD in the Workplace.* Wichita, Kan: Via Christi Health Systems; 1996.

62. Melhorn JM. CTD solutions for the 90's: prevention. In: *Seventeenth Annual Workers' Compensation and Occupational Medicine Seminar.* Boston, Mass: Seak Inc; 1997:234–245.

63. Melhorn JM. Identification of individuals at risk for developing CTD. In: Spengler DM, Zeppieri JP, eds. *Workers' Compensation Case Management: A Multidisciplinary Perspective.* Rosemont, Ill: American Academy of Orthopaedic Surgeons; 1997:41–51.

64. Melhorn JM. Physician support and employer options for reducing risk of CTD. In: Spengler DM, Zeppieri JP, eds. *Workers' Compensation Case Management: A Multidisciplinary Perspective.* Rosemont, Ill: American Academy of Orthopaedic Surgeons; 1997:26–34.

65. Ballard M, Baxter P, Bruening L, Fried S. Work therapy and return to work. *Hand Clin.* 1986;2:247–258.

66. Bruce WC, Bruce RS. Return-to-work programs in the unionized company. *J Workers Comp.* 1996;38:9–17.

67. Burke SA, Harms-Constas CK, Aden PS. Return to work/work retention outcomes of a functional restoration program: a multi-center, prospective study with a comparison group. *Spine.* 1994;19:1880–1885.

68. Centineo J. Return-to-work programs: cut costs and employee turnover. *Risk Manage.* 1986;33:44–48.

69. Day CS, McCabe SJ, Alexander G. Return to work as an outcome measure in hand surgery. Paper presented at: Annual Meeting of the American Society for Surgery of the Hand; September 15, 1993; Baltimore, Md.

70. Devlin M, O'Neill P, MacBride R. Position paper in support of timely return to work programs and the role of the primary care physician. *Ont Med Assoc.* 1994;61:1–45.

71. Gice JH, Tompkins K. Cutting costs with return-to-work programs. *Risk Manage.* 1988;35:62–65.

72. Goodman RC. An aggressive return-to-work program in surgical treatment of carpal tunnel syndrome: a comparison of costs. *Plast Reconstr Surg.* 1989;89:715–717.

Chapter 3

73. Groves FB, Gallagher LA. What the hand surgeon should know about workers' compensation. *Hand Clin*. 1993;9:369–372.

74. Grunet BK, Devine CA, Smith CJ, et al. Graded work exposure to promote work return after severe hand trauma: a replicated study. *Ann Plast Surg*. 1992;29:532–536.

75. Kasdan ML, June LA. Returning to work after a unilateral hand fracture. *J Occup Environ Med*. 1993;35:132–135.

76. Nathan PA, Meadows KD, Keniston RC. Rehabilitation of carpal tunnel surgery patients using a short surgical incision and an early program of physical therapy. *J Hand Surg*. 1993;18A:1044–1050.

77. Bernacki EJ, Tsai SP. Managed care for workers' compensation: three years of experience in an "employee choice" state. *J Occup Environ Med*. 1996;38: 1091–1097.

78. Bigos SJ, Spengler DM, Martin NA, et al. Back injuries in industry: a retrospective study. III. Employee related factors. *Spine*. 1986;11:252–256.

79. Dworkin RH, Handlin DS, Richlin DM, Rrand L, Vannucci C. Unraveling the effects of compensation, litigation, and employment on treatment response in chronic pain. *Pain*. 1985;23:49–59.

80. Hall H, McIntosh G, Melles T, Holowachuk B, Wai E. Effect of discharge recommendations on outcome. *Spine*. 1994;19:2033–2037.

81. Strang JP. The chronic disability syndrome. In: Aronoff GM, ed. *Evaluation and Treatment of Chronic Pain*. Baltimore, Md: Urban & Schwarzenberg; 1985:247–258.

82. W. Brady, J. Bass, M. Royce, G. Anstadt, R. Loeppke, and R. Leopold. Defining total corporate health and safety costs: significance and impact. *J Occup Environ Med*. 1997;39(3):224–231.

Chapter 3

Chapter 4

Return to Work: Forms, Records, and Disclaimers

J. Mark Melhorn, MD and Mark H. Hyman, MD

The patient: "Doc, can I return to work?"

The employer: "Doc, can Joe return to work?"

Both: "If I/he can return to work, what are the 'restrictions?'"

These are but a few of the questions that are asked of health care providers who treat individuals who have injuries, which may or may not be work related, but want to get back to work. The question of work restrictions and limitations is often followed with a list of job activities, many of which may not apply to the individual being treated. Additionally, the term *work restrictions* implies a negative approach rather than the terms *work guides* or *capacity guides*, which imply a positive approach. Unfortunately, the label of "work restrictions" is ingrained into the system and therefore unlikely to change, but it is important for the health care provider to communicate to the injured worker the concept of retained capacity as discussed in Chapter 3, How to Negotiate Return to Work. So, how does the health care provider approach stay-at-work and return-to-work forms, records, and disclaimers?

Introduction

Return to work is only one part of the life history of an injury or accident. The injured worker must move through five steps: injury and the determination of a relationship to the workplace; diagnosis and treatment; possible time off work, and (if there is time off) return to work; determination of impairment and disability; and resolution of disputes and settlement of the claim. (See Chapter 3 for more information about each of these steps.) Within the current workers' compensation system, the physician can improve the quality of life for the injured worker through medical care, facilitation of stay at work or early return to work, and assistance with accident prevention.[1] As an advocate for individuals and in the best interest of society, physicians should encourage appropriate early return to work and rehabilitation, not disability. Early intervention by the physician and a rehabilitation counselor after injury can facilitate a positive attitude and empower the worker to resist the negative effect of the system reinforcers that discourage early return to work.[2]

Many consider modified work to be the cornerstone of disability management.[3–5] Returning the injured employee to work is often challenging. Many obstacles develop that involve the employee, physician, and employer. Assuming the employee is willing to return to work and the employer is willing to provide modified work, the critical element becomes the physician's ability to communicate the appropriate physical capacity guides. Work guides are commonly referred to as "work restrictions."[6,7] As reviewed in Chapter 2, the term *work restrictions* should be used to refer to those activities that the individual can do but should not do because of risk. Physicians impose work restrictions for individual safety. The term *work limitations* addresses what the individual lacks in current ability or capacity (ie, what the individual cannot do). Physicians describe what individuals are not capable of doing on the basis of capacity. The concepts of restrictions and capacity tend to focus on the loss, rather than on the retained ability of the employee.

Tolerance is whether individuals are *willing to tolerate* symptoms such as pain or fatigue. Temporary work guides (or suggestions for modified duty) during the initial phases of recovery from injury or illness are frequently appropriate on the basis of symptom tolerance, but these should not become permanent. If incomplete recovery occurs, ultimately the individual must decide if the rewards of work outweigh the symptoms. The term *work guides* allows a physician to suggest appropriate levels of activity without having to specify whether the "guides" are restrictions, limitations, or statements about a believable tolerance for activity. As time for healing passes and the individual reaches maximum medical improvement (MMI), a physician should clarify for all concerned whether at this point the "guides" are work restrictions (based on risk), work limitations (based on capacity), or suggestions. But the issue of tolerance is the basis, and, ultimately, the decision to work at jobs that exceed the "guides" is the individual's. Unfortunately, the incorrect use of the term *work restrictions* (wrongly applied to restriction, capacity, and tolerance) is unlikely to disappear anytime soon, but it is important for all parties to understand and focus on the concept of retained ability.

Although a physician must consider all three parts of the return-to-work formula (risk, capacity, and tolerance) from the individual worker's point of view, perhaps the greatest amount of guesswork expected of the physician is in the determination of capacity. At the same time, this decision also has the greatest effect on the individual. Appropriate capacity or work guides require an understanding of the injury, the individual, and the job. Fortunately, physicians can make a fair estimate of the time required for healing on the basis of empiric knowledge of specific injuries. Also, individuals possess unique knowledge of their job and therefore need to actively participate in a functional capacity guide. The physician must then blend the individual's information with the employer's information while factoring in the science of the injury.

Employers often request detailed charts of "restrictions" based on ability to lift, push, pull, climb, bend, stoop, crawl, kneel, and other activities. When presented in a form, it is often difficult for the physician to differentiate what a normal healthy person of similar age, sex, education, and body build would be capable of doing. Standards created by the US Department of Labor, found in *The Dictionary of Occupational Titles*—Physical Demands of Work (Table 4-1) and Physical Demand Characteristics of Work (Table 4-2)—are a helpful starting point.[8] Millender and Conlon expanded on these guides by matching possible additional job activities to eight general job categories (Table 4-3).[9]

Chapter 4

Table 4-1 Physical Demands of Work[8]

Physical Demand Level	Lb Lifting (Frequent/ Occasional)	Lb Carry (Frequent/ Occasional)	Lb Push/ Pull	Climbing	Bend, Stoop, Twist/h	Sit/ Stand (min)	Walk (h/d)
Sedentary	0/10	0/10	100	None	0	30	1
Sedentary-light	5/15	5/15	125	Ramp	<10	30	2
Light	10/20	15/20	150	Stairs	15	45	3
Light-medium	20/35	20/35	200	Stairs	20	60	3+
Medium	20/50	25/50	250	Ladder	30	90	4
Medium-heavy	35/50	40/75	300	Ladder	40	120/120	4+
Heavy	50/100	50/100	350	Scaffold	50	180/150	5
Very heavy	50/100+	75/100+	400+	Pole/Rope	60+	210/180+	7

Table 4-2 Physical Demand Characteristics of Work[8]

Physical Demand Level	Occasional (0% to 33% of Workday)	Frequent (34% to 66% of Workday)	Constant (67% to 100% of Workday)	Typical Energy Required (Metabolic Equivalents)
Sedentary	10 lb	Negligible	Negligible	1.5–2.1
Light	20 lb	10 lb	Negligible	2.2–3.5
Light-medium	35 lb	20 lb	5 lb	3.6–4.5
Medium	50 lb	20 lb	10 lb	4.6–6.3
Medium-heavy	75 lb	35 lb	15 lb	6.4–7.0
Heavy	100 lb	50 lb	20 lb	7.1–7.5
Very heavy	>100 lb	>50 lb	>20 lb	>7.5

Communication: The Issues That Should Be Documented in Physician Records

In workers' compensation cases, and in non–workers' compensation cases in which private disability insurance or social security disability are likely to be involved, copies of the physician's records are likely to end up in the legal system. There should be a database in the records to support return-to-work decision making.

Initial Medical Record

The physician's initial medical record should include the following traditional medical information:

- Chief complaint

- History of present illness

- Review of systems

- History of previous illnesses

- Family and social history

- Physical examination, which should include:

  —general constitutional items

  —specific findings from pertinent organ system examination

Table 4-3 Guidelines for Tasks by Job Categories

Job Category	Job Description	Weight Lifted, lb*	Weight Pushed or Pulled, lb*	Weight Carried, lb*	Climbing†	Body Motion‡	Sitting-Standing Transition§	Walking (% of Day)
1	Sedentary	10/0	150/0	≤10/0	Ramp/none	<10	30 min	10
2	Sedentary-light	15/≤5	200/100–125	15/≤5	None/ramp	<10	30 min	20
3	Light	20/≤10	250/125–150	20/10–15	Stairs/none	10–15	30–45 min	30
4	Light-medium	35/≤20	300/200–250	35/20	None/stairs	15–20	45 to 60 min	40
5	Medium	50/≤35	350/250–300	50/25–30	Ladder/stairs	20–30	1–1.5 h	50
6	Medium-heavy	75/≤50	400/300–350	75/30–40	Scaffold/ladder	30–40	1.5–2 h	60
7	Heavy	100/≤50	450/350–400	100/40–50	Poles/scaffold	40–60	2–2.5 h	70
8	Very heavy	>100/>50	>450/>400	>100/>60	Rope/poles	>60	>2.5 h	80

* Values are expressed as weight infrequently (0%–33% of time)/weight frequently (67%–100% of time).
† Descriptions are expressed as type of climbing infrequently/frequently.
‡ Values are number of instances of body motion (bending, kneeling, squatting, or reaching) per hour.
§ Values are time spent in continuous transition between sitting and standing positions.
Reproduced with permission from Millender and Conlon.[9]

- A working diagnosis

- Plans for further testing

- A medical treatment plan

- Administrative issues, which should include:

  —a description of the onset of symptoms and their relationship to the workplace

  —a statement establishing causation, aggravation, or exacerbation and any relationship to the workplace injury or illness

  —details of the job at the time of onset of symptoms; interval jobs and work capacity guides; current job and current work capacity guides; and a list of what job activities the employee currently can do without symptoms plus a list of jobs the employee believes he or she could perform without symptoms

  —suggestions for workplace modifications, accommodations, or ergonomic issues

- Functional capacity guides, which should include:

  —current ability to work, regular or modified, full time or part time

  —estimated time to maximum medical improvement (MMI)

  —specific functional capacity guides as listed in the next section

Interval Report

Each follow-up office visit note should contain the interval history, including the following:

- The response to treatment (have symptoms and findings improved?)

- Any administrative and legal actions or conflicts that are of medical importance (employer refuses to accept causation, a lawyer has been retained, medical referrals, worker not receiving benefits)

- Treatment options, treatment changes, and medical testing decisions

- Work guides (these may be restrictions, limitations, or suggestions to minimize symptoms)

Final Report

When the individual has reached MMI, the physician's record should include the following:

- A summary of treatment and the response to treatment

- A declaration of MMI, in the form of a statement that the individual has reached a medical end result and that no significant change in physical findings or activity levels is expected in the foreseeable future. No significant further treatment changes or diagnostic testing should be anticipated; maintenance treatment may be ongoing, but there is no plan for a future trial of a treatment that might decrease the impairment or increase the individual's function. This means that the work status is no longer temporary, but is now permanent. A need for vocational rehabilitation may be mentioned if appropriate.

- An administrative progress statement detailing the ability to work and giving final work guides, but clearly stating whether the "guides" are work restrictions (based on risk), work limitations (based on capacity), or suggestions about the level of symptoms the individual is likely to tolerate to facilitate return to work.

- A determination of permanent impairment, usually expressed as a percentage, and most frequently obtained from the AMA *Guides to the Evaluation of Permanent Impairment*,[10] with the edition dependent on the jurisdiction of the claim.

Physicians should address these issues in individual records. Having a template or outline for dictation or recording of the visit may be helpful.

Four Screening Tests for Establishing Functional Capacity Guides

Four questions have been developed by Christian[3] to help the physician understand return to work, accommodations for the workplace, and the likelihood of successful return to work. Christian used these questions to develop a physicians' training course for work fitness and disability.

Question 1: Return to Work

The individual is asked the following questions in relation to his or her job:

- Is your injury going to make it hard for you to do your usual job the regular way?

- Are you going to have any problems with your boss or coworkers about your injury?

- Have you figured out a way to work despite your injury while you recover?

If the answers are "yes," "yes," and "no," returning to work will be difficult.

Question 2: The Grocery Store

If the individual owned his or her own grocery store, would he or she be able to find a way to work safely? If the answer is "yes," then absence from work is probably not medically required. Therefore, a nonmedical aspect (or psychosocial issue) of the injury to this individual, and *not* the medical condition, is creating the disability.

Question 3: The Molehill Sign

Is the individual making a mountain out of a molehill, or is an apparently minor health condition having a major effect on the individual's daily life and functions? This assessment requires the physician to mentally compare this individual to other individuals with similar injuries or illnesses by objective disease or injury criteria. If the answer is "yes," motivation is the issue creating disability, and the physician's job is to find the source: worker, supervisor, employer, etc.

Question 4: The Obstacle

What is the specific obstacle preventing the individual from working today? This question may uncover situational or environmental obstacles to returning to work.

Establishing Reasonable Functional Capacity Guides or Work Guides

Physicians who treat work-related injuries realize that there is no easy reference for developing work guides. By combining the elements of the injury, the individual, and the job; safe and reasonable functional capacity guides can be provided. Ideally, these guides will allow the injured employee an opportunity to return to appropriate work, while using the workplace as an integral part of the therapy program. Combining a job with rehabilitation should be the most cost-effective program possible.

It may be useful to consult published disability durations such as those in *The Medical Disability Advisor/MDGuidelines* by the Reed Group, the Work Loss Data Institute's *ODG Treatment in Workers' Comp 2004*, or L. S. Glass's *Occupational Medicine Practice Guidelines*: *Evaluation and Management of Common Health Problems and Functional Recovery in Workers*.[11–13] If the individual has exceeded the recommended maximal disability duration for the illness or injury in question, that fact can be shared with the individual and used to support written decisions by the physician encouraging a prompt return to work.

Work characteristics, including frequency of task performance and weight, should be discussed. Weight guides are based on the US Department of Labor's *Dictionary of Occupational Titles* (Tables 4-1 and 4-2).[8]

Total activities should be considered next. These may include lift, push-pull, carry, climb, body motion, sitting, standing, and walking (Table 4-3). Total activities occur in three domains: activities of daily living (ADLs), therapy (occupational and physical), and workplace activities. After arriving at a general range for total activities, the physician should apportion a percentage to home, therapy, and work.

The graph in Table 4-4 shows how to balance the amount of time and activities for therapy and work, because home usually remains fairly constant. As each individual is unique, the general approach to balancing activities is to gradually increase work while gradually decreasing therapy. Some individuals may be able to tolerate therapy and a regular workday. Others may require work guides that limit work activities, especially work hours, on therapy days. These individuals may benefit from a more frequent and active therapy program. As endurance for work activities improves, the frequency and level of activity of the therapy program can be decreased. Each individual will start this graph at a different location.

Chapter 4

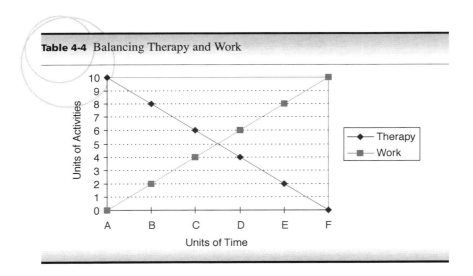

Table 4-4 Balancing Therapy and Work

Units of Activities (y-axis): 0–10
Units of Time (x-axis): A B C D E F

Legend: ◆ Therapy, ■ Work

Work characteristics can be provided in both frequency ("limited" at 0% to 12% of the work day, "occasional" at 13% to 33%, "frequent" at 34% to 66%, and "constant" at 67% to 100%) and time (0, 2, 4, 6, or 8 hours per workday). The activities that can be performed, eg, repetitive grasping, pushing, pulling, fine manipulation, vibratory tools, power tools, and hand over shoulder, should be stated.

On follow-up visits, it is important to record the individual's current working status. The medical status can simply be "yes" or "no" for presently working. If not working, the examiner has to consider why the individual is not working. It could be that no work is available from the employer, the individual does not want to work, or the individual and employer are uncertain as to work guides. Expected future changes in work guides should be discussed. For example, the physician might say: "Today you are available for light work; if you continue to do well, we will consider light-to-medium work at your next follow-up visit." This communication allows the individual time to consider the physician's recommendations. The individual may even try testing a weight level a few times to see if he or she can do it before the next visit. This home effort can allow time to build confidence, and the physician has emphasized the plan of continued improvement, not continued disability. By using the same work guides form, the physician has developed a communication tool, a record of the improvement, and the successful transition from alternative work to regular work. In addition, the last work guide can be used to complete information contained in the permanent physical impairment report.

Another opportunity for communicating in advance is the section for individuals undergoing elective surgery. This section encourages discussion about early return to work and includes the following:

> Before surgery—same work pattern. After surgery—you may return to modified light work the day after surgery (maximum 20 lb or less lift/carry; frequent at 10 lb for both arms, possible cast or dressing on, no large power or vibratory tools, limit extremity use on operated side). Your work production may initially be decreased in the postoperative period. In general, you should gradually increase your activities at home and at work. Please provide these guides to your employer prior to surgery. These workplace guides have been reviewed with me.

Physicians may have the individual sign as needed for confirmation. This section helps to stimulate communication between the individual and the physician and allows for a mutual effort to write reasonable work guides. It is important for both individual and treating physician to realize that the company physician may modify the work guides further on the basis of special knowledge of the workplace.

Sample Linkage Forms

Linkage, or the ability to combine the elements of the injury, the individual, and the job for the development of safe and reasonable work guides, occurs by using standard functional capacity forms. It is nearly impossible to remember each of the required elements each time functional capacity or work guides are being considered. To make the process manageable, reliable, readable, and consistent, *each physician should develop a standard return-to-work form based on his or her specific practice*. This creates familiarity and allows for linkage with science.

Tables 4-1 through 4-6 are the starting points. Standard forms also allow for negotiation of functional capacity with the individual. To be effective, the

Table 4-5 Epidemiologic Evidence for Work-Related Musculoskeletal Disorders*

Body Part and Risk Factor	Strong Evidence (+++)	Evidence (++)	Insufficient Evidence (+/0)	Evidence of No Effect (−)
Neck and neck/shoulder				
Repetition		X		
Force	X			
Posture	X			
Vibration			X	
Shoulder				
Repetition		X		
Force			X	
Posture		X		
Vibration			X	
Elbow				
Repetition			X	
Force		X		
Posture			X	
Combination	X			

(Continued)

Table 4-5 *(Continued)*

Body Part and Risk Factor	Strong Evidence (+++)	Evidence (++)	Insufficient Evidence (+/0)	Evidence of No Effect (−)
Hand/wrist				
Carpal tunnel syndrome				
Repetition		X		
Force		X		
Posture			X	
Vibration		X		
Combination	X			
Tendinitis				
Repetition		X		
Force		X		
Posture		X		
Combination	X			
Hand-arm vibration syndrome				
Vibration	X			
Back				
Lifting/forceful movement	X			
Awkward posture		X		
Heavy physical work		X		
Whole body vibration	X			
Static work posture			X	

* Strong epidemiologic evidence (+++) indicates that the consistently positive findings from a large number of cross-sectional studies, strengthened by the limited number of prospective studies, provide strong evidence of increased risk of work-related musculoskeletal disorders for some body parts based on the strength of the associations, lack of ambiguity, consistency of the results, and adequate control or adjustment for likely confounders in cross-sectional studies and the temporal relationships from the prospective studies, with reasonable confidence levels in at least several of those studies. Epidemiologic evidence (++) indicates that some convincing epidemiologic evidence shows a causal relationship when the epidemiologic criteria of causality for intense or long-duration exposure to the specific risk factor(s) and musculoskeletal disorders are used. A positive relationship has been observed between exposure to the specific risk factor and musculoskeletal disorders in studies in which chance, bias, and confounding factors are not the likely explanation. Insufficient epidemiologic evidence (+/0) indicates that the available studies are of insufficient number, quality, consistency, or statistical power to permit a conclusion regarding the presence or absence of a causal association. Some studies suggest a relationship to specific risk factors, but chance, bias, or confounding may explain the association. Either there is an insufficient number of studies from which to draw conclusions or the overall conclusion from the studies is equivocal. The absence of existing epidemiologic evidence should not be interpreted to mean that there is no association between work factors and musculoskeletal disorders. No epidemiologic evidence (−) indicates that there have been no adequate studies to show that the specific workplace risk factor(s) is not related to development of musculoskeletal disorders.

Table 4-6 Workplace Risk Factors

Stressor	Attributes	Work Factors
Repetition	Exertion frequency	Production standard
	Recovery time	Pacing
	Percentage recovery	Incentives
	Cycle time	Work quantities/unit time
	Velocity and acceleration	Methods/materials
	Force	Work rotation
	Posture	Manufacturing process
		Mechanical aids
		Quality control
		Machines
Force	Amplitude probability	Friction
	Distribution	Weight of work objects
	Peak	Balance
	Average	Reaction forces/torques
	Static vs dynamic	Drag forces
	Smooth vs jerky	Mechanical aids
		Gloves/handles
		Quality control
		Machines
Posture	Range of motion	Work location
	Average	Work orientation
	Time position	Work object shape
		Methods/materials
		Machine
		Environment
Vibration	Frequency	Abrasive
	Displacement	Tool drive train
	Velocity	Bit condition
	Acceleration	Isolation/dampening
	Duration	Gloves
Temperature	Low temperature	Temperature of air
	Conductivity	Work object temperature
	Duration	Air exhaust
		Gloves
		Protective clothing

(Continued)

Chapter 4

Table 4-6 *(Continued)*

Stressor	Attributes	Work Factors
Contact stress	Force	Force factors
	Area	Area of contact
	Location	Location of contact
	Duration	Gloves
Unaccustomed activities	Duration	Work schedules
	Hours	Work standards
	Days	Incentives
	Percentage of time	Methods/environment

information must be transferred to the employee and employer with every office visit.

Table 4-7 is an example of an office encounter form or charge ticket. Each office will need to modify its encounter form to accommodate its specialty. There are several important sections that all forms should have. It is very efficient and effective to have all the information for one visit on one page. This form has a carbonless copy that is given to the individual at each office visit to be taken to the employer. This makes for immediate communication between the individual and employer.

The top of the form shows the services provided during the office visit. The practice may decide to place this section on a separate form, as it is used in billing for the physician's service. The second area deals with the diagnosis. Employers may (workers' compensation) or may not (private disability) have a right to know the diagnosis without individual consent. The third area is the functional capacity guides section. The fourth contains the next appointment. The fifth is the section on individual demographics, and the last contains the individual's and/or physician's signature.

Table 4-8 is an enlargement of the functional capacity or work guides section from Table 4-7. There are two key points to include:

- "Please consider this individual to be off work until the next appointment unless alternative or transitional work is available as circled or checked below."

  ___ work status, hours of work and type of work, work characteristics

  ___ preoperative and postoperative guides

  ___ physician and individual signatures

Table 4-7 Encounter Form

The Hand Center
ORTHOPAEDICS OF THE HAND & UPPER EXTREMITY

625 N. Carriage Parkway
Suite 125, Wichita, Kansas 67208
FAX (316) 683-8787

J. Mark Melhorn, M.D.
(316) 688-5656 Appointments
(316) 688-5757 Patient Accounts
(316) 688-5454 Medical Records

PLEASE RETURN TO FRONT DESK FOR SCHEDULING

OFFICE		CAST			X-RAYS	CODE	OTHER	CODE
INITIAL 99201-5	Before surgery—same work pattern.	Short Arm	29075	R L	Cervical Spine 7v	72052	Hosp Care Init	99221-3
	After surgery—you may return to modified light	Long Arm	29065	R L			Hosp Care Subs	99231-3
	work the day after surgery. (Max. 20 lbs. or less	Thumb Spica (TS) Short Long		R L	Shoulder 3v	73030	R L Consult Init Inpat	99251-5
	lift/carry; frequent at 10 lbs. for both arms),				Shoulder 2v	73020	R L Consult FU Inpat	99261-5
FOLLOWUP 99211-5	possible cast or dressing on, no large power or	Dressing/Splint			Scapula	73010	R L	
	vibratory tools, limit extremity use on operated	Short Arm	S	R L	Clavicle	73000	R L	
	side. Your work production may initially be	Long Arm	L	R L	Humerus	73060	R L Emerg. Room	99281-5
Consult 99241-5	decreased in the post-operative period. In gen-	Thumb Spica Short Long		R L				
	eral, you should gradually increase your activi-				Elbow 4v	73080	R L	
Consult Confirm 99271-5	ties at home and at work. Please provide these	Splint DIP PIP MCP	29130	R L	Elbow 2v	73070	R L IME / CIE	
	guides to your employer prior to surgery.	Wrist Brace (WB)	99070	R L	Forearm	73090	R L	
INJECTION (ITS) 20550 R L	These work guides have been reviewed with me.				Wrist 3v	73110	R L Med Mgmt Conf	99361
		MRI		R L	Wrist 3v Grip	73110G	R L Med Mgmt Phone	99371
Sm. 20600 R L		3 Phase Scan		R L	CT	73110C	R L Rehab-consult	
Med. 20605 R L		Arthrogram		R L	Scaphoid	73110S	R L X-Ray Review	76140
Lg. 20610 R L		EMG/NCT		R L	Wrist 2v	73100	R L	
					Hand 3v	73130	R L Review Records	
c/c/t xero so/ss	Patient Signature	*Remove Implant	20670	R L	Hand 2v	73120	R L Release of records	
		Suture Tray(ST)			Fingers	73140	R L Authorization	
DIAGNOSIS	DOI or DOO MO_____DAY_____YR_____ LWD MO____DAY____YR____				Thumb	73140	R L	
	Auto Work Home School Other _____						XTP	
					G	95832		

CODES

Professional fees are charged according to services provided.
Insurance companies require this billing format, but each establish their own guides for reimbursement limits.

PLEASE CONSIDER OFF WORK UNTIL NEXT APPOINTMENT UNLESS ALTERNATIVE OR TRANSITIONAL WORK IS AVAILABLE AS CIRCLED OR CHECKED BELOW:

	TOTAL HOURS AT WORK PER WORK DAY	0 2 4 6 8 +
Unchanged from previous visit	repetitive grasping	0 2 4 6 8
Regular	Right / left hand only	pushing/pulling	0 2 4 6 8
No restrictions	with coban wrap/glove on	fine manipulation	0 2 4 6 8
As Tolerated	with buddy tape	Post Op Gradual Increasing Work Load	
Modified	with cast on ___ off	limit vibratory tools	0 2 4 6 8
No work until next visit	with splint on / AS NEEDED / off	limit power tools	0 2 4 6 8
Pt. says no work available	w/splint Work Sleep Both ↑ ↓	limit hands over shoulders	0 2 4 6 8

Driving if ok by DOT

WORK CHARACTERISTICS: Limited (0-12), Occasional (0-33), Frequent (34-66), Constant (67-100)

SEDENTARY WORK: max. 10 lbs or less lift/carry; occasional lift/carry   task rotation ergo workplace
LIGHT WORK: max. 20 lbs or less lift/carry; frequent at 10 lbs   job rotation rom ointment
LIGHT MEDIUM: max. 35 lbs or less lift/carry; frequent at 20 lbs   heat am cool pm contrast bath
MEDIUM WORK: max. 50 lbs or less lift/carry; frequent at 25 lbs   exercise stretch strength
MEDIUM HEAVY: max. 75 lbs or less lift/carry; frequent at 35 lbs   splint coban scar management
HEAVY WORK: max. 100 lbs or less lift/carry; frequent at 50 lbs
Pt. says presently working: yes no Trial regular work.

Repetitive Lift Carry 30/hr
Repetitive Grasp 250/hr or 2000/8hr

If you are not satisfied with the work restrictions above, please see your company physician.
This physician may modify these restrictions further based on their special knowledge of your work place.

A minimum of (5) working days written notice is required to send out x-rays or medical records from this office.

IF WORK COMP, YOU ARE REQUIRED TO GIVE THIS WORK STATUS TO YOUR EMPLOYER IMMEDIATELY AFTER EACH VISIT.

Physician's Signature

NEXT APPOINTMENT	M T W T F Days ____ Weeks ____ Months ____	As Needed PPI	Set

DATE	TIME	PATIENT	REASON	PRIOR BALANCE	This time is scheduled for you.

TICKET NO.	DR. #	DOCTOR	LOCATION	D.O.B.	TODAY'S CHARGE	

PATIENT NO.	RESPONSIBLE PARTY	PH#	REFERRING DR.	COPAY CHARGE	**YOU MAY BE CHARGED A FEE IF YOU FAIL TO KEEP THIS APPOINTMENT.**

This fee will not be billed to work comp or insurance and will be due before your next office visit. 48 hours notice to change your appointment is required to avoid this fee. Calls for appointment changes must be made during office hours at 688-5656 Monday - Friday 8:15-4:30.

S E X	M F	ADDRESS	CITY/STATE	ZIP CODE	
A C C T	OVER 90 OVER 60 OVER 30 CURRENT TOTAL DUE	PT BC CS PAY CHOICE	TODAY'S PAYMENT	Arrived ____ In ____ Out ____

Medicare will be filed.

INSURANCE COMPANY	BA SCT	POLICY I.D.	RELATIONSHIP TO INSURED	**BALANCE DUE**
			S E L F S P O U S E C H I L D O T H E R	

I hereby authorize my insurance benefits to be paid directly to the above signed physician, realizing I am responsible to pay non-covered services and I hereby authorize the release of pertinent medical information to insurance carriers.

Patient Signature

If your insurance policy requires a referral, it is your responsibility to call your primary physician prior to your next appointment. Co-pays are due at time of check-in. Thank you.

Copyright © 1991 The Hand Center, Wichita, Kansas. Reproduced with permission.

Chapter 4

- "If you are not satisfied with the work restrictions above, you should see your company physician. This physician may modify these restrictions further based on his or her special knowledge of your workplace."

Table 4-8 Functional Capacity or Work Guides

PLEASE CONSIDER OFF WORK UNTIL NEXT APPOINTMENT UNLESS ALTERNATIVE OR TRANSITIONAL WORK IS AVAILABLE AS CIRCLED OR CHECKED BELOW:

		TOTAL HOURS AT WORK PER WORK DAY	0	2	4	6	8	+
Unchanged from previous visit		repetitive grasping	0	2	4	6	8	
Regular	Right / left hand only	pushing/pulling	0	2	4	6	8	
No restrictions	with coban wrap/glove on	fine manipulation	0	2	4	6	8	
As Tolerated	with buddy tape	Post Op Gradual Increasing Work Load						
Modified	with cast on off	limit vibratory tools	0	2	4	6	8	
No work until next visit		limit power tools	0	2	4	6	8	
Pt. says no work available	with splint on / AS NEEDED / off	limit hands over shoulders	0	2	4	6	8	
Driving if ok by DOT	w/splint Work Sleep Both ↑ ↓							

WORK CHARACTERISTICS: Limited (0-12), Occasional (0-33), Frequent (34-66), Constant (67-100)

SEDENTARY WORK: max. 10 lbs or less lift/carry; occasional lift/carry	task rotation ergo workplace
LIGHT WORK: max. 20 lbs or less lift/carry; frequent at 10 lbs	job rotation rom ointment
LIGHT MEDIUM: max. 35 lbs or less lift/carry; frequent at 20 lbs	heat am cool pm contrast bath
MEDIUM WORK: max. 50 lbs or less lift/carry; frequent at 25 lbs	exercise stretch strength
MEDIUM HEAVY: max. 75 lbs or less lift/carry; frequent at 35 lbs	splint coban scar management
HEAVY WORK: max. 100 lbs or less lift/carry; frequent at 50 lbs	Repetitive Lift Carry 30/hr
Pt. says presently working: yes no Trial regular work.	Repetitive Grasp 250/hr or 2000/8hr

If you are not satisfied with the work restrictions above, please see your company physician.
This physician may modify these restrictions further based on their special knowledge of your work place.

Copyright © 1991 The Hand Center, Wichita, Kansas. Reproduced with permission.

Additional Forms

The sample forms illustrated in the previous section are specific to the hand and upper extremity. Additional sample tables are provided to assist in the development of other practice-specific forms and include general workplace conditions (Table 4-9), lower extremity and back (Table 4-10), and specific job tasks (Table 4-11). Not all of this information is routinely required but is presented for completeness to help physicians develop their practice-specific work guide forms. In the occupational health setting, several pages of guides may be required on the initial visit, with only updates of the changed area(s) provided on follow-up visits. Although many employers will provide their company's forms, it is often easier for physicians to use their own forms, with which they are more familiar. A copy of the functional capacity or work guides should be retained in the medical chart.

Writing Functional Capacity and Return-to-Work Guides

After reviewing the information and examples in this chapter, the physician should be ready to write the actual functional capacity or return-to-work guide. In doing so, he or she must consider the individual's symptoms, signs, risk, capacity, and tolerance; and the job description,

Table 4-9 General Workplace Conditions

	None	Infrequent	Limited	Occasional	Frequent	Continuous
Unlevel surfaces	0	1	2	4	6	8
Unprotected heights	0	1	2	4	6	8
Isolated areas	0	1	2	4	6	8
Operating cab cranes	0	1	2	4	6	8
Operating hazards, moving machinery	0	1	2	4	6	8
Dry areas only	0	1	2	4	6	8
Limit temperature <40°F or >100°F	0	1	2	4	6	8
Use of personal protective equipment	0	1	2	4	6	8
Isolated areas	0	1	2	4	6	8
Operation of company vehicles	0	1	2	4	6	8
Dry areas only	0	1	2	4	6	8
Dust >2.5 mg/cc	0	1	2	4	6	8
Respirator	0	1	2	4	6	8
Temperature <40°F or >100°F	0	1	2	4	6	8
High magnetic fields	0	1	2	4	6	8
Chemicals						
Solvents	0	1	2	4	6	8
Sealants	0	1	2	4	6	8
Skin irritants	0	1	2	4	6	8
Irritant fumes	0	1	2	4	6	8
Hearing						
Hearing ability required	0	1	2	4	6	8
Hearing aid	0	1	2	4	6	8
High noise area >85 dB	0	1	2	4	6	8
Hearing protection	0	1	2	4	6	8
Vision						
Eye goggles	0	1	2	4	6	8
Normal color vision	0	1	2	4	6	8
Peripheral vision	0	1	2	4	6	8
Depth perception	0	1	2	4	6	8
Specific visual acuity	0	1	2	4	6	8

Chapter 4

Copyright © 1991 The Hand Center, Wichita, Kansas. Reproduced with permission.

Table 4-10 Lower Extremity and Back

	None	Infrequent	Limited	Occasional	Frequent	Continuous
Bend	0	1	2	4	6	8
Twist	0	1	2	4	6	8
Stoop	0	1	2	4	6	8
Squat	0	1	2	4	6	8
Kneel	0	1	2	4	6	8
Crawl	0	1	2	4	6	8
Sit	0	1	2	4	6	8
Stand	0	1	2	4	6	8
Bench work	0	1	2	4	6	8
Walk	0	1	2	4	6	8
Climb stairs	0	1	2	4	6	8
Climb ladders	0	1	2	4	6	8

Copyright © 1991 The Hand Center, Wichita, Kansas. Reproduced with permission.

Table 4-11 Specific Job Tasks

	None	Infrequent	Limited	Occasional	Frequent	Continuous
Keyboard	0	1	2	4	6	8
Writing	0	1	2	4	6	8
Knife	0	1	2	4	6	8
Hook	0	1	2	4	6	8
Scissors	0	1	2	4	6	8
Pliers	0	1	2	4	6	8
Clamps	0	1	2	4	6	8
Pressure hoses	0	1	2	4	6	8
Telephone dialing	0	1	2	4	6	8
Drilling	0	1	2	4	6	8
Sanding	0	1	2	4	6	8
Bucking	0	1	2	4	6	8
Riveting	0	1	2	4	6	8
Deburring	0	1	2	4	6	8
Other	0	1	2	4	6	8
Above-shoulder lift in lb and time	0	1	2	4	6	8
Forward reach >18 in from body	0	1	2	4	6	8

Copyright © 1991 The Hand Center, Wichita, Kansas. Reproduced with permission.

essential functions of the job, accommodation options, employer willingness, employee willingness, previous work guides (by the family physician, company physician, or other), response to work activity, and current work status.

The art of medicine requires a blending of these factors with appropriate input from the individual. The process is easier when the individual and physician work together. The first decision is whether to recommend regular work, modified work, or no work. This decision is made by considering the injury, the individual, and the job. In cases in which the physician and the individual disagree about work guides, the negotiation strategies discussed in Chapter 2 and Chapter 3 may be helpful.

Nonmusculoskeletal Return-to-Work Forms and Records

As seen above, structured methods to record individual evaluation and progress are key. Companion resources explore this further. In particular, an examiner may want to have a Activities of Daily Living Questionnaire or Pain Questionnaire, especially in delayed recovery or issues of tolerance.[12] Finally, see also Chapter 14, Table 14-6, which provides guidance on translating capacity to activity when considering. Additional specifies are included in Table 14-2 and Table 14-3 cardiopulmonary status.

A Note About Disclaimers

As America is one of the most litigious countries in the world, physicians should have standard "disclaimers" to attach to return-to-work certification forms. These may not prevent the physician from being sued, but they may make a successful suit less likely. One example of such a disclaimer, printed here, is discussed in Chapter 8:

> The above statements have been made within a reasonable degree of medical probability. The opinions rendered in this case are mine alone. Recommendations regarding treatment, work, and impairment ratings are given totally independently from the requesting agents. These opinions do not constitute per se a recommendation for specific claims or administrative functions to be made or enforced.

This evaluation is based upon the history given by Mr/Ms ___, the objective medical findings noted during the examination,

Chapter 4

and information obtained from the review of the prior medical records available to me, with the assumption that this material is true and correct. If additional information is provided to me in the future, a reconsideration and an additional report may be requested. Such information may or may not change the opinions in this report.

Medicine is both an art and a science, and although Mr/Ms ___ may appear to be fit to work with the abilities and restrictions described above, there is no guarantee that he/she will not be injured or sustain a new injury if he/she chooses to return to work.

Summary

In today's environment, where outcomes are important and economics matter greatly, the treating physician is in a unique position to provide better management of work-related injuries. Improved outcomes are possible when the treating physician treats the whole individual. This whole-individual approach requires an understanding of the factors that contribute to the poorer outcomes, medical treatment plans that include options to address the biopsychosocial issues, and early return-to-work guides. These inclusive medical treatment plans aid in the individual's recovery and rehabilitation while avoiding many of the pitfalls of the workers' compensation system. This approach requires a team effort on the part of the individual, physician, employer, insurer, and government. Many physicians choose not to participate in early return to work because of concerns about liability. Therefore, appropriate legislation should be enacted in all jurisdictions to protect physicians from liability associated with appropriate return-to-work decisions.

Communication and education are key to avoiding unnecessary lost work time. The work guides must be safe and allow for speedy return to work, with the best interests of the individual being the primary responsibility. This means that at times paternalism/beneficence (physician directive: "Return to work is good for you") trumps autonomy (individual choice: "I don't want to work"). Ultimately, physicians are asked for their *medical advice* as to proper work guides. Physicians are not asked to function as secretaries by recording individual preferences for work activity. To accomplish these goals, the work guides must be consistent and precise. With each visit, the treating physician should understand the current influences of the workers' compensation system; must maintain return to work as a priority in the treatment plan; and must report the diagnosis, treatment plan, disability status, and expected period of disability. These guides allow the support staff to work closely with the treating physician to provide the necessary direction and continuity to lead the worker along the complicated path of returning to work. The physician must maintain the leadership role to resolve the many barriers to early return to work. The process of developing functional capacity guides is slow, time consuming, and often frustrating for both the individual and the physician, but the benefits to the individual are significant and, therefore, worth the effort.

References

1. Melhorn JM. Upper limb conditions—stay at work and return to work. In: Melhorn JM, Barr, Jr. JS, eds. *11th Annual Occupational Orthopaedics and Workers' Compensation: A Multidisciplinary Perspective*. Rosemont, IL:American Academy of Orthopaedic Surgeons, 2009: 127–146.

2. Mundy RR, Moore SC, Corey JB, Mundy GD. Disability syndrome: the effects of early vs delayed rehabilitation intervention. *AAOHN J*. 1994;42:379–383.

3. Christian J. Reducing disability days: healing more than the injury. *J Workers Comp*. 2000;9:30–55.

4. Atlas SJ, Chang Y, Kamman E, et al. Long-term disability and return to work among individuals who have a herniated lumbar disc: the effect of disability compensation. *J Bone Joint Surg Am*. 2000;82A:4–15.

5. Burton WN, Conti DJ. Disability management: corporate medical department management of employee health and productivity. *J Occup Environ Med*. 2000;42:1006–1012.

6. Melhorn JM. *Reducing Unnecessary Workplace Disability—Treating More Than the Injury*. Sacramento, CA: California Industrial Medicine Council; 2003.

7. Melhorn JM. Return to work: the employer's point of view. In: *2003 Safety and Health Conference*. Topeka, KS: Kansas Department of Human Resources; 2003.

8. US Department of Labor. *The Dictionary of Occupational Titles*. Washington, DC; 1991:1012–1014. Available at: www.oalj.dol.gov/libdot.htm. Accessed October 21, 2010.

9. Millender LH, Conlon M. An approach to work-related disorders of the upper extremity. *J Am Acad Orthop Surg*. 1996;4:134–142.

10. Cocchiarella J, Andersson G, eds. *Guides to the Evaluation of Permanent Impairment*. 5th ed. Chicago, IL: AMA Press; 2001.

11. Reed P. *The Medical Disability Advisor: Workplace Guidelines for Disability Duration*. 5th ed. Westminster, CO: Reed Group, Ltd; 2005, or at www.mdguidelines.com.

Chapter 4

12. Denniston Jr PL. *ODG Treatment in Workers' Comp 2004*. Encinitas, Calif: Work Loss Data Institute; 2004. Available in printed form or online at www.disabilityduration.com.

13. Glass LS. *Occupational Medicine Practice Guidelines*: *Evaluation and Management of Common Health Problems and Functional Recovery in Workers*. Beverly Farms, MA: OEM Press; 2004. Available in printed form or online at www.acoem.org/practiceguidelines.aspn.

14. Genovese E and Hyman M. Chapter 5, Activities of Daily Living and Psychometric Questionnaires. In: Genovese E and Galper JS eds. *Guides to the Evaluation of Functional Ability How to Request, Interpret, and Apply Functional Capacity Evaluations*. Chicago, IL: AMA Press; 2009:61–90.

Chapter 5

Evidence-based Medicine and Causal Analysis

J. Mark Melhorn, MD, Kurt T. Hegmann, MD, MPH and Elizabeth Genovese, MD, MBA (posthumous)

> When I am a patient, that's what I want MY physician to do for me.
>
> When I am a physician, that's what I should do for my patients.[1]

Evidence-based Medicine

"The conscientious, explicit, and judicious use of current best evidence in making decisions about the care of patients."[2] "As such, it means "integrating patient clinical expertise with the best available clinical evidence from systematic research."[3]

A second definition is "[a] set of principles and methods intended to ensure that to the greatest extent possible, medical decisions, guidelines, and other types of policies are based on and consistent with good evidence of effectiveness and benefit."[4] These definitions require understanding critical evaluation of the studies and knowledge of the basic epidemiologic principles of study design, point estimates, relative risk, odds ratios, confidence intervals, bias, and confounding. Too often, however, evidence-based medicine is incorrectly taken as the search for evidence to support one person's point of view or a specific clinical decision.[5]

An Internet search on April 23, 2010 for the phrase "evidence-based medicine" returned 14,200,000 Web pages, and a similar search for the phrase "practice guideline" returned 51,500,000 Web pages. The current medical literature is replete with references to "evidence-based medicine" and "practice guidelines" articles. Yet, the quality range among guidelines is marked, ranging from low to high. Thus, utilizing these words in a title or including them in an article does not render the article's conclusions scientifically based or evidence based.

The practice of true evidence-based medicine requires that every aspect of the patient's medical care should always be based on the highest quality studies.[6] For treatment purposes, this further implies the results or conclusions must be obtained from a careful, graded assessment of a comprehensive search of the entire body of evidence from patient-oriented quantitative research (especially randomized clinical trials and randomized crossover trials)[6–8] rather than from clinical experience, animal studies, or expert opinion.[9] Patient-oriented quantitative research is commonly referred to as *clinical epidemiologic research*. For causal analyses, the approach is similar but requires a graded assessment of a comprehensive search of the entire body of epidemiological evidence with particular emphasis on prospective cohort studies[6,7,9,10] as randomized trials are viewed as unethical or impractical for many exposures. Thus causal analyses rely on a completely different research database.

Evidence-based clinical decision making requires answering four questions, although more commonly, only three are addressed:

1. What is the illness or disorder of the patient given the history, physical examination, and supporting studies?

2. What is the anticipated course of the patient's illness or disorder?

3. How can I as a physician, improve the outcome(s) for this patient?

However, there is a fourth question that is usually necessary to address yet is usually overlooked or minimized in patient evaluations and is primarily addressed from population-based epidemiological studies:

4. Why did this illness or disorder occur in this patient at this time?[11,12]

In medical practice, few outcomes are certain. Therefore, the objectives of clinical epidemiologic research are to provide probabilistic knowledge on diagnosis, treatment, prognosis, and economic/decision analyses to enhance the outcomes for the patient. Population-based epidemiological research is utilized to develop knowledge on etiology (causation) to answer why the disorder may have occurred, as well as to address secondary and tertiary prevention issues.

Evidence-based Medical Research

Evidence-based medical research, whether clinical or population based, is often divided into four types: etiology (causation), diagnosis, treatment, and prognosis. Although each study type will have its own requirements, every research question will have four design characteristics. The four main design characteristics are: domain (the theoretical population to whom the study results can be applied); determinant(s) (the factor[s] under study that are related to the outcome occurrence); outcome (the health parameters under study); and occurrence relation (the association between the outcome occurrence and the determinant[s]).

A major distinction should be made between clinical and population-based epidemiologic research. The difference is determined by the determinant(s) under study. Population-based epidemiological studies quantify whether a specific determinant is associated with an outcome; for example, trauma as a causal factor (determinant) for wrist fractures or the association between childhood exposure to aerosolized enteric bacilli and subsequent reduced risk of asthma. The purpose of a causal study is to explain (prove or attempt to disprove) the occurrence of an outcome in relation to a purported risk factor to ascertain causal determinant(s). Clinical epidemiological research studies are also causal, but in a different way. In those studies, the goal is to explain (prove or disprove) that the treatment affected or changed the outcome (in other words, it is hoped that the treatment reduced or prevented the occurrence of unwanted outcomes from the illness).

Application of Evidence-based Medical Research to Return to Work

There have been attempts to formulate practice guidelines regarding return to work by organizations such as the American College of Occupational and Environmental Medicine[13] and, abroad, the United Kingdom Stationary Office[14] and Australia's Return to Work Matters.[15]

These guidelines are based primarily on consensus rather than high- or moderate-quality evidence, which is largely lacking aside from a few participatory ergonomics programs primarily involving chronic spine patients.[6]

Chapter 5

However, with the increasing number of preliminary studies suggesting considerable benefits of early return to work for the patient,[6] most physicians are gradually reducing time off from work to improve outcomes and prevent disability. How does one evaluate study quality?

Study Types

Population-based and clinical epidemiologic research require specific study designs. Experimental, blinded, randomized studies are the best way of assessing whether a treatment decision or exposure leads to a given outcome. One can standardize and randomize patients to a specific exposure (or treatment) and thus control for other factors through randomization. This allows for the strongest conclusions on whether the experimental factor (exposure or treatment) is responsible for differences between the groups of patients. One can also control the intensity and duration of determinant exposure, as well as whether the study is *single-blinded* (eg, either the subject does not know whether he or she is receiving the intervention or use of a third party blinded assessor) or *double-blinded* (generally neither the subject nor the treating provider knows who received the intervention and who did not).

There are a number of issues that make it difficult to apply experimental study designs to the evaluation of human populations. For some exposures where a hazard is believed to be present (eg, smoking), these studies are unethical.* A related issue is for exposures where hazard is unclear (eg, high versus low perceived ergonomic hazard), randomization may be difficult if not impossible as some workers lack capability to perform the job(s). Other challenges include difficulty in disguising the active intervention so that subjects cannot distinguish it from the control (eg, return to work trials). This requires utilization of other study types to determine effects, treatments, and differences in durations off work for injured workers.

Epidemiologic Studies

Epidemiology is "the science concerned with the study of factors determining and influencing the frequency and distribution of disease, injury, and other health-related events in a defined human population."[16] Epidemiology is primarily descriptive and identifies the presence or absence of associations between disease and exposure in the population(s) studied. As with experimental studies, observational epidemiologic studies are only as good as their design and analysis. It is consequently mandatory for those involved in the assessment of causality to be able to critically evaluate these studies

---

* Prospective cohort studies are the strongest study designs for such circumstances.

before automatically accepting their conclusions as valid. Furthermore, "as confident as one might be that the conclusions of an epidemiological study are scientifically sound, there is always a possibility that new discoveries or even new analyses of old data will alter those conclusions."[5]

Epidemiologic studies are usually considered to be only observational rather than experimental. Subjects are *not* randomly selected, and the exposure cannot be controlled. The simplest studies, case reports and case series, are not epidemiological, rather they are purely descriptive. They simply *describe* the occurrence of a given event in a group of patients, along with a description of the interventions or exposures they shared. While this may suggest a need for further evaluation of the potential relationship between the exposure or treatment and the observed outcome (which can be tested in future studies), case reports are hypothesis generating, not testing.

There are four main types of epidemiological studies: cross-sectional, case-control, retrospective cohort, and prospective cohort studies. (Table 5-1 provides an understanding of quality of a study. Table 5-2 provides insight into the strengths and weaknesses each study design.) While not a rigid hierarchy (a key weakness can invalidate *any* study), this classification is

Table 5-1 Study Design Pyramid

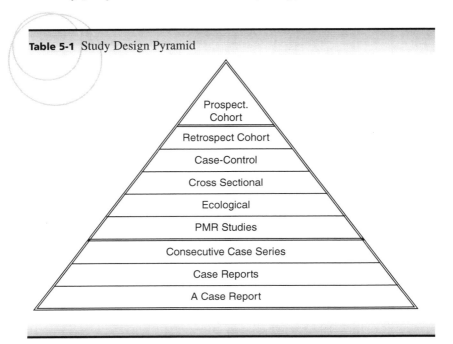

Prospect. Cohort

Retrospect Cohort

Case-Control

Cross Sectional

Ecological

PMR Studies

Consecutive Case Series

Case Reports

A Case Report

Chapter 5

Source: J. Mark Melhorn and William Ackerman. *Guides to the Evaluation of Disease and Injury Causation.* American Medical Association, 2008.

Chapter 5

Table 5-2 Comparison of Study Types

Study Characteristics	Experimental	Cross-Sectional	Case-Control	Historical Cohort	Nested Case-Control	Prospective Cohort
Blinded, single	Generally	No	No	No	No	No
Blinded, double	Sometimes	No	No	No	No	No
Investigator controls treatment or exposure	Yes	No	No	No	No	No
Data collected at single point in time	Sometimes	Yes	Yes (no)	Yes	Yes/no: cases are incident	No
Data collected longitudinally	Sometimes	No	Yes/no: incident	Yes	Yes	Yes
Work backward to identify exposures	No	Yes	Yes	Yes	No	No
Used to calculate disease incidence	No	Yes	No	Yes	Yes	Yes
Recall bias	No	Yes	Yes	No (?)	No	No
Nonresponse bias	Yes	*No	No	No	No	Yes
Likely confounders	Sometimes	Yes	Yes	No	Sometimes	Sometimes
Suitable for rare disease processes	If designed appropriately	Yes	Yes	Yes	Yes	No
Appropriate for diseases with long latency	Not really	Yes	Yes	Yes	Yes	No
Expense	Varies	Low	Low	Low	Medium	High
Strength of evidence	No	Low	Low	Medium	Medium	Good

generally reliable. Only the prospective cohort study is considered hypothesis testing.[6,9,†] An additional type of study, proportionate mortality study, is the weakest of the epidemiological studies and is performed only for analyses of mortality risks in populations, thus it is irrelevant to the discussion of return-to-work issues and will not be discussed further.

Cross-Sectional (Prevalence) Studies

Cross-sectional (or prevalence) studies are the weakest form of epidemiologic study. Data on both exposure and disease are collected at a single point in time. The main measures are prevalence rates (disease rate divided by the population at risk) and odds ratios (ratio of disease rate between the exposed and unexposed groups). These studies allow one to conclude that there may be a potential relationship between exposures and diseases that appear at a higher rate compared with another population. These studies do *not* allow one to make conclusions regarding cause and effect, because (among other weaknesses) the cases included are prevalent (have already occurred) and not incident cases (those occurring during the study). Therefore, it is inappropriate to conclude anything but the possibility of a relationship between the exposure and disease using a cross-sectional study.

Case-Control Studies

The next higher level of evidence is derived from *case-control studies*. In these studies a more direct evaluation of hypotheses is usually reported, generally based on better control of potentially confounding factors. These studies compare exposures between cases and controls. They also do *not* control the exposure of subjects to the factor or factors under evaluation, so addressing potential confounders is essential. Confounders are usually addressed through matching, exclusions, stratification, or statistical adjustment. When well designed, these studies bring supportive evidence for the relationship between the exposure and disease, although these studies can never test the hypothesis due to the weaknesses that include the use of retrospective methods. When confounders are inadequately addressed, the value of these studies is quite limited and the conclusions may be invalid.

Retrospective Cohort Studies

The next strongest observational studies are *retrospective cohort studies*, which are longitudinal analyses of how disease develops (or has responded to treatment) in a well-defined source population for which prior records are available. These studies are typically performed in occupational or insured populations in whom there is control over at least: (1) the population over

Chapter 5

[†] An additional factor is that all of these studies are retrospective studies, with the exception of prospective cohort studies.

time (including in and out migration); and (2) prior exposures captured on a reliable basis. These studies have the potential to define incident cases of disease (new cases), although this ability is more limited for less severe or nonfatal outcomes. Retrospective cohort studies are retrospective; however, where exposures are well measured, they have the ability to better identify risks of disease through better control over weaknesses, including recall bias.

Prospective Cohort Studies

The strongest observational studies are *prospective cohort studies*, which are longitudinal analyses of how disease develops (or responds to treatment) in a well-defined source population. These studies begin at a point in time and follow the population forward in time. Exposures and diseases are measured at baseline. Thus, through following the population, risks of disease (or factors bearing favorable prognoses) can be better defined. Weaknesses are still possible and there can be fatal study flaws (eg, failure to measure a risk factor or confounder, failure to adequately ascertain disease status at baseline, inadequate measurement of exposure, etc).

Compared to other observational epidemiological studies, prospective cohort studies offer the best evidence regarding cause and effect, as they most closely approximate the experimental randomized controlled trial, although they fail to randomize the exposure. Because observing large populations to see what develops over time is expensive, it is generally more efficient to evaluate retrospective epidemiological studies to first generate hypotheses.

Potential Flaws in Study Types

Study outcomes and conclusions can be strongly influenced, strengthened, or invalidated by study design and flaws. Understanding how these can affect the results may assist in better assessing the reliability and validity of the studies as well as in interpreting the conclusions.

Bias

As noted earlier in this chapter, epidemiological studies demonstrate association, not cause and effect. Researchers are generally unable to control exposure or other factors (confounders) and must, instead, collect and evaluate existing data, which makes these studies more likely to be subject to bias than experimental trials. *Bias* is a systematic or measurement error in the design or analysis of a study that leads to an overestimation or underestimation of the strength and significance of a given association. *There are three main categories of bias: (1) selection, (2) information, and (3) publication*, along with multiple subcategories that are discussed below.‡ Selection biases involve how patients were selected for the study. Information biases involve measurements of characteristics such as exposure, disease, or confounders. A bias can modify an association, artificially create a positive result, create a protective result, or produce a statistically negative result when there is actually an association. Bias can occur in both experimental and observational studies but is more common in the latter. *Channeling bias* is the tendency to prescribe (or channel) treatment in a nonrandom manner. Physicians may expect lower toxicity from COX-2 inhibitor medications and thus preferentially prescribe those medications among those at higher risk. Subsequent analyses may show elevated bleeding risk, but this could potentially be artificially elevated by demographic factors rather than a characteristic of the medication.

Publication bias is the tendency of publications to print positive study results and preclude publication of negative results. This type of bias affects the accuracy of a synthesis of the literature. Attempts are being made to register randomized clinical trials, however recent reports indicate most trials continue to go unpublished.

Detection or surveillance bias is a selection bias that results from the unequal determination of case status due to ascertainment, diagnosis, or verification problems. Examples include populations under scrutiny (eg, post-ionizing radiation exposures, known HIV-positive populations, insured vs. noninsured populations).

Health worker bias (or healthy worker effect) is a type of selection bias and describes the tendency for working populations to have fewer health problems than unemployed groups.

Lead time bias is a type of selection bias and describes the probability of a false conclusion of improved survival from early detection of disease. For example, surveillance with X rays will tend to identify earlier cases of lung cancer, but overall longevity will not be increased by surveillance.

Length time bias is a form of selection bias and results from increased identification of patients with long disease duration (often milder disease), particularly when measuring prevalence data in cross-sectional studies. The average case of a fatal or severe disease will be biased toward those lasting longer periods of time or milder cases.

_____

‡ There are multiple types of bias described, and the terms are not universally agreed upon. This text attempts to describe the most common types of bias and the more common definitions used.

Chapter 5

Migration bias is a type of selection bias in which patients relocate (or self-refer) on the basis of their disease state. For example, those with a complex disease may migrate to larger metropolitan areas (eg, multiple sclerosis) or patients may migrate to warmer climates (eg, osteoarthrosis).

(Non)response bias is a type of selection bias and involves differences in response rates between the two groups (eg, low rates of responding to questionnaires among those without a disease compared to those with a disease). This bias can occur in both epidemiological and treatment studies.

Procedure bias is a type of selection bias and involves patients not receiving identical treatment, usually due to failure to blind researchers. Procedure bias can be nothing more than an evaluator devoting a little more time or attention to patients compared with controls. This is, however, often all that is needed to shift the balance toward finding a positive effect of treatment or negative effect of exposure in a study that would otherwise have been neutral.

Sampling bias is a selection bias and is the systematic inclusion or exclusion of certain groups from a study. For example if random digit dialing is used to identify controls, those who do not have telephones will be automatically excluded and those with more than one telephone number will be over-sampled.

Reporting bias is a type of information bias and involves differential reporting of data on an exposure among those with the outcome than in patients without the outcome. For example, smoking status is more likely to be recorded on those who are admitted with a smoking-related disease compared with those who are thought to have an unrelated outcome.

Compliance bias is a type of information bias and involves differential rates of compliance with a treatment in the experimental and control groups.

Detection bias is a type of information bias and involves the detection of a disease at an earlier stage in the group that is screened than it would have been otherwise.

Measurement bias is a type of information bias and involves the use of testing to measure the results of an exposure or treatment that differs between the cases and controls. For example, job physical exposures may be measured in more detail in cases than controls.

Recall bias is a type of information bias and may occur in any study whenever a factor is recorded from memory, most commonly from the patient (eg, recall of a physical exposure after development of a musculoskeletal disorder, but even prospective cohort studies may require recall of prior exposures such as smoking at baseline). It reflects the tendency of those who have a condition, or have undergone a particular treatment, to be more likely to recall an exposure or to focus on potential side effects of the procedure than do those who did *not* experience the condition or treatment.

Confounding

Studies can also be flawed because of *confounding*, the presence of a third, or "confounding," factor that was not accounted for in either the study design or analyses (ie, matching, exclusions, stratification, or statistical adjustment). For example, the association between disabling back pain and decreased aerobic capacity (a measure of fitness) may reflect an increased prevalence of "fear-avoidance" behaviors and an external rather than internal locus of control in both groups.[17–23]

It is clear that assessing the significance of findings from a given study requires understanding of the strengths and weaknesses of various forms of study design, as well as a careful critique of the methods used in the study. One also must understand the strengths and weaknesses of the statistical analyses used.

Statistical Analysis

Quantifiable results from a study are generally characterized by a *mean* (or *median* if non-normally distributed), or average value, around which most values tend to cluster, with all other values (by definition) either larger or smaller. *Standard deviation* is a measure of the dispersion, or spread, of measurements around the mean value. Standard deviation is directly related to variance in that greater degrees of variance in results will increase the standard deviation, which, conversely, decreases when the variance is low. One standard deviation encompasses approximately 67% of the values, while two standard deviations encompasses 95% of the values.

Study analyses begin with the null hypothesis, ie, that a given intervention or exposure will not make a meaningful difference. A test statistic (eg, t-test, chi-square) is calculated on the basis of the observed data. When the statistic is so extreme there is a $\leq 5\%$ probability of results this extreme by chance alone, the result is termed statistically significant and is taken to reflect a true effect of the treatment or exposure under investigation.[24]

This information is classically communicated via the *P value*. In general, a *P* value of ≤ 0.05 is considered significant, as it indicates that the likelihood of error in classifying the observed findings as reflecting a true difference from the expected finding of no difference (the null hypothesis) is ≤5%. (The 5% level of significance is arbitrary, but widely accepted throughout the sciences). A *P* value of 0.01 decreases the chances that findings will be erroneously classified as significant (when they were not) to ≤1%.

Confidence Intervals

The preferred method to represent data is by calculating confidence intervals, which provides more information than a *P* value. Confidence intervals (aka, confidence bounds) represent the spread of data, as well as its statistical significance. Convention is to report 95% confidence intervals, which are the range of estimates that, if the study were repeated, 95 out of 100 times the results would fall within that confidence interval.

Odds Ratios

For crosssectional studies, the odds ratio is most commonly calculated, indicating the ratio between risk of disease in the exposed and unexposed populations.

Relative Risk

Relative risk is the most common measurement of cohort studies and is the ratio between the incidence rate in the exposed people compared with the incidence rate in the unexposed people. A relative risk of 2 means those exposed are twice as likely to get the disease than those unexposed.

Survival Analyses

Survival analyses are increasingly used to describe differences in survival between two groups of patients or populations followed longitudinally. These analyses may not only address fatal outcomes. Survival of prosthetic joints and development of low back pain or heart attacks are all examples of successful use of this analytical strategy.

Power is the ability of a test to appropriately reject the null hypothesis when it is false. In other words, power describes the ability of a study to detect a given difference of a given size between two outcomes if the difference really exists.[16,25,26]

All of these factors should be kept in mind when designing and interpreting results from a study.

Meta-analysis

Meta-analysis is a frequently controversial secondary analysis tool that has been applied in evidence-based medicine. In meta-analysis the results of multiple studies are pooled. The best use of meta-analysis is to combine multiple homogeneous studies of small sample sizes to gain sufficient statistical significance to render appropriately powered results. Unfortunately, the technique is most frequently used in musculoskeletal disorders studies to summarize multiple heterogeneous studies (eg, differing populations assessed, different methods of measuring disease, different methods to measure results) resulting in a summary statistic of uncertain utility as a whole. Previously, meta-analysis and systematic reviews[§] have been accorded relatively high status in evidence-based medicine. However, more recently, these studies have either been discounted largely or entirely because of these considerable limitations resulting in increasing reliance on original data.[6,8]

Analyzing and Applying Study Results for Purposes of Treatments

Original data from high- and moderate-quality studies are required for formulation of the highest quality evidence-based guidelines. Even if meta-analyses and reviews are included, many available studies evaluating exposure or the effects of diagnostic or therapeutic options have results that should be inconclusive due to reasons including weak study design, bias(es), confounding, inadequate blinding, or lack of power. There are multiple steps required for developing quality evidence-based guidance, which include: (1) development of a detailed methodology (or adoption of an existing methodology); (2) comprehensive, exhaustive literature searches for original studies; (3) critiquing of each article; (4) grading of each article (for strengths and weaknesses, which helps sort the evidence into high, medium and low quality); (5) compilation of tables of evidence; (6) synthesizing of the evidence; (7) development of guidance; (8) use of a panel of diverse multiple-specialty group of providers who are involved in this topical area; (9) external peer review; and (10) publication after review and revisions.

In many cases, the evidence is rated on a scale of A through D. Level A evidence represents "strong and research-based evidence provided by generally consistent findings in multiple high quality randomized control trials (RCTs)," while evidence is classified as level D (or I, Insufficient) when there are no randomized controlled trials of quality (or equivalents). The

---

[§] Systematic reviews have also been previously accorded a relatively high rating in evidence-based medicine; however, these studies have increasingly been recognized as frequently suffering from considerable flaws including: incomplete literature searches, lack of objective grading and critiquing of original data, and biases that are compounded or not discussed.[6] (REF: APG-I Occupational Medicine Practice Guidelines Online, Methodology for the Update of the Occupational Medicine Practice Guidelines, 3rd Edition. http://www.acoem.org/apg-i.aspx. Accessed January 10, 2011.)

United States Preventive Services Task Force and the Agency for Health Care Research and Quality have used a slightly modified version that includes levels I, II-1, II-2, II-3 and III, respectively ranging from RCTs to nonrandomized trials to expert opinion.[27] While this may be adequate to categorize the quality of the evidence, the scale does not include judgments regarding the risk of harm from interventions and may thus be somewhat limited in practical use.

The *Clinical Evidence* series from the BMJ Publishing Group[28] attempts to increase the practical application of categorized data by classifying interventions as "beneficial," "likely to be beneficial," "representative of trade off between benefit and harms," of "unknown effectiveness," "unlikely to be beneficial," or "likely to be ineffective or harmful." This goes beyond a simple analysis of the evidence per se. The American College of Occupational and Environmental medicine uses three domains for this step: (1) invasiveness, (2) adverse effects, and (3) cost.

Invariably, there are areas where quality evidence is lacking and consensus is required. Some state that support for or advice against a particular intervention may be based predominantly on expert opinion, or expert opinion plus fair evidence that the intervention is beneficial or carries risk in excess of benefit. As evidence-based medicine is, in its essence, the "ability to track down, critically appraise, and incorporate evidence into clinical practice,"[29] it would appear that categorization schemes that take into account research evidence, consensus opinion, and patient clinical experience optimally synthesize available information.

Even when studies are well designed and allow for the generation of conclusions that are statistically sound, there are other questions that still must be answered before these conclusions are used to shape clinical practice. For example, some trials of opioids last hours to days to a few weeks, while stating long-term safety is documented. Yet, these trials are of insufficient length to support such statements as applied to use of opioids over many months to years. Another important question relates to the clinical relevance of the outcomes, even if the treatment or exposure *does* have an affect on the outcome measured: does this change in outcome materially alter the expected overall clinical course, in the absence of the exposure or intervention, or result in a significant improvement or decrease in function? If the answer to this question is "yes," one should also ask whether the change in outcome was of such magnitude as to mandate an immediate reconsideration of current practice patterns.

Issues of cost vs benefit should be considered simultaneously, as one should be able to assess the costs (both direct and indirect) that would be associated with adoption of a new test, procedure, or means of reducing or mitigating exposure. This includes assessment of the cost of any additional testing or treatment that would not have been required otherwise. Overall, the incremental cost of adopting an intervention must be justified by the clinical benefit gained. Proponents of new tests and treatments may overlook this concept. Unfortunately, there is no consensus on how to unequivocally incorporate costs into decision-making. When applied to the analysis of the risk of returning to work, the risk of returning patients to work when the evidence is not clear should be weighed against the cost to the patient of not doing so and the cost to society of not suggesting return to work to patients for whom the literature suggests there is no or little risk.

Evidence-based Medicine Summary

Evidence-based medical guidance is increasingly recognized as valuable to summarize the rapidly escalating body of quality literature that physicians cannot possibly have sufficient time to collate, critique, grade, analyze, and summarize. Challenges include: (1) lack of incentives to change practices; (2) exceedingly difficult work required to (re)learn true quality evidence-based guidance; (3) resistance among some practitioners to changes in practices; and (4) large volumes of low quality guidelines, including many with disparate recommendations providing confusion.

Additional challenges include overall limitations of available studies including: (1) limiting numbers of high or moderate quality studies; (2) study biases; (3) confounding; and (4) power and sample size considerations. However, quality guidance is available on many subjects and can be supplemented by consensus guidance where quality evidence is lacking.

The area of helping patients return to work is one in which there is a particular dearth of quality evidence. There are few randomized trials that directly or indirectly address this subject. However, there are multiple other trials suggesting early return to work is not harmful and may provide superior outcomes. Increased interest in this area should spur additional research that is critical to providing quality evidence-based guidance regarding return to work decision-making.

Summary

How do evidence-based medicine and causal analysis affect the health care providers' ability to determine stay at work and return-to-work options? There are three elements involved: capacity, tolerance, and risk.

Chapter 5

Capacity is the objective ability of the worker to perform work and is generally given as upper limits (eg, 50 pounds maximum lifting from floor to waist). Capacity can be objectively and accurately measured in most situations in which motivation is good, although there are many variables that affect capacity including job variables (eg, size of the object, horizontal distance of the hands while lifting [moment], vertical location, hand coupling [hand holds], frequency of lifts, ability of the weight to shift while lifting [asymmetry], as well as individual variables (eg, age, gender, anthropometry, conditioning, and past or current injury status). To effectively measure a worker's capacity requires detailed knowledge of the job and/or the worker's tasks.

Tolerance involves capacity, but by extension includes the element of subjective capability. In noninjury settings, psychophysical testing has been used to develop worker tolerances (eg, maximum pushing limits for 95% of males). Practically, capacity and tolerance are often inseparable in clinical situations as most injured workers will demonstrate a capacity that is equivalent to the tolerance (eg, a demonstrated lifting limit is 25 pounds from the floor, and the existence of greater capacity is unknown unless objective behaviors are observed that counter that assessment).

Risk associated with return to work involves use of evidence-based medical principles, knowledge of job tasks, and causal analysis. Causation is integrally involved in estimates of job injury recurrence(s). Once capacity, tolerance, and job demands are known in detail, an estimate of the worker's ability to return to work is possible. It is important to recognize there is no absolutely perfect assessment that completely eliminates the chance of associated risk for either return to work or remaining off work. The physician should include all these elements in arriving at the best determination for each patient. Practically, the worker's stated desire and ability to return to work is often the central issue. Functionally, returning workers to modified duty (or "light") jobs and transitioning them up results in effective on-the-job conditioning and normally results in successful return to work. To make credible statements regarding return to work, it is important to take all these factors into account and be particularly knowledgeable regarding literature addressing whether returning the injured worker with a known condition to a specific form of work activity places him or her at undue risk of reinjury or harm, and conversely, whether keeping him or her off work is associated with adverse risks that are increasingly recognized, including increased disability and shortened longevity.

References

1. American College of Occupational and Environmental Medicine. ACOEM Consensus Opinion Statement: The attending physician's role in helping patients

return to work after an illness or injury. Available at: http://acoem.org/guidelines/
pdf/Return-to-Work-04-02.pdf. Accessed January 10, 2011.

2. Sackett DL, Rosenberg WM, Gray JA, Richardson WS. Evidence-based medicine:
   what it is and what it isn't. *BMJ*. 1996;312:7172.

3. Genovese E. Chapter 5. Evidence-based Medicine. In: *A Physician's Guide to
   Return to Work*. Talmage JB and Melhorn JM, eds. AMA Press, 2005.

4. Eddy DM. Evidence-based medicine: a unified approach. *Health Affairs*.
   2005;24(1):9–17.

5. Williams JK. Understanding evidence-based medicine: a primer. *Am J Obstet
   Gynecol*. 2001;185:275–278.

6. American College of Occupational and Environmental Medicine's Occupational
   Medicine Practice Guidelines, 2nd ed., Update, 2008.

7. Harris J, Sinnott P, Turkelson C, Weiss M, Hegmann KT. Methodology to
   Update the Practice Recommendations in the American College of Occupational
   and Environmental Medicine's Occupational Medicine Practice Guidelines,
   J Occup Env Med. 2008;50:282–295.

8. AAOS Guideline Development Process and Procedures. www.aaos.org/research/
   guidelines/Guideline_Development.asp. Accessed June 25, 2010.

9. Hegmann KT and Oostema SJ. Chapter 3. Causal Associations and Determination
   of Work-Relatedness. In: *Guides to the Evaluation of Disease and Injury Causation*.
   Melhorn JM, Ackermann WE III, eds. Chicago, IL: AMA Press, 2008.

10. Melhorn JM, Hegmann KT. Chapter 4. Methodology. In: *Guides to the
    Evaluation of Disease and Injury Causation*. Melhorn JM, Ackermann WE III,
    eds. AMA Press, 2008.

11. Sackett DL: Clinical epidemiology: what, who, and whither. *J Clin Epidemiol*.
    2002;55:1161–1166.

12. Karel GMM and Grobbee DE. *Clinical Epidemiology: An Introduction*.
    Orthopaedic Knowledge Update 8. Vaccaro AR, ed. Rosemont, IL: AAOS, 2005.

13. American College of Occupational and Environmental Medicine's Occupational
    Medicine Practice Guidelines, 1997;2004;2008:1.

14. The United Kingdom, The Stationary Office (TSO) Days Off Work and
    Prediction of Return to Work, The Back Book 2nd Edition, and Tackling
    Musculoskeletal Problems: A Guide for Clinic and Workplace—Identifying
    Obstacles Using the Psychosocial Flags Framework.

15. www.rtwmatter.org, the Web site of Australia's Return to Work Matters, The
    Power of Partnerships.

16. Dawson-Saunders B, Trapp RG. *Basic and Clinical Biostatistics*. 2nd ed.
    Norwalk, CT: Appleton and Lange; 1994.

17. Al-Obaidi SM, Nelson RM, Al-Awadhi S, Al-Shuwaie N. The role of anticipa-
    tion and fear of pain in the persistence of avoidance behavior in patients with
    chronic low back pain. *Spine*. 2000;25:1126–1131.

18. Buer N, Linton SJ. Fear-avoidance beliefs and catastrophizing: occurrence
    and risk factor in back pain and ADL in the general population. *Pain*.
    2002;99:485–491.

Chapter 5

19. Fritz JM, George SZ, Delitto A. The role of fear-avoidance beliefs in acute low back pain: relationships with current and future disability and work status. *Pain.* 2001;94:7–15.

20. Fritz JM, George SZ. Identifying psychosocial variables in patients with acute work-related low back pain: the importance of fear-avoidance beliefs. *Phys Ther.* 2002;82:973–983.

21. Klenerman L, Slade PD, Stanley IM, et al. The prediction of chronicity in patients with an acute attack of low back pain in a general practice setting. *Spine.* 1995;20:478–484.

22. Mannion AF, Junge A, Taimela S, Muntener M, Lorenzo K, Dvorak J. Active therapy for chronic low back pain, part 3: factors influencing self-rated disability and its change following therapy. *Spine.* 2001;26:920–929.

23. Waddell G, Newton M, Henderson I, Somerville D, Main CJ. A Fear-Avoidance Beliefs Questionnaire (FABQ) and the role of fear-avoidance beliefs in chronic low back pain and disability. *Pain.* 1993;52:157–168.

24. Pocock SJ, Hughes MD, Lee RJ. Statistical problems in the reporting of clinical trials: a survey of three medical journals. *N Engl J Med.* 1987;317:426–432.

25. Moher D, Dulberg CS, Wells GA. Statistical power, sample size, and their reporting in randomized controlled trials. *JAMA.* 1994;272:122–124.

26. Freiman JA, Chalmers TC, Smith H Jr, Kuebler RR. The importance of beta, the type II error and sample size in the design and interpretation of the randomized control trial: survey of 71 "negative" trials. *N Engl J Med.* 1978;299:690–694.

27. Agency for Health Care Research and Quality. Clinical Practice Guidelines Online. Available at: www.ahrq.gov/clinic/cpgonline.htm. Accessed January 10, 2011.

28. British Medical Journal. Clinical Evidence. Available at: http://www.clinicalevidence.com/ceweb/conditions/index.jsp. January 10, 2011.

29. Rosenberg WM, Sackett DL. On the need for evidence-based medicine. *Therapie.* 1996;51:212–217.

Chapter 5

Functional Capacity Evaluation in Return-to-Work Decision Making: Risk, Capacity, and Tolerance

Douglas P. Gross, PhD, BScPT
and Michiel F. Reneman, PhD, PT

Functional capacity evaluation (FCE) has been defined as an activity assessment that is used to make recommendations for participation in work while considering the person's body functions and structures, environmental factors, personal factors, and health status.[1] These evaluations are commonly used internationally as measures of occupational capability. Within insurance and workers' compensation systems, FCEs are used to inform decisions regarding return to work.[2] As such, they have extremely important consequences in the lives of injured workers, employers, and professionals such as physicians who base decisions on FCE findings.[3] This chapter will explore the role of FCE in return-to-work decision making from a risk, capacity, and tolerance perspective. Practical considerations when interpreting assessment results will also be highlighted.

Historical Perspective and Current Uses

Standardized functional assessment protocols have been used clinically for decades, and proprietary FCE protocols have been on the market for a number of years.[4,5] Developers of such assessments have used a number of formats (ie, one-day, two-day, or longer protocols) and included a wide variety of assessment strategies ranging from self-report questionnaires to more-or-less standardized performance-based measures.[6] Some have aimed at measuring all required activities of daily living (ADLs) and work, while others have been largely focused on identifying occupational performance capabilities. A comprehensive review of all aspects of FCE has recently been published that includes a discussion of the main elements of various FCE protocols as well as practical advice on administering and interpreting assessment results.[7]

Currently, FCEs play a major role in many insurance and workers' compensation systems worldwide.[3,8,9] These assessments are relied on to inform return-to-work decision making, including the critically important decision of whether an injured worker has sufficient functional ability to safely perform required job demands.[10] Demonstrated performance during assessment is compared to physical job demands, and if subjects meet or exceed required demands they are typically deemed fit or "safe" to return to regular duties.[11] If the injured worker does not demonstrate adequate abilities, results are often used to set activity limitations (temporary or permanent), inform prescriptions for accommodated work, or guide the development of rehabilitation and functional restoration programs. Inconsistent, erratic, or sub-maximal performance during assessment is also frequently used as evidence regarding sincerity of effort although published evidence to support such claims is scarce.[2,7]

Given the many roles played by FCE in the management of injured workers, it is very important to know the validity of these assessments and what exactly is being measured. As with any clinical or diagnostic test, FCE has strengths and limitations. Knowing the strengths and limitations will allow clinicians to be aware of when they can place their trust in assessment results and when additional information should be sought. Next we will discuss the strengths and limitations of FCE from the perspective of the risk, capacity, and tolerance framework.[12]

Risk

Risk refers to the chance of harm to a patient.[12] Risk is relevant to FCE administration from two perspectives:

1. Can FCE identify occupational activities that place workers at risk?

2. Does participating in FCE itself pose substantial risk?

Can FCE Identify Activities that Place Workers at Risk?

According to Talmage, risk is linked to the concept of *work restrictions*, which are activities a patient/worker can do, but should not do.[12] One example is the restriction from piloting aircraft in patients with seizure disorders. Flying is an activity with inherent risk for individuals with this condition. In such situations, the prescription of work restrictions is based entirely on the medical diagnosis. However, many conditions are not as clear-cut, and the prescription of necessary work restrictions is associated with a high level of uncertainty. This is the case in many musculoskeletal conditions such as knee meniscus lesions, diagnoses involving spinal nerve compression, or regional or widespread pain disorders.[13]

Prescribing work restrictions is also challenging in disorders such as some rheumatologic and neurological conditions, which are at times seen in FCE practice. For example, one of the authors recently conducted an FCE on a subject recovering from Guillain-Barre syndrome with the referral question of whether the individual's balance was good enough to return to work safely in the construction industry. In such cases, the fundamental purpose of FCE is to determine whether or not an individual is capable of working and to identify what activities are risky and should be avoided.

When uncertainty arises from the medical diagnosis regarding what work restrictions are necessary, participation in functional assessment may provide some additional information beyond that obtained from diagnostic imaging studies, although little relevant research has been conducted. One study of workers undergoing low back rehabilitation found that work restrictions based on FCE findings actually inhibited successful return to work.[14] Another series of studies in subjects with low back or upper extremity conditions have found that FCE results, while providing some information for predicting time to return to work, do not provide accurate information regarding risk of future recurrence.[15-18] These observations may reflect the nature of musculoskeletal disorders, which are often fluctuating and recurrent. However, no research has been published on restrictions based on FCE in specific nonmusculoskeletal conditions.

Does Participating in FCE Itself Pose Substantial Risk?

When restrictions do not obviously flow from a medical diagnosis, FCE may be conducted to determine safe ability for work. In this situation, participation in FCE itself potentially comes with a certain level of risk. Safety has been researched to determine whether evaluators could apply operational definitions of safety during FCE.[19-21] Definitions of safety have included biomechanical, metabolic, and psychophysical responses to the activity in an attempt to ensure that patients remain within defined limits. Patients are considered safe if they do not exceed strength and heart rate limitations or perform beyond the point at which they feel safe or willing to proceed.

In studies conducted evaluating the safety of patients with chronic back pain and healthy workers undergoing FCE, results indicate that these evaluations appear safe when used on healthy subjects and subjects with chronic low back pain.[20,21] After participating in FCE, no formal complaints of injury were filed, and increased symptoms associated with participation with the FCE consistently returned to pre-FCE levels. Specifically, 99% of healthy subjects had symptoms return to pre-FCE levels within one week (mean of 3 days), while only 1% had increased symptoms lasting for as long as 3 weeks. The pattern of pain responses of patients with back pain resembled the pain responses of healthy subjects. The authors concluded that a temporary increase in symptom intensity following FCE is common, but that FCE is safe within the operational definition of safety used which involved formal reports of injury having occurred during the FCE. A pain response following FCE can be expected, and this pain response is most likely a normal reaction of the musculoskeletal system after intensive exercise. Research in populations other than those reported above is lacking, and generalizations of these results may not be valid.

Other researchers have also reported findings of pain exacerbation after FCE. It has been reported that some patients refuse to undergo a second test session because they do not feel capable of participation in manual handling activities due to increased pain following the first session.[22] In a study in which patients with chronic back pain were retested on the day following FCE, up to 21% of patients performed worse on the second day of testing.[23] The altered performance was likely due to natural variance in performances caused by pain exacerbation, training, or other factors, but it was unlikely that altered performance was due to musculoskeletal injury.

From a biomechanical or ergonomic perspective, it has been demonstrated that during FCE some subjects may lift more than 22.5 kg and experience spinal loads that are considered potentially hazardous according to published lifting guidelines.[24] Some clinicians have also voiced their opinion that medium-to-heavy lifting is potentially unsafe.[19] However, despite exceeding "safe" lifting guidelines derived from the National Institute for Occupational Safety and Health recommendations, subjects with chronic back pain have participated in FCE without evidence of reinjury or harm.[22,24]

Capacity

Capacity has been defined as the highest probable level of functioning that a person may reach in a domain at a given moment in a standardized environment[1] and includes concepts such as aerobic capacity, strength, flexibility, and endurance. While maximum aerobic capacity is rarely required in the occupational setting, maximum strength, flexibility, and agility may be required in some occupations. Identifying a workers' capacity for various occupational activities leads to the identification of *work limitations*, which are activities the patient/worker cannot physically do.[12] Clinical measurement of capacity would require subjects to perform to physiological maximum levels and should logically lead to accurate prescriptions of work ability and limitations, optimally defined in terms of intensity, frequency, and duration. However, whether actual capacity testing can be done in a clinical setting and within the populations typically referred for FCE is a matter of debate.

The *kinesiophysical* method of FCE assessment has been proposed based on the assumption that indicators of maximum physiological effort can be observed in the clinic. Research has examined therapist judgments of maximum effort using this method and found acceptable reliability for various lifting and carrying activities.[22,23] However, consistency is lower for positional and mobility activities.[25] Some validity evidence of therapist judgments of maximum effort using this approach has also been published.[26] Other research on the accuracy of therapist determinations of maximal or sub-maximal effort during FCE has shown mixed results.[2,27]

Studies examining factors influencing performance or attempting to identify sources of variation have also raised questions regarding whether FCE actually measures capacity. In one of the first studies to investigate determinants of performance during kinesiophysical FCE, physiological indicators explained some variance in FCE results (younger males lifted to higher levels), yet a larger component of variance was explained by nonphysiological factors such as self-reports of disability.[28] Other studies in workers' compensation claimants have shown that factors such as expectations of recovery, self-efficacy, or pain intensity associate with FCE results, yet most variance remains unexplained.[29–31] Other than pain intensity, which has shown some association across different studies, attempts to replicate associations of psychological variables such as pain-related fear-avoidance beliefs, distress, self-efficacy, self-confidence, or coping style across different settings have shown inconsistent results.[32–35]

While capacity is often linked to maximal limits of the anatomical system only, within the broader view of the World Health Organization's International Classification of Functioning,[36] *capacity* is defined as the highest probable level of functioning that a person may reach in a domain at a given moment in a standardized environment. This definition also considers the complex interactions between the domains of body functions and structures, activities, and participation. Thus, capacity and willingness to work to full effort or demonstrate actual capacity is dependent on the environmental context. The only study published to date examining the association between setting and FCE performance found wide variability across settings and jurisdictions.[37] Subjects in settings where FCE results were explicitly being used to inform decisions regarding compensation

Chapter 6

claim status (and termination of wage replacement benefits depending on performance demonstrated during FCE) performed to much lower levels than subjects in a setting where such decisions were not being made. Subjects in this study had lower back pain, and related research is needed in other populations. Potentially, the reasons for FCE referral and decisions being made based on results are of great influence on performance and may differentiate whether subjects are willing to demonstrate actual physical capacity or merely levels of tolerance.

Tolerance

Tolerance is the ability to endure sustained work or activity.[12] Tolerance is therefore largely dependent on patient self-reports of pain, discomfort, fatigue, or other limits of performance. As such, determination of tolerance levels can be done by means of a simple self-report questionnaire, with performance assessment at the workplace (work trial) or during functional assessment.[11,38] While capacity assessments have a shared responsibility between worker and health care provider for determining maximal abilities, assessing tolerance and appropriate work levels may be more the responsibility of the injured worker by him- or herself. One benefit of determining tolerance using some form of functional assessment is the systematic underestimation that has been observed when subjects are asked to estimate ability.[30] As demonstrated in a study in which the abilities of healthy persons to endure sustained work (static overhead work and static forward bending) were tested using both performance-based and self-report measures, neither self-estimation nor prediction formulas were accurate in the prediction of actual capacity.[39]

The FCE approach that has been proposed with the aim of measuring tolerance levels is entitled *psychophysical*.[40] In psychophysical assessment, subjects are asked to perform various activities, but only to the levels at which they feel they need to stop for some reason. The performance level and reason for stopping is recorded and becomes the basis for setting return-to-work recommendations. It has been suggested that psychophysical FCE is limited by symptoms and psychological factors such as pain intensity, in contrast to kinesiophysical FCE.[31] However, little differences in performance outcomes have been observed in direct comparisons between psychophysical and other methods of assessment.[41] This is not surprising because in most kinesiophysical FCEs subjects are also instructed to stop activities whenever they feel the need (which is ethically appropriate). While evaluators may select either the psychophysical or kinesiophysical approach, the distinction between physiology and psychology is not likely to be made by injured workers.

Practical Considerations

There are a number of issues physicians should consider when debating whether or not an FCE is indicated and when interpreting FCE results. Cost is a critical issue but is very context dependent and will therefore not be considered here. When considering whether to refer a patient for an FCE, the physician should initially decide whether functional assessment would provide important information to augment findings from the medical examination. Are the necessary work restrictions already obvious, or is there some uncertainty due to the diagnosis? The decision of whether or not an FCE is warranted and would be beneficial is very context specific, but depends on factors such as the nature of the diagnosis, patient factors such as willingness to participate, employer willingness to incorporate assessment findings into the worksite, and the characteristics of the insurance/payer organization.

Secondly, the physician should weigh the risk versus benefit ratio for FCE. Because injured workers are often participating in strenuous physical activity during FCE, the test comes with an inherent risk of pain exacerbation or injury. While the risk of injury is no higher than participation in an exercise or rehabilitation program (possibly lower during FCE because the patient is constantly monitored by a trained evaluator), the number of patients reporting increased pain following FCE is substantial. One alternative to full FCE protocols that may further reduce risk while still providing important information for predicting return to work is a short-form FCE.[42] A short-form protocol has been shown to achieve comparable return-to-work outcomes and is associated with future return to work but has a much lower administrative burden.[43] Fewer activities are tested, therefore inherent risk is greatly reduced.

If the benefits of functional assessment do appear to outweigh the associated risks, physicians should provide some education to patients related to the likelihood of increased symptoms following FCE without provoking fear. For example:

> "During the FCE you will be assessed performing activities you often do at work to see if you have the ability to perform your regular work. Because you may not be used to this level of activity, the FCE may result in soreness or extra pain. While it is likely that you may experience more pain after FCE, this is most likely not a sign of injury. ("It may hurt you, but it will not harm you.") The risk is similar to participating in an exercise session. The soreness typically goes away within a few days, but the assessment will provide us with some information about whether or not you can perform your job."

Chapter 6

When faced with interpreting results from an FCE, a number of issues must also be considered. Physicians should understand the nature of the assessment protocol used. Was it a customized or standardized proprietary protocol? While the FCE field of research is in early stages, some protocols have been investigated more thoroughly than others in regards to reliability and validity.[44] In addition to having some knowledge of the FCE methods, physicians should determine the nature and level of the workers' compliance and participation during assessment. These details are frequently described in the full FCE report, but physicians are also able to interview patients after the FCE to determine their perceptions regarding the assessment.

The key result from FCE is the level of performance, often presented in comparison to required physical job demands. In addition to knowing how the level of performance was determined, physicians should understand how job demands were identified. Were these reported by the worker, or available from a job description or worksite visit? Validity of the methods of determining job demands is just as important as validity of FCE. Recently, a normative database consisting of 702 healthy workers (180 occupations, 4 physical demand classes) has also been published so that individuals interpreting FCE can compare results to occupation matched controls.[45] The basic assumption is that when functional capacity of healthy workers is equal to or exceeds their workload, the functional capacity of healthy workers may be considered the "norm" to which the functional capacity of patients can be compared. As it is currently unknown how this Dutch database compares to normative values, generalizations must be made with care to other groups of healthy workers.

Unanswered Questions

As mentioned above, despite widespread use of FCE our understanding of their measurement properties is still in early stages. The majority of research conducted to date has been on injured workers with musculoskeletal conditions. While this represents the largest group undergoing FCE, additional work is needed to evaluate FCE within other populations and clinical groups in which they are used. Further research is needed on the determinants of performance during FCE to more clearly elucidate what exactly is being measured, especially within the framework of the World Health Organization's International Classification of Functioning.[36] More work is also needed on how best to integrate FCE information into return-to-work decisions, recognizing the strengths and limitations of these tests. Lastly, the influence of assessment setting on performance also needs further study, including the effect of cultural setting, type of insurance system, and nature of the clinical practice in which the assessment is conducted. It is also not known whether the extra costs of FCE outweigh the potential benefits, thus cost-effectiveness studies in different settings would be beneficial.

Summary

FCEs are frequently used to inform return-to-work decisions despite an evidence base that is in early stages. We have discussed some of the strengths and limitations of FCE within the risk, capacity and tolerance framework. When making return-to-work recommendations, physicians should interpret FCE results within the workers' broader personal and environmental context as opposed to merely relying on recommendations in the FCE report.

References

1. Soer R, van der Schans CP, Groothoff JW, Geertzen JH, Reneman MF. Towards consensus in operational definitions in functional capacity evaluation: a Delphi Survey. *J Occup Rehabil.* 2008;18:389–400.

2. Pransky GS, Dempsey PG. Practical aspects of functional capacity evaluations. *J Occup Rehabil.* 2004;14:217–29.

3. Strong S, Baptiste S, Clarke J, Cole D, Costa M. Use of functional capacity evaluations in workplaces and the compensation system: a report on workers' and report users' perceptions. *Work.* 2004;23:67–77.

4. Isernhagen SJ. Return to work testing: functional capacity and work capacity evaluation. *Orthop Phys Ther NA.* 1992;1:83–98.

5. Matheson LN, Mooney V, Grant JE, et al. A test to measure lift capacity of physically impaired adults. Part 1—Development and reliability testing. *Spine* 1995;20:2119–29.

6. Innes E, Straker L. A clinician's guide to work-related assessments: 2-Design problems. *Work.* 1998;11:191–206.

7. Genovese E, Galper JS, American Medical Association. Guide to the evaluation of functional ability: how to request, interpret, and apply functional capacity evaluations. Chicago: American Medical Association; 2009.

8. Wind H, Gouttebarge V, Kuijer PP, Sluiter JK, Frings-Dresen MH. The utility of functional capacity evaluation: the opinion of physicians and other experts in the field of return to work and disability claims. *Int Arch Occup Environ Health.* 2006;79:528–34.

9. Innes E, Straker L. Workplace assessments and functional capacity evaluations: current beliefs of therapists in Australia. *Work.* 2003;20:225–36.

10. Innes E, Straker L. A clinician's guide to work-related assessments: 1-purposes and problems. *Work.* 1998;11:183–9.

Chapter 6

11. Gross DP. Measurement properties of performance-based assessment of functional capacity. *J of Occup Rehab*. 2004;14:166–74.

12. Talmage JB, Melhorn JM, American Medical Associates. A physician's guide to return to work. [Chicago, Ill.]: American Medical Association AMA Press; 2005.

13. Hadler NM. Occupational musculoskeletal disorders. 3rd ed. Philadelphia: Lippincott Williams & Wilkins; 2005.

14. Hall H, McIntosh G, Melles T, Holowachuk B, Wai E. Effect of discharge recommendations on outcome. *Spine*. 1994;19:2033–7.

15. Gross DP, Batti MC. Does functional capacity evaluation predict recovery in workers compensation claimants with upper extremity disorders? *Occup Environ Med*. 2006.

16. Gross DP, Battie MC. The prognostic value of functional capacity evaluation in patients with chronic low back pain: part 2: sustained recovery. *Spine*. 2004;29:920–4.

17. Gross DP, Battie MC. Functional capacity evaluation performance does not predict sustained return to work in claimants with chronic back pain. *J Occup Rehabil*. 2005;15:285–94.

18. Streibelt M, Blume C, Thren K, Reneman MF, Mueller-Fahrnow W. Value of functional capacity evaluation information in a clinical setting for predicting return to work. *Arch Phys Med Rehabil* 2009;90:429–34.

19. Gibson L, Strong J. Safety issues in functional capacity evaluation: findings from a trial of a new approach for evaluating clients with chronic back pain. *J Occup Rehabil* 2005;15:237–51.

20. Reneman MF, Kuijer W, Brouwer S, et al. Symptom increase following a functional capacity evaluation in patients with chronic low back pain: an explorative study of safety. *J Occup Rehabil* 2006;16:197–205.

21. Soer R, Groothoff JW, Geertzen JH, van der Schans CP, Reesink DD, Reneman MF. Pain response of healthy workers following a functional capacity evaluation and implications for clinical interpretation. *J Occup Rehabil* 2008;18:290–8.

22. Gross DP, Battié MC. Reliability of safe maximum lifting determinations of a functional capacity evaluation. *Phys Ther* 2002;82:364–71.

23. Reneman MF, Dijkstra PU, Westmaas M, Goeken LN. Test-retest reliability of lifting and carrying in a 2-day functional capacity evaluation. *J Occup Rehab* 2002;12:269–75.

24. Kuijer W, Dijkstra PU, Brouwer S, Reneman MF, Groothoff JW, Geertzen JH. Safe lifting in patients with chronic low back pain: comparing FCE lifting task and Niosh lifting guideline. *J Occup Rehabil* 2006;16:579–89.

25. Brouwer S, Reneman MF, Dijkstra PU, Groothoff JW, Schellekens JMH, Goeken LNH. Test-retest reliability of the Isernhagen Work Systems Functional Capacity Evaluation in patients with chronic low back pain. *J Occup Rehab* 2003;13:207–18.

26. Reneman MF, Fokkens AS, Dijkstra PU, Geertzen JH, Groothoff JW. Testing lifting capacity: validity of determining effort level by means of observation. *Spine* 2005;30:E40–6.

27. Jay MA, Lamb JM, Watson RL, et al. Sensitivity and specificity of the indicators of sincere effort of the EPIC lift capacity test on a previously injured population. Spine 2000;25:1405–12.

28. Gross DP, Battie MC. Construct validity of a kinesiophysical functional capacity evaluation administered within a worker's compensation environment. J Occup Rehabil 2003;13:287–95.

29. Gross DP, Battie MC. Factors influencing results of functional capacity evaluations in workers' compensation claimants with low back pain. Phys Ther 2005;85:315–22.

30. Asante AK, Brintnell ES, Gross DP. Functional Self-Efficacy Beliefs Influence Functional Capacity Evaluation. J Occup Rehabil 2007.

31. Gross DP, Bhambhani Y, Haykowsky MJ, Rashiq S. Acute opioid administration improves work-related exercise performance in patients with chronic back pain. J Pain 2008;9:856–62.

32. Reneman MF, Schiphorts Preuper HR, Kleen M, Geertzen JH, Dijkstra PU. Are pain intensity and pain related fear related to functional capacity evaluation performances of patients with chronic low back pain? J Occup Rehabil 2007;17:247–58.

33. Reneman MF, Jorritsma W, Dijkstra SJ, Dijkstra PU. Relationship between kinesiophobia and performance in a functional capacity evaluation. J Occup Rehab 2003;13:277–85.

34. Reneman MF, Jorritsma W, Schellekens JM, Goeken LN. Concurrent validity of questionnaire and performance-based disability measurements in patients with chronic nonspecific low back pain. J Occup Rehab 2002;12:119–29.

35. Reneman MF, Geertzen JH, Groothoff JW, Brouwer S. General and specific self-efficacy reports of patients with chronic low back pain: are they related to performances in a functional capacity evaluation? J Occup Rehabil 2008;18:183–9.

36. Towards a common language for Functioning, Disability and Health: ICF. Geneva: World Health Organization; 2002.

37. Reneman MF, Kool J, Oesch P, Geertzen JH, Battie MC, Gross DP. Material handling performance of patients with chronic low back pain during functional capacity evaluation: a comparison between three countries. Disabil Rehabil 2006;28:1143–9.

38. Roland M, Fairbank J. The Roland-Morris Disability Questionnaire and the Oswestry Disability Questionnaire. Spine 2000;25:3115–24.

39. Reneman MF, Bults MM, Engbers LH, Mulders KK, Goeken LN. Measuring maximum holding times and perception of static elevated work and forward bending in healthy young adults. J Occup Rehabil 2001;11:87–97.

40. Snook SH. Future directions of psychophysical studies. Scand J Work Environ Health 1999;25 Suppl 4:13–8.

41. Soer R, Poels BJ, Geertzen JH, Reneman MF. A comparison of two lifting assessment approaches in patients with chronic low back pain. J Occup Rehabil 2006;16:639–46.

42. Gross DP, Battie MC, Asante A. Development and validation of a short-form functional capacity evaluation for use in claimants with low back disorders. J Occup Rehabil 2006;16:53.

Chapter 6

43. Gross DP, Battie MC, Asante AK. Evaluation of a short-form functional capacity evaluation: less may be best. J Occup Rehabil 2007;17:422–35.

44. Gouttebarge V, Wind H, Kuijer PP, Frings-Dresen MH. Reliability and validity of Functional Capacity Evaluation methods: a systematic review with reference to Blankenship system, Ergos work simulator, Ergo-Kit and Isernhagen work system. Int Arch Occup Environ Health 2004;77:527–37.

45. Soer R, van der Schans CP, Geertzen JH, et al. Normative values for a functional capacity evaluation. Arch Phys Med Rehabil 2009;90:1785–94.

The Medical and Legal Aspects of Return-to-Work Decision Making

David J. DePaolo, JD, MBA

Medical-legal is the intersecting subset where medical considerations and legal considerations overlap. Occupational medicine practitioners are familiar with this area—an area to the medical mind that is obfuscated in gray, and an area to the legal mind that is constricted by science. This chapter will explore the increasingly complex considerations of return to work amid the various laws that govern and regulate return to work.

What is Disability?

The key return-to-work issue in the medical-legal context is the level of disability a person experiences. But defining disability in an objective manner is illusive and subject to conflicting exceptions. A prime example of this is the American Medical Association's attempt to standardize the elements of interference with the activities of daily living (ADLs) and any resultant "permanent impairment." While the *Guides* attempt "a standardized, objective approach to evaluating medical impairments,"[1] the authors acknowledge that standardization cannot be followed in all cases, for instance those cases in which "the medical evidence appears insufficient to verify that an impairment of a certain magnitude exists."[2] The *Guides*, Fifth, offers that just because a person may have an impairment that interferes with ADLs, there may be no diminution in the ability to perform productive work, or alternatively may be completely disabled from working.*,3

The practitioner is also going to experience frustration because of the inherent conflict embodied in the concepts of "return to work" and "disability." This is a chapter about the application of law, and in the practical context we are concerned with a fiction constructed in a political climate. Thus, it is useful for the practitioner to temper the concept of disability with the practical construct of "productivity." For instance, is a former professional motorcycle racer who is paralyzed from the neck down from a race crash disabled if he goes on to a successfully manage a professional race team for several years?** In other words, while the law may require an opinion on disability, the practical application in the return-to-work context is what productive work activities the injured person can do. Nevertheless, when dealing with return to work, the practitioner must first deal with the legal fiction of disability. The particular definition of disability is different from one legal system to another, if there is any definition at all. Understanding how disability is defined in the law is therefore critical to understanding the role in returning an injured person back to work. Finally, it is important for the physician to be mindful of the legal system for which a return to work opinion is sought. An opinion in one setting, for example workers' compensation, can affect the rights of either the employer or the injured worker in another setting, such as under the Americans with Disabilities Act (ADA) or the Employee Retirement Income Security Act (ERISA).

Workers' Compensation

Workers' compensation is a legislatively created benefit delivery system in which fault or negligence is generally irrelevant. Typically, some form

---

* "For example, an individual who receives a 30% whole person impairment due to pericardial heart disease is considered from a clinical standpoint to have a 30% reduction in general functioning as represented by a decrease in the ability to perform activities of daily living. For individuals who work in sedentary jobs, there may be no decline in their ability although their overall functioning is decreased. Thus, a 30% impairment rating does not correspond to a 30% reduction in work capability. Similarly, a manual laborer with this 30% impairment rating due to pericardial disease may be completely unable to do his or her regular job and, thus, may have a 100% work disability."

** Wayne Rainey, Monterey, CA – 500cc World Road Racing Champion 1990–1992, crashed in the 1993 Italian Grand Prix while leading the race and the championship series, breaking his neck. He then went on to manage the Marlboro Yamaha team 1994–1998 when he retired.

of administrative dispute resolution process is attached. One of the most fundamental, and yet most difficult precepts of workers' compensation law, is that it is generally regarded as a "disability program with a medical component."[4] For a "disability program with a medical component" one would think that the term *disability* would be defined, yet this term is curiously absent from most workers' compensation systems. For example, California's workers' compensation laws[5] do not define disability. That state's Unemployment Insurance Code does provide us with a definition, though it is unworkably vague: "An individual shall be deemed disabled on any day in which, because of his or her physical or mental condition, he or she is unable to perform his or her regular or customary work."[6] The California Unemployment Insurance Code defines an "industrially disabled person" as "an individual who has received or is entitled to receive benefits under Division 4 (commencing with Section 3201) of the Labor Code, and who is unable to perform his regular or customary work for 60 consecutive days or more, but not to exceed two calendar years from the date of commencement of his industrial disability."[7]

The definition of disability may be found in state resources that are not in either statute or regulations. California's permanent disability rating manual (PDRS) states "[t]he calculation of a permanent disability rating is initially based on a [sic] evaluating physician's impairment rating, in accordance with the medical evaluation protocols and rating procedures set forth in the American Medical Association (AMA) *Guides to the Evaluation of Permanent Impairment*, 5th Edition, which is hereby incorporated by reference."[8] This medical determination affects the legal status of the injured worker and, as a consequence, his or her return-to-work status.

Disability in workers' compensation is generally defined within the sole context of the injured worker's usual and customary occupational duties at the time of injury. For instance, champion motorcycle racer Wayne Rainey would be considered 100% permanently disabled as a consequence of his total paralysis from the neck down, yet he went on to work as a race team manager. Again, we are dealing with the contradiction between medical science (obviously Mr. Rainey retained some medical ability to engage in gainful employment) and legal fiction (disabled legally because Mr. Rainey could not race a motorcycle again).

To make matters a bit more complex, workers' compensation systems generally recognize four different types of disability: temporary partial disability, temporary total disability, permanent partial disability, and permanent total disability. These disability classifications are provided for administrative benefit determination and require a supportive medical opinion. Consequently, it is of import to understand each of these types of disabilities.

Chapter 7

The assumption in workers' compensation schemes is that the injured worker will have a difficult time assimilating to occupational duties that deviate from those that the worker has long practiced and trained, and that there will be a negative wage gap. In many cases this is a correct assumption, and that is why most states provide for "temporary partial disability" indemnity. This indemnity benefit is generally designed to provide a wage gap replacement when the injured worker's status does not permit return to usual and customary duties on a fulltime basis or permits return to restricted duties only, and thus to a lower-wage occupation.

"Temporary total disability," again generally not defined in state workers' compensation systems (perhaps because it is assumed that this is a medical status), implies that the injured worker cannot engage in any productive activity. Many states put time limits on the total amount of time that an injured worker can be "temporarily totally disabled." After such time then it is assumed that the injured worker has some permanent disability.

When an injured worker experiences some lasting consequence of his or her injury, then it is generally regarded as a "permanent disability." This may be either "partial" or "total."

Permanent total disability is fairly easy to comprehend. In the legal context, this means that the injured worker is completely unable to engage in *any* of the injured worker's usual and customary occupational duties whatsoever. This is dependent not only on the injured worker's medical status but also the availability of work to accommodate that medical status.

Permanent partial disability generally assumes that the injured worker has incurred a prolonged disability that interferes with his or her ability to make the same wages as before. Some states define this condition as inability to compete in the open labor market, some define the status as a diminution in earning capacity, and other states have even different criteria. In each of these cases, the test is whether the injured worker can do the same work as he or she was able to prior to the injury and consequential disability.

Texas is the only jurisdiction in the United States where workers' compensation insurance is optional. An employer without workers' compensation coverage in Texas is called a nonsubscriber, or "going bare." Going bare in Texas subjects the employer to civil liability for work injuries. Approximately 30% of Texas' employers, representing 20% of Texas' work force, are outside of that state's workers' compensation system.[9]

Typically a nonsubscriber Texas employer establishes its own ERISA Benefit Plan (see end of chapter) to address workplace injuries in place of workers' compensation coverage. These plans are typically constructed by specialty insurance brokers and incorporate medical, disability, and liability policies to cover work injuries and, often, injuries, diseases, and disabilities outside of work. The definition of disability in a nonsubscriber situation is going to depend on the benefit plan contract language.

Longshore and Harbor Workers Compensation Act

The Longshore and Harbor Workers Compensation Act (LHWCA) provides a workers' compensation system for maritime workers who are not "seamen" and thus who don't fall within the jurisdiction of the Jones Act (discussed later in this chapter). Like state workers' compensation, the LHWCA is a no-fault system (not dependent on a finding of fault or negligence), and a claimant under the LHWCA can seek medical and disability benefits. LHWCA fills the gap between state workers' compensation systems, which generally don't protect workers on navigable waters, and the Jones Act that protects seamen.

Disability is defined in the LHWCA as "incapacity because of injury to earn the wages which the employee was receiving at the time of injury in the same or any other employment …"[10] The LHWCA gives us something to work with regarding return to work because of this definition. The first element is "incapacity." Incapacity is not defined by the LHWCA, but the courts have interpreted this, and it requires an inquiry as to whether someone having both the injury and a similar background (age, education, and work experience) would be able to find work in the relevant geographical area.[11] The second element of disability under LHWCA, also within the purview of the physician, is "because of injury." "Injury" is defined, somewhat redundantly, as "accidental injury … arising out of and in the course of employment, and such occupational disease or infection as arises naturally out of such employment or as naturally and unavoidably results from such accidental injury. …"[12] For occupational diseases that do not immediately result in disability, the Act defines "time of injury" as the date the claimant becomes aware or should have been aware of the relationship between his employment, the disease, and the disability.[13] Unlike occupational diseases, the LHWCA does not define time of injury for accidental injuries. The courts have recognized, however, that in most cases of traumatic injury the date of injury and the date of disability coincide.[14]

Thus, a return-to-work opinion under the LHWCA is done within the context of whether the reason the claimant can or cannot work is a product of an injury caused by or arising out of work and whether this causes an inability to obtain employment.

Maritime and Railroad Workers

The advent of the railroad age in conjunction with the industrial revolution prompted the federal government to create protections for railroad workers. This law is called the Federal Employer's Liability Act. Soon thereafter Congress elected to codify and secure remedies inherent in traditional maritime law by extending FELA's jurisdiction through the Jones Act.

Federal Employers' Liability Act

The rights of railroad company employees who suffer a railroad injury are protected under the Federal Employers Liability Act (FELA).[15] This act, passed by Congress in 1908 (after the first law passed in 1906 was declared unconstitutional by the US Supreme Court), was designed to provide compensation when an employee suffers a railroad injury as a result of the railroad company's negligence.

FELA court cases involve traditional civil structure, with a judge and jury to decide questions of fact. Unlike workers' compensation or LHWCA cases, the FELA claimant must initiate a civil court action and must first prove that the railroad was negligent before obtaining the ability to recover any remedy.

Note that a FELA case involves damages and is not limited in the type of recovery that the injured worker can obtain. This means that any opinion or recommendation on return to work is going to be essentially an opinion on the injured worker's failure to return to work, and so his or her future earning capacity. There is no direct discussion of the type of disability in a FELA case. Damages may be comprised of work that was missed as a consequence of the injury and tempered by work that should not have been missed (ie, plaintiff's failure to mitigate his or her damages).

Jones Act

The Jones Act extended FELA statutory protection to mariners who previously had only common law remedies (ie, the traditions of maritime law) and allows qualifying seamen the same protections afforded railroad employees under FELA.[16]

Like a FELA case, actions under the Jones Act involve a civil jury trial and the injured seaman must prove negligence first.

And, like a FELA case, the Jones Act does not deal directly with disability, but rather a more traditional sense of "damages."[†] Thus return to work in the Jones Act context does not take into account one's disability, but rather the impact the effects of an injury have on a seaman's earning capacity, and the plethora of other objective and subjective factors of damages.

Jones Act damages are typically for "Maintenance" and "Cure." These two terms, age-old maritime terms, are usually tied together, though they represent independent damages. Both maintenance and cure extend during the period when the seaman is incapacitated to do a seaman's work and continues until maximum medical improvement status is attained.[17]

Cure refers to reimbursement of reasonable medical expenses that are "curative" of any injury or disease that may be covered by the Jones Act.[18]

Maintenance refers to the weekly checks that an employer must pay Jones Act claimants when their regular pay is interrupted due to either an injury or disease—a daily "subsistence" to the injured seaman for the reasonable expenses of room and board while ashore until such time as the seaman is found fit for duty or found to have reached maximum medical improvement (MMI) by a physician.[19]

Return to work in both FELA and Jones Act cases require an assessment of whether the injured worker can return to a work capacity sufficient to support pre-injury earnings, and if not, what the effect of the incapacity or impairment is on future earnings capacity.

[†] The jury has exclusive obligation to compute damages, and that computation need not conform to strict arithmetical calculations but may be in form of lump sum award. *McDonald v Federal Barge Lines, Inc.* (1974, CA5 La) 496 F2d 1376. In action brought under 46 USCS Appx § 688, assessment of damages is primarily question of fact for jury. *Baldwin v Huffman Towing Co.* (1977, 5th Dist) 51 Ill App 3d 861, 9 Ill Dec 469, 366 NE2d 980. In action to recover damages under 46 USCS Appx § 688, judge may award damages without specifically detailing basis for arriving at figure; medical and funeral expenses would be in addition to general, undifferentiated award. *Williamson v Western-Pacific Dredging Corp.* (1969, DC Or) 304 F Supp 509, affd (CA9 Or) 441 F2d 65, cert den 404 US 851, 30 L Ed 2d 91, 92 S Ct 90.

Chapter 7

The Americans with Disabilities Act

The Americans with Disabilities Act (ADA) was enacted in 1990 for the purpose of ensuring that those with disabilities were not discriminated against. In practical terms it is the employer who makes the ultimate decision regarding return to work. The physician's role is simply to provide the employer with guidance as to applicable restrictions that may need to be observed in the work place, or reasonable medical accommodations that can be made—ideas that facilitate the return to work process.

The ADA applies to employers with 15 employees or more. It prohibits discrimination in all employment practices, including job application procedures, hiring, firing, advancement, compensation, training, and other terms, conditions, and privileges of employment. It applies to recruitment, advertising, tenure, layoff, leave, fringe benefits, and all other employment-related activities.

Only "qualified individuals with disabilities" are protected under the ADA; thus, for the return-to-work determination, a "disability" is a critical concept and must be dealt with.

The ADA defines disability as "a physical or mental impairment that substantially limits one or more of the major life activities of such individual; a record of such an impairment; or being regarded as having such an impairment."[20]

The Equal Employment Opportunity Commission (EEOC) through the Department of Justice has responsibility for establishing and enforcing regulations that implement the provisions of the ADA.[21]

EEOC regulations make a distinction between impairment and disability. A disability under the ADA requires an impairment, a record of impairment, or being regarded as having an impairment; however, impairment does not necessarily rise to the level of disability.[22] Impairment is specifically defined in the regulations.[23] The impairment must substantially limit a major life activity such as seeing, hearing, speaking, walking, breathing, performing manual tasks, learning, caring for oneself, and working.[24] Note that the standard is "substantially limit." Conditions such as epilepsy, HIV infection, mental retardation, or paralysis are examples of impairments that "substantially limit" major life activities. Broken bones, sprains, and short term illnesses don't qualify.

The ADA is to be interpreted in light of its pending application. For example, an individual with a severe facial disfigurement may be protected from being denied employment because an employer fears the "negative reactions" of customers or co-workers. But if such condition were related to the safety of the employee or the public, then there may not be protection. To fall within the ADA, one must be a *qualified individual*, defined as a person with a disability "who meets legitimate skill, experience, education, or other requirements of an employment position that s/he holds or seeks, and who can perform the 'essential functions' of the position with or without reasonable accommodation. Requiring the ability to perform 'essential functions' assures that an individual with a disability will not be considered unqualified simply because of inability to perform marginal or incidental job functions. If the individual is qualified to perform essential job functions except for limitations caused by a disability, the employer must consider whether the individual could perform these functions with a reasonable accommodation."[25] While it is the employer who makes the ultimate determination as to whether a particular individual with a disability can be accommodated for work, the physician can and will be called upon to assist in the decision-making process. Thus it is important for the physician to understand the parameters of the employer's legal constraints. We'll break this down as simply as possible by providing lists of what an employer can and cannot do under the ADA.

What an employer can do under the ADA:

1. An employer may ask questions about the ability to perform specific job functions and may, with certain limitations, ask an individual with a disability to describe or demonstrate how he or she would perform these functions.

2. An employer may condition a job offer on the satisfactory result of a post-offer medical examination or medical inquiry if this is required of all entering employees in the same job category. A post-offer examination or inquiry does not have to be job related and consistent with business necessity.

3. If an individual is not hired because a post-offer medical examination or inquiry reveals a disability, the reason(s) for not hiring must be job related and consistent with business necessity. The employer also must show that no reasonable accommodation was available that would enable the individual to perform the essential job functions or that accommodation would impose an undue hardship. A post-offer medical examination may disqualify an individual if the employer can demonstrate that the individual would pose a "direct threat" in the workplace (ie, a significant risk of substantial harm to the health or safety of the individual or others) that cannot be eliminated or reduced below the "direct threat" level through reasonable accommodation.

4. An employer may conduct employee medical examinations in cases in which there is evidence of a job performance or safety problem, examinations required by other federal laws, examinations to determine current

"fitness" to perform a particular job, and voluntary examinations that are part of employee health programs.

5. An employer may consider health and safety when deciding whether to hire an applicant or retain an employee with a disability. The ADA permits employers to establish qualification standards that will exclude individuals who pose a direct threat—ie, a significant risk of substantial harm—to the health or safety of the individual or of others, if that risk cannot be eliminated or reduced below the level of a "direct threat" by reasonable accommodation.

What an employer *cannot* do:

1. An employer may not ask or require a job applicant to take a medical examination before making a job offer. It cannot make any pre-employment inquiry about a disability or the nature or severity of a disability.

2. A post-offer medical examination may not disqualify an individual with a disability who is currently able to perform essential job functions because of speculation that the disability may cause a risk of future injury.

3. An employer may not simply assume that a threat exists; the employer must establish through objective, medically supportable methods that there is significant risk that substantial harm could occur in the workplace.

Family and Medical Leave Act (FMLA)

FMLA needs to be understood in three different contexts: the federal statute, state statutes, and collective bargaining agreements (see ERISA). Each of these build on the other and, though each may refer generally to the FMLA, there are inherent differences that the physician should be aware of.

Federal

The Federal FMLA[26] was passed by the 103rd US Congress and subsequently was signed into law on August 5, 1993. It requires employers having 50 or more employees to provide job-protected unpaid leave due to a "serious health condition" that makes the employee unable to perform his or her job, among other qualifying events.

The term *serious health condition* means an illness, injury, impairment, or physical or mental condition that involves inpatient care in a hospital, hospice, or residential medical care facility; or continuing treatment by a health care provider.[27] It can also mean an injury or illness incurred by a covered service member in the line of duty that may render the service member medically unfit to perform the duties of the member's office, grade, rank, or rating.[28]

A physician must "certify" an employee for leave under the FMLA. If the employer is not satisfied with the employee's presentation of an FMLA certification, then the employer may pay for a second opinion. If the second opinion conflicts in any way with the first opinion, then the employer may pay for a third opinion, which shall be final.[29] Federal regulations specify exactly what the "certification" must contain in order to comply with FMLA requirements.[30] Remember that the FMLA, like the ADA, is about discrimination. The physician's duty under the FMLA is to provide a certification about the ability, or inability, of the employee to perform a job. It is up to the employer ultimately to decide if the employee's job can be held open for the employee's ultimate return to work.

State

Most state FMLA statutes operate similarly to the federal statute but provide broader protection. For instance, the state of California's FMLA statute[31] provides that the term *parent* includes any "other person who stood in loco parentis to the employee when the employee was a child." Because the federal FMLA law is primary, the federal law will supercede any state law unless provisions of state law are more generous or liberal. The physician should understand to what extent the particular state's FMLA provisions provide greater protection than the federal law.

ERISA

The Employee Retirement Income Security Act of 1974 (ERISA) is a federal law‡ that sets minimum standards for retirement and health benefit plans in private industry. ERISA does not require an employer to establish a plan. It only requires that those who establish plans must meet certain minimum standards.

ERISA covers retirement, health, and other welfare benefit plans (eg, life, disability, and apprenticeship plans). Among other things, ERISA provides

---

‡ Portions of ERISA are codified in various places of the US Code, including 29 U.S.C. ch.18, and Internal Revenue Code § 219 and § 408 (relating to the Individual Retirement Account) and § 410 through § 415, and § 4971, § 4974, and § 4975.

that those individuals who manage plans (and other fiduciaries) must meet certain standards of conduct. Enforcement and regulatory oversight of ERISA plans is the province of the US Department of Labor, Employee Benefits Security Administration.[32]

A return-to-work analysis in an ERISA situation requires knowledge of the employee disability benefit system. But, while the specifics of a return-to-work opinion will depend upon the details of the disability program in question, all employers subject to its ERISA's provisions must comply with it's broad guiding principles.

ERISA governs disability plans provided by employers, so the return-to-work opinion of the physician is based on "disability." A benefit is a "disability benefit" under the regulation, subject to the special rules for disability claims, if the plan conditions its availability to the claimant upon a showing of disability. It does not matter how the benefit is characterized by the plan or whether the plan as a whole is a pension plan or a welfare plan. If the claims adjudicator must make a determination of disability in order to decide a claim, the claim must be treated as a disability claim for purposes of the regulation.

Disability is defined differently by different plans. Likewise, many plans also define modified work and return-to-work requirements. Because the definition of disability and requirements for return to work are contractually defined, the physician should seek this information from the employer to ensure that opinions are consistent with the employer's plan. Texas nonsubscribers who elect to provide protection to their employees for work injuries and disability benefits will be governed by ERISA. In addition, heightened FMLA rights are also the subject of ERISA when a part of a collective bargaining agreement. Such plans are typically benefit programs provided by private-sector employers for their employees (or by unions, acting either independently or jointly with employers, for their members).

Physician Liability

In both Jones Act cases and FELA cases, return-to-work assessments take on greater significance because of the inherent dangerous nature of maritime and railroad activities. The physician, in returning an injured seaman or railroad worker to work, needs to be concerned not only with the worker's ability to perform the duties of the work assignment, but also whether that seaman poses a threat or safety hazard to the vessel and co-seamen. Indeed, the physician may be held liable for damages to third parties in situations in which an unfit injured worker was returned to work.[§,33] Jurisdictions vary on physician liability to third parties depending on specific law applicable to the jurisdiction, but the fundamental issue is whether it is foreseeable that third parties could be injured or killed as a result of the return to work of an injured worker.[34]

In an Arizona appellate case involving an exam of a workers' compensation claimant, Ritchie v. Krasner,[35] the court held that an Independent Medical Examiner owed a duty of reasonable care to the patient even absent a formal doctor-patient relationship. Ritchie sustained a work injury, and the carrier referred him to Krasner for an independent medical examination. Krasner failed to diagnose a compressed spinal cord causing part of the cord to die. Eventually, after treatment by another doctor, Ritchie died from an accidental drug overdose. The court first found that Krasner owed Ritchie a duty, despite having no formal doctor-patient relationship, because Ritchie relied on Krasner's original misdiagnosis and thus did not procure an alternative opinion or treatment.[§,36] After the Ritchie decision, the Arizona legislature in 2010 introduced House Bill 2465 and Senate Bill 1214, which would limit the liability of physicians who conduct evaluations for third parties, such as insurance companies; however, these bills were not passed and there are no current plans to introduce similar legislation in 2011.

Summary

Return to work necessarily involves an opinion regarding disability. Disability can mean different things depending on the legal system in which the issue arises. Understanding your role as a physician in rendering a return-to-work opinion is dependent upon the applicable legal system and a thorough understanding of all the facts that can affect a return to work opinion. Thus, like all areas of professional life, there remains the potential for liability despite the lack of a direct physician-patient relationship. The careful physician will scrupulously review all provided medical records and question not only the patient but also the referable laws and records.

---

§ "Where a physician certifies the employee as fit to return to heavy labor, it is not the employee's burden to show malpractice by the examining physician, rather it is sufficient to show that the railroad knew or should have known that the employee was unfit for the work because of his condition." *Fletcher v. Union Pacific R.R. Co.*, 621 F.2d 902, 909 (8th Cir. 1980). "Most such cases find that the examining physician was an agent of the railroad. ... However, such a finding is not essential." Ibid at n. 10.

§ "We too cannot envision a public benefit in encouraging a doctor with specific individualized knowledge not to investigate the symptoms of a cervical spine injury."

References

1. American Medical Association. *Guides to the Evaluation of Permanent Impairment*, 5th ed., Chicago, Ill: American Medical Association; 2001:1.

2. Ibid., 19.

3. Ibid., 5.

4. Quote attributed to Bruce Wood, associate general counsel and director of workers' compensation for the American Insurance Association – "Debating 'Compcare': How Federal Healthcare Legislation Might Affect Workers' Compensation"; Thorness, Bill, *National Council on Compensation Insurance Issues Report 2010*.

5. See generally Division 4, Part 1 starting with section 3200 of the California Labor Code.

6. California Unemployment Insurance Code § 2626(a).

7. Ibid., § 2776(a).

8. *Schedule for Rating Permanent Disabilities*, January 2005, 1–2.

9. University of Texas, Austin McCombs School of Business, *A Texas Workers' Compensation System Overview*, available at http://www.mccombs.utexas.edu/dept/irom/bba/risk/rmi/arnold/downloads/A%20Texas%20Workers.doc. Accessed 02/09/2009.

10. 33 U.S.C. 902(10).

11. See *Hairston v. Todd Shipyards Corp.*, 849 F.2d 1194 (9th Cir. 1988) (criminal record is relevant part of background); *Trans-State Dredging v. Benefits Review Board*, 731 F.2d 199, 201 (4th Cir. 1984). See also *Rivera v. United Masonry* (DC Cir., 1991) 948 F. 2d 774.

12. 33 U.S.C. 902(2).

13. 33 U.S.C. 910(i).

14. *Port of Portland v. Director, Office of Workers Compensation Programs, etc.*, 192 F.2d 933 (1999).

15. Generally at 45 U.S.C. 51, et. seq.

16. 46 U.S.C. 688.

17. *Vaughan v. Atkinson*, 369 U.S. 527 (1962).

18. *Vella v. Ford Motor Co.*, 421 U.S. 1 (1975).

19. Ibid.

20. 42 U.S.C. § 12102(2).

21. See http://www.ada.gov/publicat.htm.

22. Code of Federal Regulations, Part 36, Subpart A, § 36.104.

23. Ibid.

24. See generally the U.S. EEOC ADA website at http://www.ada.gov.

25. http://www.ada.gov/q%26aeng02.htm.

26. 29 U.S.C. 2601, et seq.

27. 29 U.S.C. 2611(11).

28. 29 CFR 825.800.

29. 29 U.S.C. 2613.

30. See 29 CFR 825.306(c) & (d) for the actual specific certification guidelines.

31. The California Family Rights Act, CA. Gov. Code §§ 12945.1–12945.2.

32. See http://www.dol.gov/ebsa/aboutebsa/main.html for more information.

33. *Fletcher v. Union Pacific R.R. Co.,* 621 F.2d 902, 909 (8th Cir. 1980).

34. Leonardo, Suffolk University Law Review [Vol. XLII:277].

35. *Ritchie v. Krasner* (2009) 211 P.3d 1272.

36. *Ritchie v. Krasner* at 1281.

Chapter 8

Disability Determinations and Return to Work

Les Kertay, PhD

> I'm a great believer in luck and I find the harder I work, the more I have of it.
>
> —Thomas Jefferson

> If a drug were associated with the level of mortality found in work absence, we would consider it malpractice to prescribe it.
>
> —Gordon Waddell, MD

A fundamental assumption of *A Physician's Guide to Return to Work* is that work is central to human well-being. We need to feel productive, valued, and engaged in order to function at the highest level of health. Because of this, one of the key outcomes for measuring quality health services should be the patient's ability to remain at work, to be fully productive while at work, and to return to work as promptly and safely as possible in the event that a work absence becomes medically necessary. To effectively achieve these outcomes for a patient, the physician who becomes involved in the care of the injured worker or in disability evaluation and management must learn skills beyond the basic requirements of traditional medical practice. These additional skills include the ability to evaluate functional impairment; the ability to translate a medical understanding of impairment into a clear statement of functional limitations and medically necessary work restrictions; and the ability to effectively negotiate between the patient, employer, and insurers. It is to this last skill that the present chapter turns.

What does a physician need to know about how disability insurance works? How does the insurer determine disability, and how does that determination relate to the concerns of the patient, the employer, and the physician?

Most importantly, how does everyone involved in the determination of compensation for disability most effectively cooperate to enhance health outcomes? This chapter is about understanding the importance of these questions and includes a strategy for answering them.

What Is a Disability Determination?

It is important to recognize that a *disability determination* differs from an *impairment evaluation*, and the distinction between these two concepts is one of the most difficult for both physicians and disability insurers to grasp. Communications and forms from disability insurance carriers, both public and private, can contribute to the confusion. A physician often assumes he or she is being asked whether his patient in disabled, and then is confused and sometimes affronted when the insurer challenges the physician's opinion. Fundamentally, this miscommunication is rooted in the fact that, whereas an impairment evaluation is a medical procedure, a disability determination is a contractual, medicolegal process for which medical information is a necessary, but not a sufficient condition.

The key to ensuring clear communication between medical providers and disability insurers is to understand and resolve the confusion between impairment evaluation and disability determination. There are three key sources of confusion. First, the term *disability* is used in multiple contexts, and each context has its own set of definitions and rules. Second, each of the key players in determining disability brings a different mindset to the process. Finally, the definition of terms used in determining disability overlaps with, but does not necessarily precisely coincide with, either their colloquial definitions or their more precise medical definitions.

Contexts

In broadest terms, the concept of disability represents the recognition that some individuals have decreased abilities in circumscribed domains and that these decreased abilities present barriers to functioning normally in the world. This is an extremely broad concept that is applied differently depending on the context.* One application of the disability construct

---

* The 1980 World Health Organization (WHO) defines disability as ". . . any restriction or lack of ability to perform an activity in the manner or within the range considered normal for a human being." (World Health Organization. *International Classification of Functioning, Disability, and Health*. Geneva, Switzerland: World Health Organization, 2001.) This deliberately broad definition allows the WHO to pursue its broad agenda to apply medical concepts and conduct epidemiological analysis across many cultures, countries, and individual circumstances, but it is ill-suited to a more precise application, such as disability insurance.

involves recognizing and overcoming barriers to normal functioning in society. In the United States, a prime example of this context is the Americans with Disabilities Act (ADA), both in its original 1990 form and as modified by the ADA Amendments Act (ADAAA) of 2008. Fundamentally, the ADA extends the protections of the Civil Rights Act of 1964 to individuals with recognized disabilities and prohibits, under particular circumstances, discrimination based on a disability, where *disability* is defined by the ADA as "a physical or mental impairment that substantially limits a major life activity."** Recently, the definition of "major life activities" was broadened by the 2008 ADAAA to include "caring for oneself, performing manual tasks, seeing, hearing, eating, sleeping, walking, standing, lifting, bending, speaking, breathing, learning, reading, concentrating, thinking, communicating, and working."[1] The critical point is that, in the context of the ADA and the principle of access and civil rights, disability determinations are made in order to ensure that individuals are afforded access to important activities, including work, through reasonable accommodations or modification of duties. Where the ADA applies, the individual who is defined as "disabled" is assisted in his or her efforts to maintain employment, and the motivation of the disabled individual is to demonstrate that he or she can continue to do a job if given the appropriate assistance to do so. Here the role of the physician is to help evaluate the nature of the impairment and the accommodation required to overcome that impairment and to certify the medical ability to remain employed if provided with an appropriate accommodation.

Contrasted with this situation is the context in which an individual seeks compensation, rather than accommodation.† Here, the definition of *disability* is narrowed to reflect the inability to earn a living as a result of an illness or injury that leads to functional impairment. This can occur in multiple settings including Social Security, workers' compensation, and private disability insurance, each with its own set of rules, regulations, definitions, and contracts.

Across these varied settings, however, the key element is that the individual seeks compensation because he or she has difficulty or is unable to perform the important functions of his or her occupation. In order to qualify for

---

** Importantly, the interpretation and implementation of the ADA was determined by rules and regulations created by the Equal Employment Opportunity Commission (EEOC) which, among other changes in meaning, restricted *substantially limits* to mean "significantly or severely restricts."

† Seeking compensation is not necessarily incompatible with seeking accommodation, and returning an individual to work is often an important focus for disability insurers. Here the discussion is focused on the contrasting motivations involved, for illustrative purposes.

compensation, the individual must demonstrate that he or she *cannot* continue to work even with accommodation. The role of the physician is also altered. The physician's evaluation of impairment is used to demonstrate risk and/or a lack of ability, and the physician is most often asked to certify that the patient is unable to continue working. In other words, the requirements of two main contexts in which the term *disability* is applied can be diametrically opposed: in the ADA context the patient and physician are motivated to demonstrate capacity, whereas in the disability insurance context the patient and physician are often required to demonstrate the lack of capacity.

Mindsets

Disability is a biopsychosocial phenomenon.[2-4] In broad terms and across multiple settings, statistical regressions have shown that a number of factors consistently appear as critical variables in understanding absence from and return to work. These are, in descending order of effect: (a) the extent of physical findings demonstrating impairment; (b) the employee's attitude toward work and disability;[5-8] (c) the attending physician's attitude toward work and disability;[8-9] (d) the employee's perception of workplace support for staying at, or returning to, work;[8] and (e) the type and extent of compensation available while away from work. Although a full discussion of these factors is beyond the scope of the present chapter, it is important to note that, of these five factors, four are psychosocial in nature and three involve attitudes regarding work. What follows is a brief discussion of these factors, especially as they relate to the mindsets underlying the key stakeholders in disability determinations.

The Patient: One's attitude toward work is one of the key variables in whether the individual stays at work, and whether he or she returns to work following an absence.[6-8] Often this is simplified to be about "motivation," but the equation is not nearly as straightforward as that. The question is not whether we are motivated; unless an organism is inert, all living beings are motivated to maximize potential benefits and minimize potential costs. With respect to motivation and work, Dr. Ken Mitchell has put forth an equation that sets out the variables:[10]

$$f(motivation) = \frac{V + Pos}{C}$$

That is, motivation with respect to work is a function of the perceived value or utility of the work (V), the perceived chance of successfully going back to or staying at work (Pos), and the real and perceived cost of returning to or staying at work (C). The individual who perceives his or her work to be of value, who feels valued by his or her employer, and who believes him- or herself to be capable of returning successfully is more likely to regain functional capacity. Ultimately, the patient must answer the question, "What's in it for me?" and his or her answer to that question will be a strong predictor of the outcome.

The Employer: The employer, too, is motivated by whatever is most advantageous. There is a cost associated with recruiting, hiring, and training an employee. There is also a cost associated with returning the employee to work, especially if the position needs to be accommodated or if the return needs to be gradual in order to allow for work restrictions and limitations. The more complex and specialized the job the trickier is this calculation, but in virtually all settings, the economics of this equation will influence employer behavior.

There are also other costs and benefits that affect the employer, and these factors are not always taken into account. Sometimes employers believe that there is a medical risk in bringing an employee back at less than 100% capacity, whether or not this is true for a specific job, and this perception will influence the availability of return-to-work programs. Even more intangibly, the employer who is perceived as supporting the employees' efforts to stay at and return to work will be rewarded by increased loyalty, which will in turn improve worker productivity. For the present discussion, the important point is to remember that an employer will need to understand the value of returning its employee to the workforce, and negotiating that value is an important part of a successful outcome.

The Insurer: The insurer, too, is motivated to obtain the greatest advantage. This is often taken to mean that the insurer is motivated entirely by profit and that profit, in turn, is driven by collecting premiums and paying out as little as possible in benefits. However, such a business model would be extraordinarily shortsighted, and it fails to take into account the fundamental role of insurance. Insurance is a promise to pay a benefit if the contractually defined terms of a claim are met; for disability, the promise is to replace a portion of income if the covered individual becomes unable to work as defined by the contract. The insurance company lives and dies by its reputation, which depends on the degree to which it is perceived to deliver on its promises.

The fundamental mindset of the insurer, therefore, is to promote its reputation by delivering on this contractual promise, whether the customer is an individual policyholder or an employer who buys a group policy to cover employees. To deliver on that contractual promise means the insurer must pay valid claims promptly and with good customer service, deny payment of any claim that is not valid, and when appropriate assist the claimant's efforts to return to work.‡

In carrying out these functions, the insurer is bound by a contract that has multiple complex provisions. Depending on whether the purchaser is an individual or an employer, different governmental regulations, taxability requirements, and litigation rules may apply. In short, the insurer must determine whether the claimant is eligible for benefits (eg, the employee was employed at the time of disability claim, the employer had paid benefits for that particular employee); whether the standard of proof for the claim has been met; and the terms under which payment is to continue.§ In the end, to understand the mindset of the insurer one must understand what the insurer needs in order to make an accurate contractual determination.

The Physician: Put simply, the physician wants what is best for his or her patient. The actions that lead to this outcome, however, occur in a context that is increasingly complex, and the physician's motivations are also affected by financial necessity and the need to prioritize limited time. In contrast to decisions regarding health care, the patient's request to complete a form in support of disability leaves the physician on unfamiliar ground. Most often, the physician will have neither the time nor the inclination to fully evaluate the health implications of what is being requested. He or she will instead either defer the form to office staff or complete the form with minimal information. It is unlikely that this occurs because the physician doesn't care about the health of his or her patient; instead, it is more likely to be that the physician fails to understand work as an important part of health, and so he or she is dispensing with an administrative detail so that he or she can get back to more familiar aspects of patient care. Unfortunately,

---

‡ If the insurer is a publicly held company, an additional motivation is to ensure an appropriate return on the investment of shareholders. Sometimes this is seen as a conflict of interest, which assumes that shareholder value is tied to denying claims. However, here too the insurer's value to the shareholder depends on the company's reputation, which means that shareholder value is tied not to a specific outcome of the contractual (eg, disability) determination but rather to ensuring that the determination is made promptly and accurately.

§ Depending on the contract, there may be additional promises. The insured individual or company may have purchased additional benefits to provide for vocational rehabilitation or other services to assist in return to work, or the employer may have purchased reporting and assessment to help reduce workplace injuries and facilitate "stay at work" or "return to work" programs. Despite the many possible nuances, the essential nature of the business transaction remains the same: in exchange for a premium the insured purchases a contract that contains a promise and the conditions under which that promise will be fulfilled; the insurer agrees to retain sufficient invested funds in order to pay on any promise made while the contract is in effect, and which meets the contractual terms under which the promise is to be fulfilled.

the patient doesn't receive a careful analysis of functional capacity and a discussion about the importance of staying at or returning to work, and the insurer doesn't receive information vital to making the best possible determination about the patient's claim.

Terminology

In addition to the complex interactions of the factors associated with determinations for disability benefits, specific terminology comes into play. At times, that terminology differs from standard medical nomenclature, and it often differs from colloquial usage. When the physician fails to understand the specific language used by the insurer, misunderstanding is common.

The physician will often be asked to complete an Attending Physician Statement (APS, see Figure 8-1) that requests information regarding the diagnosis, treatment, and functional capacity of the patient who has filed a claim for disability. In the service of having a shared language, the most commonly employed terms are defined below from the insurer's point of view and contrasted where appropriate with common medical usage.

Impairment: As a medical term, *impairment* is a loss or decline of functional capacity as a result of a medical condition or symptom. Insurers will not typically use the term because it is not specific to contractual definitions required for a disability determination. However, it may be used at times by claims specialists and, when referenced, the term *impairment* will often be used interchangeably with the more precisely defined *limitation.*

Limitation: A *limitation* is something that an individual *cannot perform* due to a medical condition. An individual who is paraplegic is limited from walking (ie, *cannot* walk). An individual who is actively having a seizure is limited from climbing (*cannot* climb) a ladder. A limitation is not a matter of motivation but is instead an impossibility. By definition, limitations are most often objectively measurable, and tests can be devised to objectively assess the limits of physical and mental capacities.

Restriction: The complement to a functional *limitation* is a *restriction* that results from a medical impairment. While the *limitation* is something the patient *cannot* do, the *restriction* is what the patient *should not* do because there is a substantial and immediate risk of demonstrable harm to him- or herself or to others. For example, whereas a person *cannot* climb a ladder during a seizure, once the seizure is over he or she is capable of doing so. However, it poses a known risk, and therefore the individual may be restricted from doing so because he or she *should not* because of the risk of injury. Because they involve an assessment of future risk, restrictions are less objectively measurable than limitations, and the degree of objectivity

Figure 8-1 Sample Attending Physician's Statement

Patient Name	Date of Birth	Social Security Number

Primary Diagnosis	Secondary Diagnosis
Objective Findings:	
Symptoms:	
Diagnostic testing	
Current treatment including medication and dosage	
Other providers	

Limitations (*what the patient cannot do*):	
Restrictions (*what the patient should not do*):	
Date restrictions and limitations began	Date you expect restrictions and limitations to end

Name	Degree	Medical Specialty
Address		Phone
Signature		Date

depends on the extent to which the risk is known from research or past experience. For example, there is a known risk for working at heights in a seizure disorder that is not yet controlled, but there is little evidence that, absent other risk factors, work-related stress increases the risk of a second heart attack once the first has been appropriately treated. "Not working at heights" is reasonably objective, whereas "avoiding stressful situations" is not.

Main Duty: A vocational rather than a medical concept, a *main duty*, some-times referred to as a *material and substantial duty*, is typically an activity that is both essential to the performance of a particular occupation and that is performed on a regular basis. Most often, *main duties* are defined specifi-cally in disability contracts, but in general terms these are the activities that define the occupation. For example, a physician might occasionally lift a 50-pound package of medical supplies; however, this would not be consid-ered a main duty because it is neither essential to being a physician nor is it an everyday occurrence in most medical practices. On the other hand the ability to think critically, solve problems, and perform patient care are main duties for a physician, because they are essential, if not definitional, activi-ties. Similarly, driving would be a main duty for a tractor-trailer operator, but not for an office worker.

Making the Disability Determination

As previously noted, a disability determination differs from an impairment evaluation in that the latter is a medical procedure whereas the former is a medicolegal process. In making a disability determination, the insurer is bound by a contract that has multiple complex provisions. Depending on whether the purchaser is an individual or an employer, different gov-ernmental regulations, taxability requirements, and litigation rules may apply. The insurer must determine whether the claimant is eligible for benefits (eg, the employee was employed at the time of disability claim, the employer had paid benefits for that particular employee); whether the standard of proof for the claim has been met; and the terms under which payment is to continue.[§§]

The Claims Specialist and Supporting Professionals
Typically, the ultimate responsibility for a disability determination falls to a *claims specialist.* Most often this is an insurance professional who is not medically trained but is instead trained in the process of interpreting and applying contractual language in the context of medical and vocational information. Sometimes, the claims specialist does have medical and/or vocational training, but even then the level of training will be less than that of the treating physician.

When a claims specialist receives a disability claim, the claim will have three main components. There will be a *Claimant's Statement*, in which

---

[§§] See preceding note.

the person filing the claim will state the condition he or she believes causes disability and will describe the activities he or she believes he or she cannot perform as the result of that condition. The claim will also contain an *Employer Statement* and/or a job description that outlines the occupational requirements of the position from which the claimant believes he or she is disabled. Finally, the claim will contain an *Attending Physician's Statement*, in which at least one treating physician will be asked to describe (at a minimum) the claimant's diagnosis and any associated functional limitations or medically necessary restrictions.

The first step for the claims specialist will be to verify certain contractual criteria, such as eligibility and coverage at the time of the claim. If the contract contains provisions regarding pre-existing conditions and the claim is filed shortly after the claimant became covered, the claims specialist will evaluate if that provision applies. The claims specialist must also determine which specific definition of disability applies in the applicable contract purchased; eg, it may be an "own occupation" definition in which the claimant must be unable to perform the main duties of his or her own occupation, or it may be an "any occupation" definition in which the claimant must be unable to perform the main duties of any occupation for which he or she is reasonably suited. Once these and any other applicable contractual factors are resolved, the benefits specialist must evaluate whether the claimant meets the definition of disability as it appears in the contract.

Because the claims determination is often complex, the claims specialist will be supported within the insurance company by a variety of technical professionals whose task is to help him or her interpret the medical, vocational, and legal nuances of each individual claim. Medical information is typically reviewed by nurses and/or physicians employed by, or consultant to, the insurer; their task is to translate the complex medical data contained in the available medical records and render it in a report that is a fair and unbiased interpretation of the available office notes, laboratory and imaging studies, and other clinical data. Increasingly, the reviewing medical professional will call or write the claimant's attending physician, if the reviewing medical professional has a question about, or disagrees with, the attending physician's opinion regarding the degree of impairment.

Paralleling the medical review of the claim file, a vocational expert may be asked to verify the main duties of the claimant's occupation, to ensure that the claims specialist has a complete understanding of the capacities that are required for the claimant to perform his or her occupation. Alternatively, if the claimant has an "any occupation" definition of disability, the vocational expert will help determine if there are occupations that the claimant would be qualified to undertake, based on an analysis of transferable skills.

Table 8-1 The Idealized Disability Determination Process

	Activities	Restrictions & Limitations	Occupational Duties
Claimed	Claimant statement, interview	Attending Physician Statement	Employer Statement, Job Description
Validated (with examples of tools for validation)	Activity logs, field visits, surveillance, interviews	Medical Records Review, AP contact, IME, FCE	Occupational analysis, Occupational databases

The Process of Claims Determination

Table 8-1 represents graphically the way in which a disability claim is validated and is an idealized version of the logic behind a disability determination for compensation.[11] As noted above, the claim consists of three parts in which the disability is asserted: the claimant's statement regarding daily activities (what the claimant states he or she can and cannot do), the employer's statement regarding the demands of the occupation (what the claimant must be able to do in order to perform his occupation), and the attending physician's statement rendering an opinion regarding functional impairment (assessed functional limitations and medically necessary restrictions). The disability insurer's task is to validate each of these aspects of the claim, and he or she does so utilizing a number of resources and tools including: interviews, activity logs, database searches, and possibly surveillance to validate claimed activity levels; vocational expertise to validate occupational demands; and medical expertise to interpret and validate the limitations and/or restrictions asserted by the attending physician. Having validated each area, the claims specialist's task is to determine, within the boundaries of the contract, whether the available information provides support for the assertion that the claimant is medically unable to perform the main duties of his or her occupation. When the answer is "yes," then the claim is valid. When the answer is "no," then the claim is not valid according to the terms of the contract. When the answer is uncertain, then additional investigation is undertaken.

Beyond the Claim Determination: Returning Patients to Work

Based on the analysis outlined above, the claim determination may be that the claim is denied pending appeal or other reconsideration of the decision. If the claim determination is that the claimant meets the definition of disability and will be paid benefits, unless the claimant is unfortunate enough to be permanently and totally disabled as a result of a catastrophic condition, the process for the claimant is far from over. Now the focus must turn to improving the claimant's level of functioning so that he or she can regain capacity and, it is hoped, return to work.

As noted in the discussion at the beginning of this chapter, most of what determines whether an individual receives disability benefits is psychosocial and revolves around the attitudes of the key players. Does the claimant believe he or she can successfully return to the workforce, and are the rewards enough to risk the loss of the partial but certain income afforded by disability payments? Does the employer have in place a program that will allow accommodations and support graduated return to work, understanding that the cost-benefit balance will ultimately be to the company's advantage? Does the insurer understand that investing in vocational rehabilitation will, in the right claims, have a high return on investment? And finally, does the physician sufficiently understand the importance of work as a part of health outcomes to play the appropriate role with the patient, the employer, and the insurer? It is to the role of the physician in relation to the insurer that we now turn in order to understand what is expected of the physician and how the physician can maximize the outcome for everyone concerned.

The Role of the Physician in Relation to Impairment Evaluation

Physicians may take three different roles in relation to disability insurance. Most often, the physician is involved as a treating provider who has been asked by the patient to complete the paperwork necessary to support an application for disability. A physician may also be employed by the insurer to help the claims specialist interpret and understand the medical information in the file and to help provide guidance. Finally, a physician may be involved with the disability insurer as the provider of an independent opinion regarding the degree of the claimant's impairment, either through an Independent Medical Records Review (IMRR) or an Independent Medical Examination (IME).

Often these roles are seen as antithetical. Typically, the attending physician is seen as the "patient advocate," by which is usually meant that he or she tries to help the claimant obtain disability benefits. The physician employed by the insurer is often seen as the "company doctor" and is often thought to be employed for the purpose of helping to deny disability benefits. Because these roles are often viewed as adversarial, the third-party physician who provides an IMRR or IME is seen as independent of influence from either the attending physician or the insurer and, therefore, the most impartial.

However, the author of this chapter believes that, if all involved physicians understood the role of medicine in determining disability, all would take the same approach to the individual filing a claim for disability. If the attending physician were truly an advocate for the patient's interests, he or she would work toward the goal with the greatest health outcome. That has been demonstrated repeatedly to be staying at work, with accommodations if necessary, for as long as possible; to be out of work only when necessary and only for as long as necessary; and to return to work as soon as medical restrictions can be accommodated or no longer apply. It has already been said that this is also the best outcome for the insurer and the employer as well. In other words, the interests of the attending physician, the insurance physician, and the independent examiner coincide.

How do physicians help to achieve this common goal? Regardless of the specific role, the physician's task in evaluating work disability is to consider all the available medical information, both subjective (symptoms) and objective (signs), both supporting impairment and not supporting impairment, and to arrive at a conclusion regarding the nature and degree of an individual's impairment, if any. This means understanding the activities involved in the occupation and determining, based on medical evidence, whether performing those activities will result in substantial harm and/ or whether the individual is unable to perform those activities based on a medical condition. In evaluating these questions, the physician will take into account any reported symptoms but will separate the symptoms from the underlying medical findings.

This is another way of stating the Risk-Capacity-Tolerance model for evaluating work restrictions. In this model, medical evidence supporting the contention that performing a work-related activity is likely to result in physical or psychological harm to the individual leads to a *restriction*, something the individual *should not* perform. If the individual is *unable* to perform an activity, this is recorded as a *limitation*. Discomfort that does not coincide with the medical need for a work restriction, or that causes an individual to stop performing an action before having reached his physical limit, is *tolerance* and should be considered as a potential barrier to remaining at or returning to work; however tolerance in itself does not constitute the basis of a workplace disability.

Of critical importance is the fact that, if all physicians involved in the disability determination apply the principles of the Risk-Capacity-Tolerance model, the process becomes not only less contentious but also maximizes the outcomes for everyone involved. To be sure, this practice creates additional responsibilities for all physicians involved in the disability determination. For the attending physician, this level of objectivity regarding a patient's application for disability requires the willingness to learn how to evaluate and estimate functional capacity, or it requires the willingness to defer such evaluation to another physician who is trained to do so. It also means explaining to the patient why work is good for his or her health, and sometimes it means risking the patient's displeasure at being told "no." Though time consuming, this should not differ from some of the tough conversations required of the physician-patient relationship with respect to health behaviors such as smoking, substance abuse, overeating, or lack of exercise. In fact, for the attending physician this is the key point: work must be on a par with more obvious health-related behaviors.

For the physician engaged by the insurer, either as an employee or as an independent examiner, the model requires that all medical information be considered objectively, including the attending physician's opinion and the symptoms reported by the patient. In making a disability determination, one does not automatically take another physician's word for something any more than would be the case in a second medical opinion. At the same time, another physician's opinion is not simply discounted or ignored. Each of these physicians has an advantage: the attending physician has the advantage of seeing and examining the patient, whereas the insurance physician has the advantage of having access to, and the time to read, all the medical records from all the providers.

Also, a physician can neither ignore patient tolerance in determining what he or she should and should not do nor simply assume that avoiding work activities because of discomfort is a good choice. Instead the physician must understand that tolerance will pose a barrier to returning the individual to work. Tolerance for activity must be addressed as a part of the medical analysis, by evaluating the consistency of symptoms with the underlying pathology and with what would be expected in the condition.

The Attending Physician's Role with the Disability Insurer

This chapter concludes with some suggestions for the attending physician as he or she communicates with the insurer. Below are some basic rules for being involved in the disability determination process and for smoothing communication with the disability insurer.

1. *Decide if the physician's involvement in the disability claim is in the patient's best interest.* This often-overlooked question is important because the treating physician must understand that involvement in the disability determination will affect his or her relationship with the patient. This effect will occur whether the disability application is supported or not. Supporting the patient's claim will have health consequences, and in order to mitigate those consequences it will be important

to be involved in the efforts to return the patient to work. The claim requires communicating with the insurer by providing forms and medical records and perhaps by speaking with employed or examining physicians. It will take time. The attending physician should also ask if he or she has the skills needed to conduct a fair and competent evaluation of impairment. If not, consider referring the patient to another evaluator for a second opinion.

The employed or evaluating physician must also determine if there is any reason that a specific conflict of interest will cloud the ability to render a fair, thorough, and objective analysis of the available medical information. For example, he may know the treating physician personally or by reputation, and that can cloud judgment. Physicians engaged by the insurer must also be able to adequately set aside any financial conflict of interest; the insurer must be, and virtually always is, paying for an objective determination, not for a particular opinion.

2. *Support conclusions with medical evidence and apply evidence-based practice wherever possible.* The attending physician who supports a claim for disability benefits will be expected to provide medical records. The more those records reflect a clinical examination that supports an opinion regarding impairment, the more likely the insurer will be to understand and accept the claimed functional limitations and work restrictions. The more the treatment plan is evidence-based and includes a focus on return to the highest possible level of functioning, the more likely it will make sense to the insurer and the more it will be in the patient's best interests. For the physicians evaluating the attending physician's information, it is likewise important to be aware of the evidence base for work-related absence and for the most appropriate treatment for the condition claimed as the basis of the disability. It isn't a question of evaluating the attending physician's competence but one of objectively assessing whether the information provided about restrictions and limitations is consistent with what would be expected given the medical information provided and of ensuring that the most appropriate outcome occurs for everyone involved.

3. *Communicate clearly and precisely*

   a. Learn the terminology: It is important to understand what the insurer means by terms such as *restriction* and *limitation*, and it is important to understand the physical demand levels from the Dictionary of Occupational Titles (DOT)[12] (see Table 8-2) because they are often used in disability forms. In the case of the Social Security Administration (a governmental body, but also the largest disability insurer in the world, by far), severity specifiers such as *mild*, *moderate*, and *severe*, and terms such as *persistence* and *pace* have specific meanings. If the form asks for specific functional capacities for sitting, standing, and walking during an 8-hour work day, the form should specify whether these are cumulative or separate.[#] If the form does not contain definitions, clarifying any uncertainties before completing the form will save time in the long run and will avoid misunderstanding that can negatively impact the claim determination.

b. Use precise language: In giving a restriction, it is better to say that the claimant "should not lift more than 20 pounds occasionally, or 10 pounds frequently" than it is to say "no heavy lifting" or "no lifting." The former is less likely to be misunderstood and is also much more easily compared to occupational demands. In addition, it is important to be clear that "frequent" and "occasional" are used in the context of the DOT as specified in Table 8-2, or to specify otherwise. Psychological or cognitive functions can be more difficult to specify, but here too it is better to say "unable to concentrate on complex problem solving for more than 20 minutes at a time" than it is to say "cannot concentrate." If it is not possible to specify functioning at this level, consider what other sources of information are needed in order to make a more accurate determination rather than guessing or making a broad statement that is more likely to be misinterpreted.[##] It may be that a second opinion, an FCE, or an IME should be recommended, or further testing may be indicated.

c. Stay within medical scope: Turning back to Table 8-1, the medical role is to determine functional limitations and/or medically reasonable restrictions and not to make occupational or contractual determinations. Physicians are concerned with the degree of medical impairment, not with the contractual determination regarding whether the individual is "disabled." Similarly, physicians are not typically trained in making occupational determinations. It is better to state

---

[#] The distinction can make a difference to the claim determination in unexpected ways. For example, if the physician indicates that the patient can sit for 4 hours, stand for 2 hours, and walk for 2 hours, he might think that this means that the patient can work 4 hours in a day if sitting, or 2 hours in a day if standing or walking; in other words, at most half-time. However, if the insurer treats this cumulatively then it will be taken to mean that the claimant has physical capacity for full-time work in which he can sit no more than 4 hours, and stand or walk no more than 2 hours each.

[##] This applies also to examining and insurance physicians. One of the keys to knowing that more information is needed, such as an IME or FCE, is that the available medical data do not allow a level of specificity from which an occupational determination can be made.

Table 8-2 Work Activity Descriptors

Work Pattern	Occasional (0%–33% of the work day)	Frequent (34%–66% of the work day)	Constant (67%–100% of the work day)
Sedentary	10 lbs; standing or walking	Sitting	
Light	20 lbs	10 lbs and/or walk/stand, push/pull, or use arm/leg controls	Push/pull or use arm/leg controls while seated
Medium	50 lbs	20 lbs	10 lbs
Heavy	100 lbs	50 lbs	20 lbs
Very Heavy	Over 100 lbs	Over 50 lbs	Over 20 lbs

a reasonable restriction and leave the determination as to whether it prevents the performance of a main duty to the appropriate resource. Along this same line, it is worth noting that the statement "no work" is both too vague to be useful and is an occupational, rather than a medical, statement. This statement is often given by attending physicians when completing a disability form, but it does not help the patient obtain disability benefits and will contribute to delays in claim processing.

d. Let the facts speak for themselves: Adjectives and adverbs rarely add much to medical determinations. One is not "more" or "less" pregnant, and in the same way one is not "profoundly" or "mildly" disabled; either the circumstances meet the contractual definition of disability or they do not. Similarly, pejoratives and confrontational statements will not help a patient obtain disability benefits and will almost never change the opinion of another physician. Almost always, a rational and evidence-based communication will carry more weight than one that is intended to arouse an emotional response.

4. *Focus on return to work as early as medically reasonable.* Throughout this chapter the focus has been on the fact that a return to work is the most advantageous outcome for patients, attending physicians, employers, and insurers. Disability insurance is not an entitlement but is instead a means of providing support in the unfortunate circumstance that an insured person is unable to perform the duties of his or her occupation. If the person is able to work, for many of the multiple reasons discussed in this chapter, every accommodation should be tried.

If a temporary accommodation is required for this to happen, it is in everyone's best interest to do so. Ultimately, if the individual must be away from work due to an illness or injury, the only true positive outcome is returning to work either in the individual's own, or another, occupation.

The author once learned a question from a former supervisor, and that question has been effective in practice, in independent evaluations conducted for insurers, and as an insurance employee: "If this person wanted to work, would you let them?" If the honest answer to this question is "yes," then any assigned limitations are not severe enough to preclude work and any assigned restrictions are not medically necessary. Put in the context of the Risk-Capacity-Tolerance model, if the physician would allow the patient to work if he or she were motivated to do so, then the claim is based on tolerance rather than risk or capacity.

Only if the answer is "no" can it be said with reasonable medical certainty that the individual is unable to, or should not, return to work due to impairment; and only if the answer is "no" should the physician sign a form in support of disability. Unless the answer to this question is unequivocally "no," the course of action that has the best health, financial, and social outcome is to work with the individual to remove any perceived barriers to return to work and to support them in doing so. This last is equally true for the treating physician, employers, insurers, and independent examiners, and most importantly, it is the right course of action on behalf of the patient.

References

1. ADA Amendments Act of 2008; 42 USCA, 12101 note: U.S. Equal Employment Opportunity Commission. Available at http://www.eeoc.gov/policy/adaaa.html.

2. Kertay L, Pendergrass TM. Biopsychosocial factors in claims for disability compensation: issues and recommendations. In: Schultz IZ & Gatchel RJ, eds. *Handbook of complex occupational disability claims: Early risk identification, intervention and prevention.* New York: Kluwer Academic; 2005.

3. Sullivan MJ, Feuerstein M, Gatchel R, Linton SJ, Pransky G. Integrating psychosocial and behavioral interventions to achieve optimal rehabilitation outcomes. *J Occup Rehab.* 2005;15(4):475–489.

4. Krause, N, Frank, JW, Dasinger, LK, Sullivan, TJ, Sinclair, SJ. Determinants of duration of disability and return-to-work after work-related injury and illness: challenges for future research. *Am J Indust Med.* 2001;40:464–484.

5. Cole DC, Mondloch MV, Hogg-Johnson S. Listening to injured workers: how recovery expectations predict outcomes—a prospective study. *Can Med Assoc J.* 2002;166:749–54.

6. Berglind H, Gerner U. Motivation and return to work among the long-term sick-listed: an action theory perspective. *Disab Rehab*. 2005;24:719–726.

7. Shaw WS, Yueng-Hsiang, H. Concerns and expectations about returning to work with low back pain: identifying themes from focus groups and semi-structured interviews. *Disab Rehab*. 2005;27:1269–1281.

8. Franche R-L, Krause, N. Readiness for return to work following injury or illness: conceptualizing the interpersonal impact of health care, workplace, and insurance factors. *J Occup Rehab*. 2002;12:233–256.

9. Dasinger LK, Krause N, Thompson PJ, Brand RJ, Rudolph L. Doctor proactive communication, return-to-work recommendation, and duration of disability after a workers' compensation low back injury. *J Occup Env Med*. 2001;43:515–525.

10. Goetzel RZ, Long SR, Ozminkowski RJ, Hawkins K, Wang S, Lynch W. (2004). Health, absence, disability, and presenteeism cost estimates of certain physical and mental health conditions affecting US employers. *J Occup Env Med*. 2004;46:398–412.

11. Mitchell K. The dance of the invisible impairments: chronic pain syndromes & the disability insurer. *Am Soc Chr Pain News*. 2000. (Reprinted in a proprietary document by Unum Group.)

12. Paul Taylor, Vice President MetLife, personal communication.

13. US Department of Labor. *Dictionary of Occupational Titles, Revised 5th Edition*. Washington, DC: US Department of Labor; 2003.

Medications, Driving, and Work

**James B. Talmage, MD, J. Mark Melhorn, MD
and Mark H. Hyman, MD**

Introduction

Health care providers must consider an individual's known medical conditions and medication use. This information is utilized when determining work guidelines and advice about complex psychomotor tasks, like work. Driving is an almost universal task, so there are studies that evaluate driving ability with various diseases or injuries, as well as while taking certain medications.[1–14]

Work is extremely variable and thus, while there are studies on medications and driving, there are few studies exploring medication effects on other work abilities. For guidance in assessing work ability for "safety sensitive" employees, whose work could result in harm to self or others if not done correctly, physicians typically refer to guidelines for driving.

In Western society, automobile use for personal transportation is common, but health care providers need to remember that some workers do not have personal vehicles or driver's licenses. Employers cannot require an employee to be able to drive (for instance, for getting to and from work) unless driving is an essential function of the employee's job. Being able to work involves:

- Being able to *travel* to and from work (not drive),
- Being able to be at work (not in dialysis or chemotherapy sessions),
- Being able to do appropriate assigned tasks and duties.

This book typically analyzes work ability questions using the Risk-Capacity-Tolerance model. In analyzing the effect of medications on work ability, the primary concern is risk. Some medications, like beta blockers for a patient with hypertension, may decrease the individual's maximal exercise capacity (by limiting heart rate increase). Some medications have fatigue as a side affect, which can be an issue of tolerance. This chapter will consider the **risk** posed by medications that might affect a discussion about work between a physician and a patient.

This chapter will focus on medical issues. Legal issues related to driving and work while taking medications are jurisdiction specific and will change over time.[15] A 2009 list indicated that some states (Arizona, Georgia, Indiana, Illinois, Iowa, Michigan, Minnesota, Nevada, North Carolina, Ohio, Pennsylvania, Rhode Island, Utah, Virginia, and Wisconsin) have "per se" laws in which it is illegal to operate a motor vehicle if there is any detectable level of a prohibited drug or its metabolites in the driver's blood (not urine, but blood).[16]

Thus, physicians will need to stay current on the legal issues in their local jurisdiction. It may be wise to document an assessment of apparent driving ability and a warning about driving while impaired in the medical record when potentially problematic medications are prescribed.

US Federal Guidance

The most frequently consulted and cited medical advice about driving, and by analogy about safety-sensitive work in general, is the US Federal Motor Carrier Safety Administration (FMCSA) rules and guidance for health care providers assessing commercial drivers, so we will consider this system in some detail. Commercial drivers, like pilots and nuclear power plant operators, are held to a higher standard than are drivers of personal vehicles, so if a driver could be certified as safe to drive commercial vehicles while taking a particular medication, it is reasonable to conclude that he or she can safely drive a private vehicle, or perform most safety-sensitive, nonfederally regulated work.

The 2006 Large Truck Crash Study Report to Congress[17] evaluated 967 large truck crashes in 17 states over a 3-year period. Twenty-three percent of these crashes resulted in a human fatality, 29% resulted in incapacitating human injury, and all resulted in some degree of human injury. (These were not minor "fender-benders.") The truck driver was felt to be at fault in 87% of these, while the vehicle (10%) and the environment (2%) were much less frequently culpable. Twenty-six percent of these crashes were believed to be at least partially caused by prescription medication use (the number one factor statistically), 17% were attributed to over-the-counter medication use (the number 4 factor), while illegal drug use (2%, factor number 25), and alcohol use (0.8%, factor 26) were infrequent causes.

The *Physician's Desk Reference* lists more than 700 medications with a warning to use with caution when operating a motor vehicle or machinery.[18]

Clearly both illegal drug and alcohol use and prescription medication use can be major factors in serious motor vehicle accidents. The National Highway Transit Safety Administration's Multiple Medications and Vehicle Crashes: Analysis of Databases Final Report (2008) lists 15 medication classes with an odds ratio of >1.5 for impairing the user enough to contribute to motor vehicle accidents in published epidemiologic studies.[19] See Table 9-1.

The FMCSA guidance also illustrates how problematic this whole topic is. The FMCSA lists methadone and insulin as logically disqualifying a commercial driver, although there is a lengthy process diabetics can pursue hoping to be exempted from the insulin restriction. The regulation on medication use states:

49 CFR §391.41 Physical qualifications for drivers.

(b) A person is physically qualified to drive a commercial motor vehicle if that person (b)(12)(i) Does not use a controlled substance identified in 21 CFR 1308.11 *Schedule I*, an amphetamine, a narcotic, or any other habit-forming drug.

(b)(12)(ii) **Exception.** A driver may use such a substance or drug, if the substance or drug is prescribed by a licensed medical practitioner who:

(b)(12)(ii)(A) Is familiar with the driver's medical history and assigned duties; and

(b)(12)(ii)(B) Has advised the driver that the prescribed substance or drug will not adversely affect the driver's ability to safely operate a commercial motor vehicle; and

(b)(13) Has no current clinical diagnosis of alcoholism.[20]

Thus, at the time of a driver's annual or biennial medical re-certification exam, if the health care provider finds the driver is using a potentially impairing medication, he or she is to delay certification until receiving a letter from the prescribing physician. There can be problems with this approach.

Table 9-1 Top 15 Medication Classes with Highest Odds Ratios (p ≤ .05)[2]

Drug Class	Odds Ratio (OR) with 95% C.I.	Possible Effects	Indication for Use
BARBITURATES	7.50 (2.35, 23.91)	Drowsiness	Nervousness, Seizures
ANTIHISTAMINES	3.00 (1.05, 8.55)	Dizziness, bronchospasm. Avoid alcohol and other medicines that affect the CNS	Asthma, Allergies
ANTITUSSIVES, NON-NARCOTIC	2.23 (1.30, 3.82)	Dizziness, drowsiness, depression	Cough
ANALGESICS, NARCOTICS	2.22 (1.98, 2.49)	Dizziness, drowsiness, blurred vision	Pain
ANTIPSYCHOTICS, ATYPICAL, DOPAMINE, & SEROTONIN ANTAG	2.20 (1.37, 3.52)	Drowsiness	Schizophrenia
SKELETAL MUSCLE RELAXANTS	2.09 (1.71, 2.55)	Dizziness, drowsiness, lightheadedness	Muscle Spasms
ANTI-ANXIETY DRUGS	2.00 (1.72, 2.31)	Drowsiness	Anxiety
ANTICONVULSANTS	1.97 (1.64, 2.38)	Drowsiness	Seizures
SEROTONIN-2 ANTAGONIST/REUPTAKE INHIBITORS (SARIS)	1.90 (1.49, 2.44)	Dizziness, drowsiness, headache, confusion	Depression
BELLADONNA ALKALOIDS	1.85 (1.08, 3.19)	Dizziness, drowsiness, confusion	GI symptoms
INSULINS	1.80 (1.45, 2.22)	Hypoglycemia	Diabetes Mellitus
HYPOTENSIVES, SYMPATHOLYTIC	1.79 (1.17, 2.74)	Hypotension, drowsiness, blurred vision	Hypertension
SEROTONIN-NOREPINEPHRINE REUPTAKE INHIB (e.g., VENLAFAXINE)	1.78 (1.19, 2.66)	Dizziness, drowsiness, hypertension, seizures	Depression
PLATELET AGGREGATION INHIBITORS	1.69 (1.17, 2.43)	Headache, weakness, shakes, aches	Stroke prevention
ANTIEMETIC/ ANTIVERTIGO AGENTS	1.63 (1.17, 2.28)	Drowsiness, dizziness	Nausea, vomiting, vertigo

The first problem is the prescriber may not be familiar with the commercial driver's assigned duties. Another problem is that the prescribing physician may not be familiar with the literature on how likely medication-induced psychomotor task impairment is to be present. Further, this impairment may be unrecognized by the patient.

Another set of problems surrounds the question: How does the prescriber know the drug will not adversely effect the driver's ability to safely drive? Instead of asking this question about use of a prescription medication, substitute the words "alcohol at a blood alcohol level of 0.12% (150% of the presumed level of intoxication for driving). This FMCSA guidance becomes:

> A driver may not drive with a blood alcohol level of 0.12% unless he or she has a letter from his or her physician stating the physician has advised the driver this will not adversely affect the driver's ability.

While some individuals recognize when they are impaired by alcohol and arrange for a designated driver (or taxi), many individuals do not recognize their own impairment, and thus drive drunk. Alcohol impairs judgment, and folks with impaired judgment do not consistently recognize their own impairment. The 2008 National Survey of Drug Use and Health (NSDUH) found that 10 million people (4% of the population) aged 12 or older reported driving in the prior year while under the influence of illicit drugs, and 31 million (12% of the population) reported driving while under the influence of alcohol.[21] If individuals consistently recognized their own medication or alcohol induced impairment, 31 million Americans would not have driven under the influence of alcohol in 2008. While driving impaired on alcohol or medication raises the risk of a motor vehicle accident, only some of those who drive while impaired have crashes.

Asking a prescription medication user to self-report impairment in driving skills is a flawed process. In addition, the prescribing health care provider frequently records in medical records what medications are being taken, occasionally records a mental status exam, but rarely records when (how many hours ago) the last dose of potentially impairing medication was taken prior to that day's examination. Thus, even if a prescriber reviews his or her records, these records do not indicate whether the patient was seen when blood levels of the potentially impairing medication were at peak, mid, or trough level. Trough level may be the time when withdrawal symptoms are present. Medical records rarely document how the patient appears if a habituating medication dose is inadvertently missed.

Thus, a health care provider can ask a patient if he or she has already had an accident or a "near miss" incident while driving on a medication or with a blood alcohol level of 0.12% and can also ask how comfortable a patient is while driving on a medication or with a blood alcohol level of 0.12%, but unless the health care provider, or a professional driving instructor/evaluator, actually rides with the individual both at peak and at trough blood levels, there is no clear way for a health care provider to know an individual's driving ability while on potentially impairing medication.

The final set of problems is medicolegal. The FMCSA seems to be saying to the examiner for a commercial driver who is using a potentially impairing medication, "Please request the prescriber of this medication to send you one of two possible letters."

- Choice #1 Letter: I am prescribing drug "A" for this individual. I know about the individual's driving duties. I have advised the individual that this drug will not affect his or her driving ability.

- Choice #2 Letter: I have been prescribing drug "A" for this individual. I didn't know that this individual was a commercial driver. He or she is impaired by this drug and should not be driving, but I negligently forgot to advise him or her of this. Please do not certify this individual as a commercial driver.

In a litigious society, every health care provider will feel compelled to send Letter #1 regardless of the medical facts, so this FMCSA requirement would appear to do nothing to bring science and logic to driving decisions.

Other Real-World Problems

A major shortcoming in the literature on medications and driving is that while there are some studies on how impairing specific medications are when used alone, there are few studies on multiple medication being used simultaneously (opioids and anxiolytics, or opioids and "muscle relaxants," for example). Some chronic pain patients daily use opioids, "muscle relaxants," anticonvulsants, antidepressants, and anxiolytics or sedative hypnotics. How such multiple medications use affects injury risk while driving is not well researched, and there are almost no studies on other safety-sensitive jobs.

Thus, there is no clearly scientific way either a prescribing physician or an evaluating physician can certify an employee or a driver as "safe" to work (risk assessment) while using a potentially impairing medication. If employers have a company policy that specifies for safety-sensitive positions what medications may not be used, health care providers should obtain and use the employer's policy. As more jurisdictions adopt "Drug Free Workplace" statutes, more employers have, or will have, such policies. Physicians should be aware of the current literature on medications and task impairment, which currently relates almost exclusively to driving.

As an interesting aside, while there is literature and discussion about potentially impairing medication use by drivers, pilots, sea captains, train engineers, nuclear power plant operators, etc, there seems to be little or no literature or discussion about use of these medications by "safety sensitive" health care providers (eg, surgeons) or law enforcement officers (who must responsibly handle weapons and motor vehicles during high-speed chases).

Specific Medications

In the National Highway Transit Safety Administration's Multiple Medications and Vehicle Crashes: Analysis of Databases Final Report (2008) is a table (Table 9-1) showing the calculated **odds ratio** for classes of medications causing motor vehicle crashes, derived from published epidemiologic literature that recorded medications found in drivers involved in crashes (numerator) and the percentage of drivers who are using a medication (denominator, based on the frequency these medications are prescribed to the population).

The FMCSA has had input from its Medical Expert Panels and its Medical Review Board. Based on this input as well as its own research, current guidance for health care providers in the FMCSA Examiner's Handbook[22] is that commercial drivers:

- May use a hypnotic with a half-life of less than 5 hours for no more than 2 weeks.

- Should not use a sedating anxiolytic (all anxiolytics except buspirone).

- Should not use a narcotic antitussive within 12 hours of commercial driving (with obvious implications for use of long-acting sustained release opioids or short-acting opioids for pain control).

- Should not use a "first generation" antidepressant (tricyclic).

- Should not use an antihistamine within 12 hours of commercial driving.

Summary

Thus, a physician can advise an employee and an employer (with patient consent) about medication use, the limitations of scientific literature, and the level of risk of motor vehicle accident while driving and taking a medication. Whether an employee is willing to do a specific job while taking one or more potentially impairing medications and whether an employer's policies permit the employee to do a specific job while taking one or more potentially impairing medications are questions a physician cannot answer.

Jurisdiction-specific laws about driving while using medications need also to be considered.

References

1. Carr DB, Ott BR. The older adult driver with cognitive impairment. *JAMA.* 2010;303(16):1632–1641.

2. Blair S, Chaudhri O, Gregori A. Doctor, can I drive with this plaster? An evidence based response. *Injury.* 2002;33(1):55–56.

3. Iverson DJ, Gronseth GS, Reger MA, et al. Practice Parameter update: Evaluation and management of driving risk in dementia. Report of the Quality Standards Subcommittee of the American Academy of Neurology. *Neurol.* 2010; 74:1316–1324.

4. Egol Ka, Sheikhzadeh A, Moghtaderi S, et al. Lower-extremity function for driving an automobile after operative treatment of ankle fracture. *JBJS-Am.* 2004;85:1185–1189.

5. Holt G, Kay M, McGrory R, et al. Emergency brake response time after first metatarsal osteotomy. *JBJS-Am.* 2008;90:1660–1664.

6. Chen V, Chacko AT, Costello FV, et al. Driving after musculoskeletal injury. addressing patient and surgeon concerns in an urban orthopaedic practice. *JBJS-Am.* 2008;90:2791–2797.

7. Tremblay M, Corriveau H, Boissy P, et al. Effects of orthopaedic immobilization of the right lower limb on driving performance: an experimental study during simulated driving by healthy volunteers. *JBJS-Am.* 2009;91:2860–2866

8. Chong PY, Koehler EAS, Shyr Y, et al. Driving with an arm immobilized in a splint: a randomized higher-order crossover trial. *JBJS-Am.* 2010;92: 2263–2269

9. Liebensteiner MC, Birkfellner F, Thaler M, et al. Driving reaction time before and after primary fusion of the lumbar spine. *Spine.* 2010;35(3):330–335.

10. Hartenbaum N, Collop N, Rosen I, et al. Editorial: truckers with osa, should they be driving? *JOEM.* 2006; 48(9):871–872.

11. Tregear S, Reston J, Schoelles K, et al. Obstructive sleep apnea and risk of motor vehicle crash: systematic review and meta-analysis. *J of Clin Sleep Med.* 2009;5(6):573–581.

12. Orth M, Diekmann C, Suchan B, et al. Driving performance in patients with chronic obstructive pulmonary disease. *J Physiol and Pharmacol.* 2008; 59-Suppl 6:539–547.

13. Alcohol and other drug use among victims of motor-vehicle crashes–West Virginia, 2004–2005. *MMWR.* 2006;55(48):1293–1296.

14. Dubois S, Bëdard M, Weaver B. The impact of benzodiazepines of safe driving. *Traffic Inj Prev.* 2008;9:404–4134.

15. Annas GJ. Doctors, drugs, and driving-tort liability for patient-caused accidents. *NEJM.* 2008;359(5):521–525.

16. Drugged Driving. National Institute on Drug Abuse Info Facts, November 2009:1–5. http://www.nida.nih.gov/PDF/Infofacts/driving09.pdf. Accessed 10/22/2010.

17. http://www.fmcsa.dot.gov/facts-research/research-technology/report/ltccs-2006. pdf. Accessed 10/22/2010.

18. Hartenbaum NP. Chapter 11, Substance abuse and medication use. In: Hartenbaum NP. *The DOT Medical Examination*, Fifth Edition. Beverly Farms, MA: OEM Press; 2010.

19. http://www.nhtsa.gov/DOT/NHTSA/Traffic%20Injury%20Control/Articles/ Associated%20Files/810858.pdf. Accessed 10/22/2010.

20. http://www.fmcsa.dot.gov/rules-regulations/administration/fmcsr/fmcsrruletext. aspx?rule_toc=760&section=391.41&section_toc=1781. Accessed 10/22/2010.

21. Substance Abuse and Mental Health Services Administration. 2008 National Survey on Drug Use and Health. Rockville, MD: Office of Applied Studies, 2009.

22. http://nrcme.fmcsa.dot.gov/mehandbook/MEhandbook.htm. Accessed 10/22/2010.

Chapter 9

Chapter 10

The Challenges to and Importance of the Primary Care Physician's Role in Return to Work

Douglas Martin, MD

The primary care physician's role in the return-to-work decision-making process has been characterized by authors who have written about the different benefit systems with a wide-ranging and conflicting set of descriptors: important, elementary, critical, mesmerizing, trivial, fundamental, demeaning, curious, and my favorite, contumelious. However you may define this role, one thing is known: it must be done appropriately in order to obtain the best outcome for the patient.

The Lack of Educational Background in Return-to-Work Decision Making for Primary Care Providers

Oversight and accreditation for medical school curricula and medical residency training is governed quite tightly.[1] Basic sciences and the fundamentals that compose each specialty's core essentials are the focus of study. There is a surprising lack of attention paid to the approach toward the injured worker and the importance of the return-to-work decision-making process. The public and our patients, on the other hand, have a belief and expectation that because we provide work-related injury and illness care, we have the expertise and core knowledge of the appropriate data and evidence to make these determinations with the same skill we use in the treatment of the injury or illness. Unfortunately, this is simply not the case. It is frequently stated by primary care physician educators that this presents a dilemma that is too simple to emphasize, yet too difficult to address.

A substantial amount of work injury and illness care is provided by primary care physicians. It is true that there are geographical differences across the country. In some Midwestern states, the frequency of workers' compensation patients who see primary care providers as opposed to occupational medicine physicians or other specialty physicians can approach 70%. It would seem intuitive that the primary care disciplines should then have a wealth of experience and expertise in dealing with return-to-work matters. Contrarily, in a survey of family physicians in Iowa, less than 20% felt that they had sufficient training and education to feel as though they were doing a "good job."[2]

Why is this so? An answer to this question may simply lie in the amount of time spent on the issue in the formalized residency training processes. The family medicine residency requirements, for example, mandate only one month within a three-year residency devoted to community medicine. Of that one-month block, only a fraction is typically devoted to the concepts of occupational medicine and its provision.[3]

The problem goes much deeper. Most primary care physicians are trained very well in the ethics and sanctity of the physician-patient relationship paradigm. Frequently, physicians in primary care disciplines are lauded for their ability to approach the patient as a whole; taking the biopsychosocial model of medical care to the ultimate level. This works well for most clinical encounters, but in actuality may be a stumbling block because the primary care physician may not take into consideration the effect of the psychosocial aspects of the other players in the system. The focus is frequently solely on the effects on the patient at the time of the clinical encounter and not upon the long-term negative effects that can occur when proper attention is not paid to the return-to-work decision-making process. The ultimate victim of this misguided focus within the workers' compensation system is the patient.

The Problem with Patient Advocacy and the Primary Care "Loyalties Bind"

One of the main problems that has occurred and has created poor outcomes in workers' compensation care delivered by primary care physicians is that the concept of patient advocacy has been altered, if not usurped, in the last few decades. For years, paternalism was a professional point of pride for physicians who felt an obligation to care for their patients with a staunch sense of parental discipline receiving a healthy dose of respect in return.[4] It used to be an accepted fact that the concept of paternalism was a good thing. In the past, when the physician said, "Jump," the response from the patient was, "How high?" When the doctor stated, "You must do this," the patient asked, "How frequently and for how long?" Now, when the provider says, "Do this," the common response from the patient is "Why should I?"

I am not suggesting that this is altogether a bad thing, but it does illustrate a significant issue and barrier to primary care physician expertise in the arena of return-to-work management. With the explosion of medical information now available on the Internet and other sources, patients are more likely to read information about their diagnosis and treatment. Some walk into a doctor's office with pages of information copied from a Web site in preparation for discussions with the doctor about their medical condition. Coupled with the information explosion is the fact that there has been a change in education of physicians that occurred in the 1980s. The idea of making the patient's beliefs a part of the medical decision-making process was added to a physician's training. Now it is recognized that compliance with medical treatments can be improved by allowing the patient to be part of the decision-making process and also by considering his or her individual life experiences in this process.[5] Autonomy has replaced paternalism.

Therefore, the return-to-work decision-making process is more complex than it was in the past. When thinking about this, please put yourself in the shoes of the injured worker. Ask yourself whether you would decide to stay home or go to work when there is a reasonable benefit system in place to cover your lost income. I believe the answer is obvious in most situations. When the patient is asked to become involved in the treatment process in this manner, the physician is presented with a dichotomy: should the patient be involved in his or her treatment plan and risk that he or she may choose a path that is not in his or her best interest medically, or do I disregard this partnership and merely become a dictator?

It has been stated that this dilemma is really an example of a change in the view of patient advocacy. There has been much discussion concerning the true definition of this term, but all would agree that patient advocacy is a good thing.[6] The problem appears to be rooted in the fact that the concept of patient advocacy is not bad but that the definition of the term has changed. *Patient advocacy* is no longer defined by the physician doing what is in the best interest of the patient (beneficence) but is now defined by the physician doing what the patient wants (autonomy).

Often the patient says that he or she want time off from work. If the physician is not in agreement with the patient's viewpoint, he or she is subject to patient scrutiny and frequently is accused of not being a patient advocate!

The workers' compensation system does not help the doctor in this area. Employers frequently want to know what an injured employee can and cannot do. Frequently, physicians are asked to fill out ambiguous forms with check boxes, lists, etc, of a variety of potential activities. Some primary care physicians would rather mark the "no work" box rather than sit down and think about the individual, the injury, and how it may affect the ability to do a certain job task. It is inherently more difficult to fill out a long series of boxes or list specific activities that a patient can perform.

Another significant issue for the primary care provider is the factors of time and money. Primary care providers are expected to see and treat a wide variety of patients, and are often compensated largely based upon volume. There is a disincentive for the primary care provider to take time to fill out these forms and deal effectively with the return-to-work decision-making process with a true advocacy viewpoint because they are not paid to do so. Why spend an extra 5 to 10 minutes with the patient to explain the benefits of return to work when it does not alter the CPT code that is billed for the encounter? Why spend an extra 5 to 10 minutes filling out the return-to-work form in detail when it takes 5 seconds to mark the "no work" box and the CPT code does not change?

Whether by tradition or reluctance by other interested parties to take the reins, the physician has been put in a precarious loyalties feud within the workers' compensation system. Insurers and employers expect doctors to provide unbiased information concerning an employee's medical condition and ability to work. This data is then used as a tool to validate claims, impose reprimands regarding work attendance, and determine the distribution of awards or benefits. The medical profession does not acknowledge nor willingly accept being assigned this third-party role as corroborator of fact, especially when the doctor's decision may have negative financial implications for the patient.[7] All physicians take to heart that this patient is the individual that, by oath, is to be advocated for and whose interests should be placed above anyone else.

A Return to Basic Scientific Principles Is Needed

Primary care physicians need to think about the return-to-work decision-making process in terms of some very basic scientific principles. Let's flash back to undergraduate training. Simple laws of physics, albeit meta-phorically, can be extremely beneficial as a mechanism of analysis for any patient.

Newton's First Law of Motion:
Things in motion stay in motion, things at rest stay at rest,
unless acted upon by an outside force.[8]

Return-to-Work Decision-Making Corollary:
Patients who are in motion continue to improve,
but those at rest without active involvement remain stagnant. Patients
who are taken off work, remain off work. Patients who continue to work,
continue to be productive.

This "law" illustrates the importance of active involvement in the man-agement of return to work by the primary care provider. When work itself is an important part of the therapeutic intervention, the patient has a ten-dency to continue to improve. A patient who is out of work because the primary care provider is unwilling to include return to work as a treatment recommendation will experience prolonged disability unless significant resources (forces) are used to move the case forward. Additionally, a company that does not have a transitional duty program and is resistant to having the employee return to work until he or she is 100% improved promotes case stagnation.

Second Law of Thermodynamics:
In the universe, there is a tendency for matter to assume its most
disorganized state whenever possible. Energy is required to maintain
order in the universe.[9]

Return-to-Work Decision-Making Corollary (Law of Return-to-Work
Management Entropy):
Patients' cases left alone, without proactive management,
become chaotic whenever possible.

If the primary care physician does not recognize that the return-to-work decision-making process is important in the resolution of the injury or illness, the primary care physician, in effect, is promoting disorganization. Because patients' workplace and work activity are part of the "order" or "normality" within their universe, the physician should strive to maintain this whenever possible, thus avoiding the negative consequences of pro-longed work inactivity and disability.

Workplace Organizational Justice Theory and the Physician's Role

The primary care provider's role and decisions affect the successful outcome of treatment of an employee's injury or illness. If the basic tenets of these selected physical laws have not adequately demonstrated the importance of the return-to-work decision-making process by the primary care provider, then one can gain further insight from other scientific disciplines. Social anthropologists and psychologists have described workplaces and relationships between employers and employees in terms of their organizational structure and managerial decision making. Successful and productive relationships have been identified by what is termed "workplace organizational justice." A wide variety of employment issue outcomes have been described in the literature as following the workplace organizational justice model, including the issues of pay, job satisfaction, and layoff.[10] Most recently, the issue of work-related disability has also been studied.[11–13]

There are three basic types of fairness principles that constitute the workplace organizational justice theory. The first, "distributive justice," is the perceived fairness of the outcomes of a decision-making, resource allocation, or dispute resolution process. The second, "procedural justice," refers to the fairness of the policies and procedures governing behaviors and decision making in the workplace. Lastly, "interactional justice," refers to the quality of the interaction between the individual and the decision maker, and specifically whether the decision maker treats the employee with respect.

As part of the original hypothesis and research on the issues described previously, it would appear that all three areas of justice would need to be at an acceptable level for an employee to have a positive outcome. In the return-to-work and work disability arena, distributive justice might be measured by a positive outcome of a work-related injury from the standpoint of function or benefit compensation. "Procedural justice" might be the presence and details of a company's transitional duty policy or the presence of a post-accident drug testing policy. "Interactional justice" would refer to the personal perception of the relationship between employee and supervisor, or employee and treating physician, when dealing with an injury under the workers' compensation system.

Research continues to show that despite all three areas of fairness being important to a certain degree; "interactional justice" has the strongest predictive value when it comes to a successful outcome. The primary care provider should, therefore, not underestimate the affect of the physician-patient relationship. Furthermore, physicians should avoid the all-too-common temptation to blame "the system" on the lack of recovery or delayed recovery that they may see in their individual workers' compensation patient cases. The primary care physician should not give up when it seem to him or her that the employer is not being fair to the patient with a work-related injury, nor should a physician retaliate when an employer does not have a transitional duty program. The physician should capitalize on the positive relationship that he or she has with the patient. This process includes setting goals for recovery and instituting return-to-work parameters while communicating with the employer the other aspects of "distributive" and "procedural justice" that might be improved.

Recently, some physicians have suggested that interactional justice may call for a return to the paternalistic role of the physician and the positive aspects of this time-honored tradition. This has led to the development of the philosophical term *pseudopaternalism*.[14] Pseudopaternalism describes the marriage of the old-school benevolent physician role with the novel findings of the significance of interactional justice.

Return to Work and the Medical Home

It would be an oversight to leave out a discussion concerning recent health care reform measures and the significance of the patient-centered medical home. Primary care physicians have long since identified that a significant barrier to a healthy population and the cost effective means to that goal is the fragmented and misaligned health care delivery system in the United States.

The current US health system contains substantial inefficiencies. Among them is the overreliance of patients on specialized practitioners. This leads to excessive and inefficient cost structures that reward duplicate X rays, unnecessary tests, and multiple consultations with differing specialists, as well as other unnecessary ancillary procedures.

Meanwhile, as specialist fees and salaries increase, those of primary care practitioners decline. The primary care physician has the ability and the need to consider the holistic health condition of his or her patients. In the health care industry it is widely agreed that recipients of primary care live longer, healthier lives.

According to the Patient Centered Primary Care Collaborative,[15] a coalition of greater than 700 major employers, consumer groups, patient quality organizations, health plans, labor unions, hospitals, clinicians and many others who have joined together to develop and advance the patient centered medical home, the PCMH will broaden access to primary care physicians while expanding and enhancing the primary care physician's role as central care coordinators. This role of care coordinator will require that the physician:

- Take personal responsibility and accountability for the ongoing care of patients;

- Be accessible to their patients on short notice, for expanded hours, and open scheduling;

- Be able to conduct consultations through email and telephone;

- Conduct regular checkups with patients to identify looming health crises and initiate treatment or prevention measures before costly, last-minute emergency procedures are required;

- Advise patients of preventive care based on environmental and genetic risk factors they face;

- Help patients make healthy lifestyle decisions; and

- Coordinate services when specialist care is needed, making sure the care is relevant, necessary, and performed efficiently.

It would seem intuitive that the primary care physician would, under the patient-centered medical home model, become even more involved in the return-to-work decision-making process. In some cases, the primary care physician may not be the one providing the occupational medical care. Clearly, the goal of the patient-centered medical home is the development of a coordination of care model. The primary care physician will, by definition, play a management role of increasing importance in the return-to-work arena.

Many large corporations have "signed on" to the patient-centered medical home model, and some have taken a leadership role in advocating for it legislatively.[16] It would appear that employers are making a point that they would like the primary care physicians to become even more involved in return-to-work decisions, whether it be in workers' compensation, personal injury/illness, or other short-term disability situations.

Indeed, one of the core principles of the patient-centered medical home model is known as "whole person orientation."[17] This is the idea that a personal physician is responsible for providing for all the patient's health care needs or takes responsibility for appropriately arranging care with other qualified professionals. This includes care for all stages of life: preventive services, acute care, chronic care, and end-of-life care. Strangely, national discussion of the patient-centered medical home has not really touched on the principles described in this chapter. It appears that the primary care physicians, despite the challenges described in this chapter, are positioning themselves for an increasing role in the return-to-work decision-making process going forward.

Disability Prevention

At least one formal survey of treating physicians and several informal polls consistently estimate that only a small fraction of medically excused days off work are medically required. Medically required would mean that all work *of any kind* is medically contraindicated. The majority of the days granted as off work are attributed to a variety of nonmedical factors such as: administrative delays, lack of transitional work, ineffective communication, and other logistical problems. Overwhelming data suggests that participants in the disability benefits system seem largely unaware that so much disability is not medically required. A doctor's signature on a form confirming that a medical condition exists is frequently accepted as "proof" that a diagnosis creates disability, and as a result, absence from work is "excused." Benefits are awarded without further inquiry.

People can generally work at something productive as long as there is no contraindication (significant risk of substantial harm), but the key question is often, "What work?" Traditionally, many barriers that look like they are medical are really situation specific. The employee with a cast on his dominant hand may not be able to swing a hammer but can likely do many other things. Someone who has had recent surgery may not be able to work a full day but might be able to work a few hours.

Many employees end up sitting at home because their employers have made the business decision to not make accommodations for their work capacity. Frequently, these decisions are classified as "medical," when, in fact, they are not. Once the decisions are labeled as "medical," they are not questioned.

There is much opportunity to reduce medically discretionary and medically unnecessary disability. There is not much that can be done to reduce medically required disability as this is within the purview of safety engineers, ergonomists, and others whose expertise is used to decrease risk. The primary care physician should contemplate the end result of his or her

Chapter 10

decision and take people off work only when the situation calls for a medically required disability. It is helpful for physicians to consider these terms using the definitions indicated below:

- *Medically required disability* is absence when attendance by the patient is required at a place of care (hospital, doctor's office) or when recovery or quarantine requires confinement to bed or to home. Absence is also appropriate when being in the workplace, or traveling to work, is medically contraindicated. Examples would be when the condition poses a direct threat to the public, co-workers, or the worker personally.

- *Medically discretionary disability* is time away from work at the discretion of a patient or an employer that is associated with a diagnosable condition that may have created some functional impairment but left other functional abilities still intact. This is most commonly due to a patient's or employer's decision to not make the extra effort required to find a reasonable accommodation for the patient to stay at work during illness or recovery.

- *Medically unnecessary disability* occurs whenever a person stays away from work because of nonmedical issues. This becomes the case when the perception that a diagnosis alone, without demonstrable significant risk or functional impairment (capacity), justifies work absence. Another example of this type of disability is when nonmedical psychosocial problems masquerade as medical issues (job dissatisfaction, fear, anger, etc). This also occurs when there is poor information flow or when there is an administrative or procedural delay.

When the primary care physician thinks in these terms, the result is that it is a rare case that medically required disability exists. Work excuse notes should be the exception.

The Three-Phase Approach and Final Words

What then should be some guiding principles for a primary care clinician? We have discussed previously the pivotal role of the physician in the initial encounter with the patient according to the workplace organizational justice theory model and how that sets the stage for a successful outcome when return to work is used as a treatment. It is helpful to think from a primary care perspective in terms of acute, subacute, and chronic phases of return-to-work decision making, regardless of the injury or illness that is being treated.[18]

The first phase, which typically occurs in the first 2 weeks of the injury or illness, is commonly referred to as the *acute phase*. The focus for primary care providers is typically on symptom relief. It is crucial to instill in the patient the importance of maintenance of activity level. Frequently, reassurance is given that activity is good and will not be harmful. Time will need to be spent giving rational explanations regarding the diagnosis at hand.

Goal setting for recovery is important. Debunking myths that the patient brings should also be addressed during the acute phase. The overwhelming majority of diagnoses will be successfully treated to resolution in these first 2 weeks.

During the second phase, commonly known as the *subacute phase*, it is even more important for the primary care provider to focus on early return to work. Reinforcement of this principle is paramount during the time frame of 2 to 12 weeks following injury. The focus for patients who receive treatment during this time frame should be on ability, not disability. Any ineffective treatments provided in the *acute phase* should be ceased. It is in the *subacute phase* that the physician should be attuned to potential red flags that might be barriers to recovery. These red flags may be nonmedical or psychological. Once identified, an appropriate discussion concerning these issues should occur with the patient or employer as appropriate. If multiple red flags present themselves, a referral to a specialty provider, such as an occupational medicine specialist or a psychiatrist, may be necessary.

In the third or *chronic phase*, a multidisciplinary program should be engaged. The chronic phase includes any injury or illness that persists past 12 weeks. Frequently this will require specialty involvement of pain management plus vocational rehabilitation. The typical primary care physician will need to ask for referrals for these services. From the patient treatment perspective, the primary care physician should emphasize self-efficacy and counsel the patient as to the known ineffective therapies using evidence-based medicine to avoid iatrogenic complications. Continued communication with the employer can facilitate the ability of the employer to provide workplace accommodations and to encourage return-to-work options. It often becomes the "tipping point" for any type of return-to-work success.

Many primary care physicians have communicated to me that one of the issues that they struggle with is they don't know how to ask for help in any given worker-care situation. While it is true that every workers' compensation case is unique, the primary care physician should acknowledge his or her level of expertise within these situations. Some family physicians are experts in the diagnosis and treatment of musculoskeletal problems, while others are better at psychiatric diagnoses.

Chapter 10

The bottom line is that early on the primary care provider needs to identify a comfort level with return-to-work decision-making issues. This includes not being ashamed or embarrassed to ask for help or guidance from employer representatives, insurance carriers, or other providers when indicated. In these situations, the incorrect decision can have a great negative implication for patients in ways that may not seem readily apparent at the time.

Summary

The primary care physician is often the first healthcare provider to see the injured worker. This presents a unique opportunity for the primary care physician to engage the injured worker in a discussion of the benefits of staying at work or early return to work. Although this task can be time consuming, the benefits to the patient's well-being can be significant.

References

1. Accreditation Council for Graduate Medical Education. Online under "ACGME Policies and Procedures" at www.acgme.org. Accessed January 21, 2011.

2. Iowa Academy of Family Physicians. 2007 Survey of Practice Demographics. Available from Iowa Academy of Family Physicians, Des Moines, Iowa.

3. http://www.acgme.org/acWebsite/downloads/RRC_progReq/120pr07012007 .pdf. Accessed January 21, 2011.

4. Edge RS, Krieger JL. Legal and ethical perspectives in health care: an integrated approach. New York: Delmar Publishers, 1998.

5. Stewart M, Brown JB, Donner A, McWhinney IR, Oates J, Weston WW, et al. The impact of patient-centered care on outcomes. *J Fam Pract*. 2000; 49(9): 796–804.

6. Weinstein J. Partnership Doctor and Patient: Advocacy for Informed Choice vs. Informed Consent. *Spine*. 2005; 30(3):269–271. http://tdi.dartmouth.edu/ documents/publications/JWPartnershipEditSpi1C28D0-1.pdf. Accessed January 21, 2011.

7. American College of Occupational and Environmental Medicine. Preventing needless work disability by helping people stay employed. 2005. http://www .acoem.org/guidelines.aspx?id=566. Accessed January 21, 2011.

8. Browne, Michael E. *Schaum's Outline of Theory and Problems of Physics for Engineering and Science*. New York: McGraw-Hill; 1999–2007:58.

9. Fermi, Enrico. *Thermodynamics*. New York: Dover Publications; 1956, 1936.

10. Colquitt, JA et al. Justice at the Millennium: a meta-analytic review of 25 yeas of organizational justice research, *J Applied Psych*. 2001;86:425–445.

11. Elovainio M et al. Does organizational justice protect from sickness absence following a major life event? *J Epidemiol Community Health*. 2010;64: 470–472.

12. Roberts K, Markel K. Claiming in the name of fairness: organizational justice and the decision to file for workplace injury compensation, *J Occup Health Psych*. 2001;6(4):332–347.

13. Liljegren M and Ekberg K. The associations between perceived distributive, procedural, and interactional organizational justice, self-related health and burnout. *Work*. 2009;33:43–51.

14. American Academy of Disability Evaluating Physicians. The Physicians Role in the Determination of Disability, Comprehensive Training Course, 2010. Chicago, IL: AADEP.

15. http//:www.pcpcc.com. Accessed January 21, 2011.

16. Abelson R. UnitedHealth and I.B.M. test health care plan. *New York Times* 2009;Feb 6.

17. Ferrante JM, Balasubramanian BA, et al. Principles of the patient-centered medical home and preventive services delivery. *Ann Fam Med*. 2010 Mar–Apr;8(2):108–16.

18. Tackling Musculoskeletal Problems—A Guide for Clinic and Workplace—Identifying Obstacles Using the Psychosocial Flag Framework. Kendall & Burton. The Stationery Office, Norwich, UK. 2009.

Chapter 10

Working With Common Spine Problems

Marjorie Eskay-Auerbach, MD, JD

Spinal conditions are one of the most common causes for work-related absences. Physicians are often asked by patients, employers, and insurers about a patient's ability to return to work and to perform a particular job. This chapter examines return-to-work issues for symptomatic lumbar disk herniation with radiculopathy and nonspecific low back pain. These conditions are commonly seen by physicians and are a frequent cause of disability in developed nations.

Presumed Disability

The Social Security Administration's (SSA's) criteria for total disability due to musculoskeletal impairments have not changed significantly over time, and include some criteria that are particularly relevant to spinal problems:

Section 1.00 Musculoskeletal System - Adult

a. General. Regardless of the cause(s) of a musculoskeletal impairment, functional loss for purposes of these listings is defined as the inability to ambulate effectively on a sustained basis for any reason, including pain associated with the underlying musculoskeletal impairment . . . must have lasted, or be expected to last, for at least 12 months. For the purposes of these criteria, consideration of the ability to perform these activities must be from a physical standpoint alone.

Spinal conditions considered and listed in the SSA information, include herniated nucleus pulposus, spinal arachnoiditis, osteoarthritis, degenerative disk disease, facet arthritis, and vertebral fracture resulting in compromise of a nerve root (including cauda equina) or the spinal cord.

Evidence of the following must be present and associated with the diagnosis:

A. Nerve root compression characterized by neuro-anatomic distribution of pain, limitation of motion of the spine, motor loss (atrophy with associated muscle weakness or muscle weakness) accompanied by sensory or reflex loss, and if there is involvement of the lower back, positive straight-leg raising test (sitting and supine); *or*

B. Spinal arachnoiditis, confirmed by an operative note or pathology report of tissue biopsy or by appropriate medically acceptable imaging, manifested by severe burning or painful dysesthesia, resulting in the need for changes in position or posture more than once every 2 hours; *or*

C. Lumbar spinal stenosis resulting in pseudoclaudication, established by findings on appropriate medically acceptable imaging, manifested by chronic nonradicular pain and weakness, and resulting in inability to ambulate effectively, as defined in 1.00B2b.

Source: Disability Evaluation Under Social Security (Blue Book, September 2008).

SSA Pub. No. 64-039 ICN 468600.

There are many individuals who meet the SSA criteria and continue to work (eg, a person who is paraplegic using a wheelchair) with or without accommodation. Therefore, while the criteria may seem reasonable at first, the variation among the clinical presentation of patients makes uniform application of the criteria difficult.

Certain phrases within the SSA criteria deserve additional attention. For example, limited range of motion (ROM) of the spine (section A) is no longer considered a criterion for impairment ratings (AMA *Guides*, Sixth).[1] It is neither predictive of a patient's ability to function nor indicative of a particular diagnosis (other than ankylosing spondylitis). A prospective clinical study comparing normal ROM and actual ROM used to perform activities of daily living (ADLs) in asymptomatic patients found that most individuals use a relatively small percentage of their full active ROM when performing ADLs.[2] The description of arachnoiditis includes mention of "severe pain resulting in the need for changes in position or posture more than once every two hours." Most normal people change position or posture more than once an hour. More frequent movement has not been shown to reduce pain in individuals with pre-existing low back pain.[3]

SSA includes in its definition, the "inability to ambulate effectively." This is clarified by the following paragraphs:

b. What we mean by inability to ambulate effectively.

(1) Definition. Inability to ambulate effectively means an extreme limitation of the ability to walk; i.e., an impairment(s) that interferes very seriously with the individual's ability to independently initiate, sustain, or complete activities. Ineffective ambulation is defined generally as having insufficient lower extremity functioning (see 1.00J) to permit independent ambulation without the use of a hand-held assistive device(s) that limits the functioning of both upper extremities.

(2) To ambulate effectively, individuals must be capable of sustaining a reasonable walking pace over a sufficient distance to be able to carry out activities of daily living. They must have the ability to travel without companion assistance to and from a place of employment or school. Therefore, examples of ineffective ambulation include, but are not limited to, the inability to walk without the use of a walker, two crutches or two canes, the inability to walk a block at a reasonable pace on rough or uneven surfaces, the inability to use standard public transportation, the inability to carry out routine ambulatory activities, such as shopping and banking, and the inability to climb a few steps at a reasonable pace with the use of a single hand rail. The ability to walk independently about one's home without the use of assistive devices does not, in and of itself, constitute effective ambulation.

Source: Disability Evaluation Under Social Security (Blue Book, September 2008).

SSA Pub. No. 64-039 ICN 468600.

Spinal disorders vary in their clinical presentation, and it is well established that physical examination findings and imaging studies do not correlate well with functional status. Individuals with minimal changes on imaging studies may report severe pain and limited ability, and others with severe changes on imaging may describe little or no pain and normal function. Each term in the SSA definition has a precise definition determined by case law, and therefore, interpretation of this section, and others, is dependent on legal precedent rather than accurate clinical information regarding the applicant's condition.

The concepts of risk, capacity, and tolerance are described in detail in Chapter 2. The application of these concepts to lumbar disk herniation and nonspecific low back pain are discussed in the following sections.

Chapter 11

Lumbar Disk Herniation Resulting in Radiculopathy

Lumbar disk herniation may be an asymptomatic radiographic finding in patients.[4] However, for the purposes of this book, discussion is limited to clinically significant lumbar disk herniation with findings of radicular pain, numbness, and weakness, with or without loss of bowel and/or bladder control.

Risk Assessment

Physician-imposed activity restrictions are frequently based on perceived risk of reinjury. The risk of recurrent symptoms or recurrent disk herniation is a concern in the patient who has been treated for symptomatic lumbar disk herniation after it has stabilized. In patients who have been treated surgically, restrictions are recommended or imposed with the intent of preventing recurrent disk herniation. In patients who have responded to nonsurgical intervention, restrictions may be recommended in an effort to prevent recurrent symptoms, usually sciatica.

The incidence of recurrent disk herniation after surgery is reported in the range of 5% to 12%.[5] Intuitively, it would seem that the risk of recurrent symptomatic disk herniation could be mitigated by appropriate restrictions on activity. This leads to the assumption that specific activities can be implicated as the cause of disk herniations. However, the series reported by Suri et al[6] found that many of the lumbar disk herniations requiring surgery did not have a patient-identified initiating event, and the events the patients did associate with the onset of their symptoms were generally not ergonomically stressful for the back.

Historically, treating physicians have empirically assigned restrictions and limitations of activity to patients after the diagnosis of and treatment for a lumbar disk herniation. The most common restriction placed on patients after treatment for this condition is related to the weight that can be "safely" lifted. Lifting restrictions are most often expressed in terms of the maximum number of pounds that can or should be lifted. However, recommendations to limit weight without considering other parameters (posture, age, gender, etc.) are not supported by scientific principles.[7,8] Placement of lifting restrictions also assumes that lifting activities are the cause of lumbar disk herniations. However, again, the majority of first-time lumbar disk herniations occur with nonlifting activities and without specific inciting events.[6]

In two studies, Carragee, et al., found that time to return to work was shortened by the absence of postoperative activity restrictions after limited diskectomy. Complication rates were comparable in cases where restrictions were imposed, and early return to work had no adverse effect on outcomes.[9] Specifically the rate of recurrent disk herniation was not increased by permitting patients to return to full duty work or unrestricted activity after lumbar diskectomy.

These findings are significant because although a causative relationship cannot be demonstrated, a patient's belief that there is a link may be sufficient to affect his or her understanding of risk of injury and in turn, hinder physical rehabilitation emphasizing function[7,8] and vocational rehabilitation. Postoperative restrictions or warning against reinjury may validate patient fears of returning to regular activity.

In this setting, as is the case with nonspecific low back pain and other musculoskeletal complaints, patient education takes on even greater importance. Patient education including consistent, evidence-based recommendations about safe ability and encouraging resumption of activity independent of pain status has been shown to result in improved disability outcomes in patients with low back pain and other disorders.[10]

Capacity

Patients with lumbar disk herniations, in most cases, will have reduced their activity after the event and prior to treatment. It can be anticipated that the accompanying deconditioned state will lead to a decreased exercise capacity in the first few months after the onset of symptoms. It has previously been reported that intensive exercise programs are more effective for improving functional status and rate of return to work (short-term follow-up).[11] Exercise programs starting 4 to 6 weeks after surgery seem to lead to a more rapid decrease in pain and disability than no treatment, and high-intensity programs are more efficient than lower-intensity programs in effecting that decrease. There is no evidence that active programs increase the reoperation rate after an initial surgery.[12]

Intervention aimed at active rehabilitation with a gradual return to regular duty, early mobilization, and education might further improve ability by providing support for increased activity.[13]

Tolerance

Tolerance in the context of return to work is the ability to put up with symptoms that accompany work activities (pain or fatigue) while performing an activity the individual clearly is able to do. The industrial engineering definition is "[a] time period during which a worker can effectively perform a task without a rest period while maintaining acceptable levels of physiological and emotional well-being."[14] This definition accounts for the intangible factors of perceived rewards from work, such as income, self-esteem, health benefits, etc, that play a role in the individual's assessment of what is tolerable.

Treatment outcomes are, in part, described as good or poor, based on the individual's return to activity. A "good" outcome describes return to preinjury activity, which implies tolerance for any residual symptoms. With a "bad" outcome, function is perhaps even more limited after surgery than before.

In general, the effect of compensation has been demonstrated to have clinical significance with respect to surgical outcomes and to be a potential confounding variable in all studies of surgical interventions.[15] In the recent SPORT study, workers' compensation patients treated for lumbar disk herniations were found to improve substantially with both surgical and non-operative treatment. However, the benefit of surgery diminished with time in the workers' compensation group. At two years, there was no significant advantage demonstrated for surgical treatment over other treatment in any outcome (pain, physical function) in the workers' compensation population, while in the nonworkers' compensation group, the advantage for surgery persisted at two years.[16]

Other studies have shown that return to work is independent of treatment and unrelated to improvement in pain, in function, or in satisfaction with treatment for lumbar disk herniation with sciatica. Individuals initially receiving workers' compensation had more disability and decreased quality of life outcomes compared to those who did not; however, long-term employment and disability outcomes were favorable for most patients with a disk herniation, regardless of initial workers' compensation status.[17] Return to work has been shown to be more closely associated with change in disability than change in pain.[18]

The SSA criteria for disability based on spinal problems require objective evidence of impairment in terms of physical or imaging study findings. However, impairment measured by objective findings clearly cannot be extrapolated to determine tolerance and/or disability. When evaluating a patient for SSA and completing forms that request information regarding work restrictions or work capacity, physicians are inclined to take into account the biopsychosocial model for disability, with acknowledgement of other factors that may play a role, including the patient's purported tolerance for activity. However, the questions raised by employers are based on the biomedical model, which equates impairment with disability. The questions ask about work restrictions based on risk and work limitations based on capacity. The forms typically do not ask about patient tolerance or comfort at work. The approach for evaluating work disability, as set out in Chapter 2 of this book, provides a framework and language that can be used to answer a "medically unanswerable question" (ie, "Should this patient have the tolerance to do this job?").

Consensus Criteria on Lumbar Disk Herniation

There are currently at least two recognized resources for consensus criteria on lumbar disk herniation. The Medical Disability Advisor from the Reed Group (www.mdguidelines.com) provides consensus return-to-work criteria for International Classification of Diseases, Ninth Revision (ICD-9) codes 722.0 (lumbar disk herniation). These criteria indicate that persisting radicular pain is still compatible with function and that most patients should eventually return to their original type of work. Data from this source indicate that most patients with lumbar radiculopathy do, in fact, return to work. The Official Disability Guidelines (www.odg.com) or ODG Guidelines provide similar data regarding return to work.

Nonspecific Low Back Pain

For 85% to 90% of patients with back pain, there is no known pathology or change in anatomy that explains the pain.[4] Physicians use a variety of terms to describe low back conditions, with no medical consensus that any given term is appropriate.[19] The term *mechanical* generally implies that the pain is musculoskeletal in origin, and typically worse with activity and better with rest. Pain that does not respond to changes in activity requires additional evaluation, and potentially serious spinal conditions such as tumor, infection, and fracture must be ruled out.[20] In order to explain low back pain to injured patients, treating physicians will often refer to back "strains" or "sprains," frequently using the words interchangeably, to describe episodes of acute pain. The term *nonspecific low back pain* may more accurately describe this condition. Using the words *sprain* or *strain* to describe nonspecific back pain that first began during a low intensity activity of daily living (ADL) or light work activity can inappropriately communicate to patients that such light routine activity can pose a risk to their spine, so the diagnostic term "nonspecific low back pain" (ICD-9 code 724.5) is preferred.

Although the specific underlying pathology is not known in most cases, many physicians attribute low back symptoms to lumbar disk degeneration.[21] Disk degeneration has been viewed as a result of aging and cumulative "wear and tear" changes from mechanical insults and injuries.[22] In this model, various occupational activities associated with physical

Chapter 11

loading have been implicated as accelerating degenerative changes in the disk. There has been an emphasis on heavy material handling, postural loading, and vehicular vibration as causally related to progressive degenerative change.[21] Contrary to these common beliefs, newer studies have found that cumulative or repetitive loading is not harmful to the disks. This is consistent with the general view that in other parts of the musculoskeletal system, repetitive activities with increased physical loading can increase the strength of bone, ligaments, muscles, and tendons.[23]

Disk degeneration is now properly viewed as being determined in large part by genetic influences. In a review article that summarizes findings of the Twin Spine Study, a multidisciplinary and multinational research project started in 1991, significant findings included the identification of the substantial influence of heredity on lumbar disk degeneration and identification of the first gene forms associated with disk degeneration. Most of the specific environmental factors previously thought to be primary risk factors for disk degeneration appeared to have modest effects, if any.[21] The authors are careful to note that disk degeneration and low back pain are not synonymous, and the relationship between the two remains poorly defined as yet.

A series of articles evaluating a number of physical activities that have been implicated in causing of low back pain used the Bradford Hill criteria for causality in an analysis of systematic reviews of the literature. These studies found strong evidence for consistency of no association between awkward occupational postures and low back pain.[24] There was conflicting evidence for any significant association between occupational bending and low back pain and a clear causal relationship could not be established. Similarly, a clear causal relationship between occupational twisting and low back pain could not be established. Based on the results of this review, the authors found it unlikely that occupational bending or twisting were independently causative of low back pain.[25] This same group of authors concluded that there was insufficient evidence to establish causality between occupational sitting and low back pain,[26] occupational standing or walking and low back pain,[27] or occupational pushing or pulling and low back pain.[28] Based on their review, it was unlikely that occupational lifting was independently causative of low back pain in the population of workers studied.[29]

Risk Assessment

For patients who have recovered from an episode of nonspecific low back pain, the risk of recurrence and/or chronicity are concerns. Recurrent low back pain has not been well studied to date, in part because of difficulty classifying repeat episodes as a recurrence or new. In addition, much of the research and literature has been aimed at primary prevention of low back pain.

The rate of recurrence of a low back disorder is estimated to range from 3% to 86% within one year; however, this wide range has been attributed to the lack of a uniform definition of the term *recurrent*.[30] Recurrences contribute disproportionately to the total burden of work-related nonspecific low back pain, both through additional care seeking and work disability.[31] Postinitial episodes account for more than two-thirds of compensated medical and lost time costs.[32]

Independent factors that are predictors for episodes of recurrent low back pain in actively employed people have been identified and include high stress, poor physical health, high back pain and back pain disability, spinal deformity, and frequent job changes (more than one job within the plant during 12 months). Of these factors, level of physical health was the best predictor of a recurrent episode of low back pain in employed persons.[33] Only one factor (deformity) is a biomedical model spinal condition.

A similar systematic review of predictors of chronic disabling low back pain found a number of factors that were weak predictors of chronic pain with activity limitation one year after the onset of low back pain. These included the presence of radiculopathy (a biomedical factor) and several psycho-social factors. Psychosocial factors with a positive likelihood ratio (>2) included nonorganic signs, psychiatric comorbidity, pain-related impairment, presence of a somatization disorder, and high fear avoidance beliefs. Compensation status, high work demands, better general health, and pain intensity had likelihood ratios, if positive, of <2.[34]

The largest prospective study of American workers' future risk of workers' compensation claims for back pain problems is still the Boeing aircraft study.[35] In this study more than 3000 workers were observed prospectively for four years. The greatest risk factors for a future claim were having current back pain or having had previous back pain (relative risk, 1.7) and not enjoying one's job (relative risk, 1.7). The low level of risk was the same regardless of whether the back pain was past pain or current pain and regardless of whether the individual's job was light or heavy.

These findings have been repeated in subsequent studies. Workers with a history of sick leave for musculoskeletal conditions in the year prior to the initial sick leave for low back pain had an almost 3-fold risk of recurrent sickness absence compared to those without. Those workers with chronic complaints also had an increased rick of recurrent absence for illness. Perceived pain, functional disability, physical health, and general health at return to work were significantly poorer among workers with recurrent sick leaves during follow-up.[36]

Chapter 11

Predictors of Work Disability

A number of factors have been identified consistently as predictive of delayed recovery or work disability. In spite of a benign initial presentation and numerous treatment interventions, 10% of occupational low back pain claims follow a course longer than 3 months and account for approximately 90% of costs for occupational low back pain.[37] Patients with similar examination findings and imaging studies have varied pain and disability outcomes, suggesting that other factors play a role.

In a large group of new workers' compensation claims for lost work time from back injuries, risk factors for chronic disability included radiculopathy, substantial functional disability (Roland disability questionnaire), more widespread pain (multiple sites), and extended time off work. In addition, workers who described their jobs as "very hectic" or received no offer of a job accommodation to facilitate return to work (eg, light duty, reduced hours) and the specialty of the first health care provider for the injury were statistically significant for predicting receipt of work disability compensation one year later.[38]

Worker expectations for recovery also play a role with respect to return to work. Workers with lower expectations and greater work fear avoidance at the time of injury are significantly more likely to receive compensation six months after injury.[39] This finding seems to be unique to low back pain claims when compared to claims for other musculoskeletal conditions.[40]

Treatment with oral opioid analgesics has become increasingly common for acute musculoskeletal pain, including acute low back pain. Recent findings indicate that early treatment with opioid medications is significantly associated with adverse outcomes including prolonged disability, higher medical costs, higher risk for surgery, and late use of opioids.[41] Analysis of data from the Washington Workers' Compensation Disability Risk Identification Study Cohort demonstrated that receipt of more than 7 days and more than one prescription of opioids within 6 weeks of the first medical visit for the injury were associated with work disability at one year. Use of prescribed opioids for more than 7 days in workers with acute back injuries has since been identified as a risk factor for long-term disability.[42]

Prevention studies are another way of looking at potential factors in causation (risk). If cigarette smoking causes disease, a decreased rate of smoking should result in less disease. In addition, if work is a toxin causing back problems, then altering work should result in fewer back problems. A systematic review of back pain prevention trials found that the only factor or intervention for which there was proof of efficacy in preventing back disorders was exercise.[43] No ergonomic intervention has been proven to decrease the incidence of "work related" back pain. This suggests that work does not put the spine at risk, but rather that once back pain develops, work-like activity may increase symptoms (tolerance, not risk).

Capacity

Decreased capacity is anticipated in patients with low back pain. As noted in the previous section, activity can increase functional level and capacity. The importance of regular exercise is recognized, although the need for a structured rehabilitation program and/or the form that exercise should take remains unclear.

Graded exercise has been applied as a rehabilitation technique for working patients with nonspecific recurrent low back pain, with emphasis on core strengthening and stabilization exercises. This technique has been shown to improve disability and other health parameters over the short term.[44] There may be a positive effect on sick leave for workers with subacute and chronic back pain, but there is conflicting evidence for the effectiveness of exercise treatment in reducing recurrent symptoms.[45]

A recent systematic review of the available evidence suggested that graded activity in the short term and intermediate term is only slightly more effective than a minimal intervention. Graded activity was not more effective than other forms of exercise for persistent low back pain.[46] Therefore, the effectiveness of physical conditioning programs in reducing sick leave, when compared to usual care or other exercises in workers with back pain, remains uncertain.[45]

Tolerance

The importance of psychosocial factors with respect to return-to-work activities is discussed in detail above. These factors are more consistent with the concept of tolerance.

Most patients with low back pain are physically capable of activity but intolerant of the associated pain and therefore choose to avoid those activities. However, tolerance appears to have a psychosocial component, as indicated by the numerous studies that address factors other than physical ability or capacity as predictive of return to work.

As outlined in Chapter 2 and in the above discussion, tolerance is not a basis for physician-imposed work restrictions (risk) or work limitations (capacity). Tolerance issues, logically, are a patient choice, and physicians should decline to certify inability to work on the basis of issues of tolerance in the absence of severe pathology that cannot be medically improved.

Chapter 11

The method of discussing this situation suggested in Chapter 2 again can be used:

> You do not appear to meet the Social Security Administration's criteria for total disability. Thus, in our society, there is some job you're expected to be able to do. Because there is no medical evidence that you are at high risk of significant harm by working, I can not certify that you're disabled for this job. There is no basis for work restrictions based on risk. Whether the rewards of working are sufficient for you to choose to remain at work, or whether the pain or fatigue you feel is sufficient for you to choose a different type of work, or not to work at all, is a question only you can answer. I can record what you feel to be your current activity tolerances, but not as work restrictions or work limitations. Your tolerances are not scientifically measurable, and they may change in the future, depending on how active you are.

The techniques discussed in Chapter 3 are also helpful when discussing return-to-work issues with patients.

Consensus Criteria on Low Back Pain

The Medical Disability Advisor provides consensus return-to-work criteria for International Classification of Diseases, Ninth Revision (ICD-9) codes 846 and 847 (lumbar strain). These criteria indicate that persisting back pain is still compatible with function, and that most patients should eventually return to their original type of work. The real-world data that appear in Tables 11-1, 11-2, and 11-3 also indicate that most patients with lumbar strain do in fact return to work. The ODG Guidelines also provide data regarding expected duration of time off work for these diagnoses.

Table 11-1 Nonspecific Treatment for Low Back Pain (Consensus)

Job classification	Duration, days		
	Minimum	**Optimum**	**Maximum**
Sedentary work	0	1	14
Light work	0	3	14
Medium work	1	14	56
Heavy work	3	28	84
Very heavy work	3	42	91

Reproduced with permission from Reed.
http://www.mdguidelines.com/

Table 11-1 (*continued*)

ICD-9-CM: 724.2

Cases	Mean	Min	Max	No Lost Time	Over 6 Months
21539	46	0	219	0.2%	1.6%

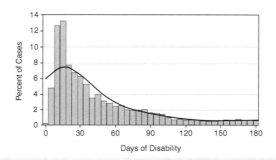

Reproduced with permission from Reed.
http://www.mdguidelines.com/

Chapter 11

Table 11-2 Medical treatment, Lumbar Disk Displacement

Job classification	Duration, days		
	Minimum	Optimum	Maximum
Sedentary work	1	7	14
Light work	1	14	21
Medium work	1	21	42
Heavy work	1	56	91
Very heavy work	1	91	156

Reproduced with permission from Reed.
http://www.mdguidelines.com/

Table 11-3 Surgical treatment, Lumbar disk diskectomy

Job classification	Duration, days		
	Minimum	Optimum	Maximum
Sedentary work	3	14	35
Light work	7	21	42
Medium work	14	42	84
Heavy work	35	49	112
Very heavy work	42	56	140

ICD-9-CM: 722.10

Cases	Mean	Min	Max	No Lost Time	Over 6 Months
6030	73	0	292	0.1%	7.4%

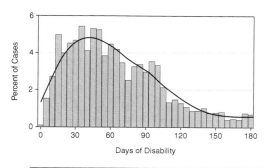

Percentile:	5th	25th	Median	75th	95th
Days:	11	33	59	97	188

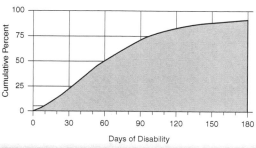

Reproduced with permission from Reed.
http://www.mdguidelines.com/

Summary

The discussions above illustrate how the principles of risk, capacity, and tolerance can be applied to return-to-work decision making for common diagnoses such as lumbar disk herniations and low back pain. Most patients with these problems are capable of remaining at work. Current work ability may increase with recreational activity, formal work conditioning therapy, and/or with return to work with gradually increasing work assignments. There is no science to support the need for activity restrictions in patients with lumbar disk herniations or low back pain, and limitations may in fact impede the patient's return to work and foster disability unnecessarily.

References

1. American Medical Association. *Guides to the Evaluation of Permanent Impairment*. 6th ed. Chicago, Ill: American Medical Association; 2008.

2. Bible J, Biswas B, Miller C, Whang, P, Grauer J. Normal functional range of motion of the lumbar spine during 15 activities of daily living. *J Spinal Disord Tech*. 2010;23(2):106–112.

3. Dunk NM, Callaghan JP. Lumbar spine movement patterns during prolonged sitting differentiate low back pain developers from matched asymptomatic controls. *Work*. 2010;35(1):3–14.

4. Deyo RA, Weinstein JN. Low back pain. *N Engl J Med*. 2001;344:363–370.

5. Errico TJ, Fardon DF, Lowell TD. Contemporary concepts in spine care: open discectomy as treatment for herniated nucleus pulposus of the lumbar spine. *Spine*. 1995;20:1829–1833.

6. Suri P, Hunter D, Jouve C, Hartigan C, Limke J, Pena E, Swaim B, Li L, Rainville J. Inciting events associated with lumbar disc herniation. *Spine*. 2010;10:388–395.

7. Magnusson M, Pope M, Wilder D, Szpalski M, Spratt K. Is there a rational basis for post-surgical lifting restrictions? 1. Current understanding. *Eur Spine J*. 1999;8:170–178.

8. Magnusson M, Pope M, Wilder D, Szpalski M, Spratt K. Is there a rational basis for post-surgical lifting restrictions? 1. Possible scientific approach. *Eur Spine J*. 1999;8:179–186.

9. Carragee EJ.; Han MY.; Yang B; Kim DH.; Kraemer H; Billys J. Activity restrictions after posterior lumbar discectomy: a prospective study of outcomes in 152 cases with no postoperative restrictions. *Spine*. 1999;24(22):2346–2351.

10. Rainville J, Pransky G, Indahl A, Mayer E K. The physician as disability advisor for patients with musculoskeletal complaints. *Spine*. 2005;30(22):2579–2584.

Chapter 11

11. Ostelo RWJG, de Vet HC, Waddell G, Kerkchoffs MR, Leffers P, van Tulder M. Rehabilitation following first-time lumbar disc surgery: a systematic review within the framework of the Cochrane Collaboration. *Spine*. 2003;28(3): 209–218.

12. Ostelo RWJG, Pena Costa LO; Maher CG, de Vet H, van Tulder M. Rehabilitation after lumbar disc surgery: an update Cochrane Review. *Spine*. 2009;34(17):1839–1848.

13. Donceel P, du Bois M, Lahaye D. Return to work after surgery for lumbar disc herniation: a rehabilitation-oriented approach in insurance medicine. *Spine*. 1999;24(9):872.

14. Parker, Sybil P. *McGraw-Hill Dictionary of Scientific & Technical Terms*. 6th ed. New York: McGraw-Hill; 2003.

15. Harris I, Mulford J, Solomon M, van Gelder JM, Young J. Association between compensation status and outcome after surgery: a meta-analysis. *JAMA*. 2005;293:1644–1652.

16. Atlas SJ, Tosteson TD, Blood EA, Skinner JS, Pransky GS, Weinstein JN. The impact of workers' compensation on outcomes of surgical and nonoperative therapy for patients with a lumbar disc herniation: SPORT. *Spine*. 2010;35(1):89–97.

17. Atlas SJ, Chang Y, Keller RB, Singer DE, Wu YA, Deyo RA. The impact of disability compensation on long-term treatment outcomes of patients with sciatica due to a lumbar disc herniation. *Spine*. 2006;31(26): 3061–3069.

18. Jensen OK, Nielsen CV, Stengarard-Pedersem K. One-year prognosis in sick-listed low back pain patients with and without radiculopathy. Prognostic factors influencing pain and disability. *The Spine Journal*. 2010;10(8):659–675.

19. Fardon D, Pinkerton S, Balderston R, et al. Terms used for diagnosis by English speaking spine surgeons. *Spine*. 1993;18:274–277.

20. Acute Low Back Pain Problems in Adults: Assessment and Treatment; Quick Reference Guide for CliniciansClinical Practice Guideline #14, U.S. Agency for Health Care Policy and Research (1994).

21. Battie MC, Videman T, Kaprio J, Gibbons LE, Gill K, Manninen H, Saarela J, Peltonen L. The Twin Spine Study: contributions to a changing view of disc degeneration. *Spine*. 2009;9:47–59

22. Battie MC, Videman T, Levälahti E, Gill K, Kaprio, J. Genetic and environmental effects on disc degeneration by phenotype and spinal level. *Spine*. 2008;33: 2801–2808.

23. Videman T, Gibbons LE, Kaprio J, Battie MC. Challenging the cumulative injury model: positive effects of greater body mass on disc degeneration. *Spine*. 2010;10:26–31.

24. Roffey DM, Wai EK, Bishop P, Kwon BK, Daganais S. Causal assessment of awkward occupational postures and low back pain: results of a systematic review. *Spine*. 2010;10:89–99.

25. Wai EK, Roffey DM, Bishop P, Kwon BK, Dagenais S. Causal assessment of occupational bending or twisting and low back pain: results of a systematic review. *Spine*. 2010;10:76–88.

26. Roffey DM, Wai EK, Bishop P, Kwon BK, Dagenais S. Causal assessment of occupational sitting and low back pain: results of a systematic review. *Spine*. 2010;10(3):252–261.

27. Roffey DM, Wai EK, Bishop P, Kwon BK, Dagenais S. Causal assessment of occupational standing or walking and low back pain: results of a systematic review. *Spine*. 2010;10(3):262–272.

28. Roffey DM, Wai EK, Bishop P, Kwon BK, Dagenais S. Causal assessment of occupational pushing or pulling and low back pain: results of a systematic review. *Spine*. 2010;10(6):544–553.

29. Wai EK, Roffey DM, Bishop P, Kwon BK, Dagenais S. Causal assessment of occupational lifting and low back pain: results of a systematic review. *Spine*. 2010;10(6):554–566.

30. Oleske DM, Lavendar SA, Andersson GBJ, Morrissey MJ, Zold-Kilbourn P, Allen C, and Taylor E. Risk factors for recurrent episodes of work-related low back disorders in an Industrial Population. *Spine*. 2006;31(7):789–798.

31. Radoslaw W, Kim J, Pransky G. Work disability and costs caused by recurrence of low back pain: longer and more costly than in first episodes. *Spine*. 2006;31(2):219–225.

32. Wasiak R, Young AE, Dunn KM, Cote P, Gross DP, Heymans MW, von Korff M. Back pain recurrence, an evaluation of existing indicators and direction for future research. *Spine*. 2009;34(9):970–977.

33. Oleske DM, Lavendar SA, Andersson GBJ, Morrissey MJ, Zold-Kilbourn P, Allen C, and Taylor E. Risk Factors for recurrent episodes of work-related low back disorders in an industrial population. *Spine*. 2006;31(7):789–798.

34. Chou, R and Shekelle P. Will this patient develop persistent disabling low back pain? *JAMA* 2010;303(13):1295–1302.

35. Bigos, SJ, Battie MC, Spengler DM, Fisher LD, Fordyce WE, Hansson TH, Nachemson AL, Wortley MD. A prospective study of work perceptions and psychosocial factors affecting the report of low back injury. *Spine* 1991; 16(1):1–6.

36. Lotters F, Hogg-Johnson S, Burdorf A. Health status, its perceptions and effect on return to work and recurrent sick leave. *Spine*. 2005;30(90):1086–1092.

37. Shaw WS, Pransky G, Patterson W, Winter T. Early disability risk factors for low back pain assesses at outpatient occupational health clinics. *Spine*. 2005;30(5):572–580.

38. Turner JA, Franklin G, Fulton-Kehoe D, Sheppard L, Stover, B, Wu R, Gluck JV, Wickizer TM, Thomas M. ISSLS Prize Winner: Early predictors of chronic work disability: a prospective, population-based study of workers with back injuries. *Spine*. 2008;33(25):2809–2818.

39. Turner JA, Franklin, G, Fulton-Kehoe D, Sheppard L. Wickizer TM, Thomas M. Worker recovery expectations and fear-avoidance predict work disability in a population-based workers' compensation back pain sample. *Spine*. 2006;31(6):682–689.

40. Gross DF, Battie MC. Recovery expectations predict recovery in workers with back pain but not other musculoskeletal conditions. *J Spinal Disord Tech*. 2010; 23(7):451–456

Chapter 11

41. Webster BS, Verma SK, Gatchel RJ, Relationship between early opioid prescribing for acute occupational low back pain and disability duration, medical costs, subsequent surgery and late opioid use. *Spine*. 2007;32 (19):2127–2132.

42. Franklin GM, Stover BD, Turner JA, Fulton-Kehoe D, Wickizier TM. Early opioid prescription and subsequent disability among workers with back injuries: the disability risk identification study cohort. *Spine*. 2008;33(2):199–204.

43. Bigos SJ, Holland J, Holland C, et al. High-quality controlled trials on preventing episodes of back problems: systematic literature review in working-age adults. *Spine*. 2009;9:147–168.

44. Rasmussen-Barr E, Äng B, Arvidsson I, Nilsson-Wikmar L. Graded exercise for recurrent low-back pain: a randomized, controlled trial with 6-, 12-, and 36-month follow-ups. *Spine*. February 1, 2009;34(3):221–228.

45. Schaafsma F, Schonstein E, Whelan KM, Ulvestad E, Kenny DT, Verbeek JH. Physical conditioning programs for improving work outcomes in workers with back pain. Cochrane Database Syst Rev. 2010 Jan 20;(1):CD001822.

46. Macedo LG, Smeets RJ, Maher CG, Latimer J, McAuley JH. Graded activity and graded exposure for persistent nonspecific low back pain: a systematic review. *Phys Ther*. 2010 Jun;90(6):860–79.

Working With Common Upper Extremity Problems

J. Mark Melhorn, MD and Shirley M. Seaman, PA-C

Upper limb musculoskeletal disorders continue to account for a signifi-cant number of work-related illnesses and disabilities in the United States. According to the US Bureau of Labor and Statistics, nontraumatic musculo-skeletal conditions account for 65% of all occupational illnesses in the United States.[1] Upper limb musculoskeletal conditions (shoulder, elbow, forearm, wrist, and hand) rank in the top 5 for financial severity and days away from work.[2] In 2005, upper limb musculoskeletal conditions accounted for 30% of all injuries and illnesses with days away from work.[3] Shoulder disorders account for 3% to 5% of total lost workdays and 10% to 11% of claims and costs in workers' compensation cases. In 2005, 31.5% of elbow injuries resulted in 31 days or more away from work with a median of 14 days. Furthermore, the state of Washington found that elbow disorders accounted for the third-highest incidence rate with 29.7 injuries per 10,000 full-time employees, while forearm, wrist, and hand injuries accounted for 7% to 8% of total lost workdays and 17% to 23% of workers' compensation claims.[4]

Time Off Work (Reducing Medically Unnecessary Disability)

Employers, patients, lawyers, and the courts often assume that time away from work after an illness or injury is necessary. They typically unquestion-ingly assume that as long as a doctor makes a medical diagnosis or verifies that there is ongoing treatment the individual should be off work. Most neglect to inquire whether the patient is actually unable to do any productive work safely. Medically necessary lost work days should only occur when the patient must remain in bed or because there is truly no way to protect the recovering worker from further harm while in the workplace. As one employer states, "We can accommodate any modified work guides short of absolute bed rest."

Educating physicians to the need to reduce unnecessary disability while providing effective methods to accomplish this goal is the key. This chapter will explore common upper limb musculoskeletal disorders by specific *International Classification of Diseases, Ninth Revision, Clinical Modification* (ICD-9-CM) diagnosis that may be associated with workplace activities and will provide appropriate suggestions on approaches for stay-at-work–return-to-work options with suggested disability durations. Each diagnosis will be discussed using the concepts of capacity, risk, and tolerance to judge the individual's readiness for return to work.

Work-related injuries continue to be a burden on society and a hardship for the individual employee-patient. In 1998, the Bureau of Labor and Statistics[5,6] reported 1996 data revealing a total of nearly 1.9 million injuries and illnesses in private industry that required recuperation away from work at an estimated $418 billion in direct costs and (using the lower range of estimates) indirect costs of $837 billion.[7]

Although efforts are being made to reduce incidence rates for musculoskeletal disorders (MSDs) commonly labeled as cumulative trauma disorders (CTDs), disproportionately higher costs are associated with this category of conditions as defined by the Occupational Safety and Health Administration (OSHA). Feuerstein et al[8] reviewed 185 927 claims in the federal workforce and concluded that upper extremity MSDs had much higher costs for direct and indirect medical care because of the longer duration of treatment and greater work disability. Webster et al[9] found that the mean cost per case for upper extremity MSDs was $8070 compared to a mean cost of $824 for all other cases. The US Bureau of Labor Statistics found the median number of lost work days for all cases in 1996 was 5 days, with carpal tunnel syndrome (CTS) at 25 days.[6] As more nations continue to experience an aging workforce, physicians are certain to be confronted with increasing return-to-work and disability determinations.

Presumed Disability

Section 2(a) of the Social Security Administration's criteria for total disability of the upper extremities[10] specifies the inability to perform fine and gross movements effectively on a sustained basis for any reason, including pain, associated with an underlying musculoskeletal impairment that has lasted or is expected to last for at least 12 months. For the purposes of these criteria, the ability to perform these activities must be considered from a physical standpoint alone; subjective complaints do not qualify. It would appear that these two statements are in conflict, which can make SSA determinations difficult.

Second, section 2(2)c states that inability to perform fine and gross movements effectively means an extreme loss of function of both upper extremities, ie, an impairment(s) that interferes very seriously with the individual's ability to independently initiate, sustain, or complete activities. To use their upper extremities effectively, individuals must be capable of sustaining such functions as reaching, pushing, pulling, grasping, and fingering to be able to carry out activities of daily living (ADLs). Therefore, examples of inability to perform fine and gross movements effectively include, but are not limited to, the inability to prepare a simple meal and feed oneself, the inability to take care of personal hygiene, the inability to sort and handle papers or files, and the inability to place files in a file cabinet at or above waist level.

Section 2(2)d states that pain or other symptoms may be an important factor contributing to functional loss. For pain or other symptoms to be found to affect an individual's ability to perform basic work activities, medical signs or laboratory findings must show the existence of a medically determinable impairment(s) that could reasonably be expected to produce the pain or other symptoms. The musculoskeletal listings that include pain or other symptoms among their criteria also include criteria for limitations in functioning as a result of the listed impairment, including limitations caused by pain. It is therefore important to evaluate the intensity and persistence of such pain or other symptoms carefully to determine their effect on the individual's functioning under these listings.

Finally, section 1.05 addresses amputations of both hands due to any cause.

Shoulder: Rotator Cuff Impingement Syndrome

Rotator cuff impingement or rotator cuff syndrome (ICD-9-CM codes 726, 726.1, 726.10, 726.11, 726.2, 840, 840.9 or ICD-10 codes M75.4. M75.8, M75.9) rarely qualifies for total upper extremity disability. Also known as impingement syndrome, subacromial impingement syndrome, and painful arc syndrome, rotator cuff impingement syndrome occurs when the musculotendinous structure that provides strength and mobility to the shoulder joint

Chapter 12

(rotator cuff) rubs against the coracoacromial arch (coracoid process, the coracoacromial ligament, the acromion, and the acromioclavicular joint capsule), especially when the shoulder is placed in the forward-flexed and internally rotated position. Impingement is thought to be a precursor to a rotator cuff tear, although the cuff tends to tear near its insertion on the greater tuberosity, and impingement tends to occur a few centimeters further medially. Impingement occurs in three stages and normally increases with age, shoulder laxity, repetitive overhead activity, sleeping with the shoulder abducted, previous injury, osteoarthritis, bone spurs, and anatomic abnormalities.

Risk Assessment

The largest meta analysis of the epidemiologic data for workplace risk factors and the associated development of musculoskeletal disorders by body part was completed in 1997 by the National Institute of Occupational Safety and Health (NIOSH).[11] Workplace risk factors include repetition, force, posture, vibration, and their combination. The analysis cautioned that the development of musculoskeletal disorders is modified by psychosocial factors. For considering risk assessment and capacity, the data can be helpful for constructing return-to-work guides for specific body parts.[12] The tables that follow for each diagnosis in this chapter are based on the criteria outlined in Table 12-1.[12]

Capacity

Chronic cases of impingement may have reduced shoulder motion. This is a limitation in capacity to do activities such as overhead work with the ipsilateral hand. If there is reduced motion, physicians need to describe the work limitations present on the basis of decreased shoulder motion. Other than decreased shoulder motion, there are no issues of capacity for shoulder impingement syndrome. The issue is usually tolerance. Patients can carry out activities involving use of the shoulder, but they dislike doing so because it hurts.

Tolerance

Tolerance is the usual issue when discussions of work ability arise in patients with impingement syndrome. When the degree of impingement is mild on imaging studies, and when limited use of the shoulder is involved, most physicians will agree that patients should be able to work despite pain. When the degree of impingement on imaging studies is severe, when nonoperative treatment has failed, and when the job requires significant use of the shoulder, most physicians would recommend surgical treatment. For these patients, most physicians would also give guidance that decreasing the use of the shoulder at work might result in decreased pain. While this is not a work limitation, the patient's decision not to do certain activities at

Table 12-1 Risk Factors for Neck and Shoulder Musculoskeletal Pain*

Body Part and Risk Factor	Strong Epidemiologic Evidence (+++)	Epidemiologic Evidence (++)	Insufficient Epidemiologic Evidence (+/0)	No Epidemiologic Evidence (−)
Neck and Neck/Shoulder				
Repetition		X		
Force	X			
Posture	X			
Vibration			X	
Shoulder				
Repetition		X		
Force			X	
Posture		X		
Vibration			X	

* **Strong epidemiologic evidence** (+++) indicates that the consistently positive findings from a large number of cross-sectional studies, strengthened by the limited number of prospective studies, provide strong evidence of increased risk of work-related musculoskeletal disorders for some body parts based on the strength of the associations, lack of ambiguity, consistency of the results, and adequate control or adjustment for likely confounders in cross-sectional studies and the temporal relationships from the prospective studies, with reasonable confidence levels in at least several of those studies. **Epidemiologic evidence** (++) indicates that some convincing epidemiologic evidence shows a causal relationship when the epidemiologic criteria of causality for intense or long-duration exposure to the specific risk factor(s) and musculoskeletal disorders are used. A positive relationship has been observed between exposure to the specific risk factor and musculoskeletal disorders in studies in which chance, bias, and confounding factors are not the likely explanation. **Insufficient epidemiologic evidence** (+/0) indicates that the available studies are of insufficient number, quality, consistency, or statistical power to permit a conclusion regarding the presence or absence of a causal association. Some studies suggest a relationship to specific risk factors, but chance, bias, or confounding may explain the association. Either there is an insufficient number of studies from which to draw conclusions or the overall conclusion from the studies is equivocal. The absence of existing epidemiologic evidence should not be interpreted to mean that there is no association between work factors and musculoskeletal disorders. **No epidemiologic evidence** (−) indicates that there have been no adequate studies to show that the specific workplace risk factor(s) is not related to development of musculoskeletal disorders.

Source: United States Department of Health and Human Services. Musculoskeletal Disorders and Workplace Factors. A Critical Review of Epidemiologic Evidence for Work-Related Musculoskeletal Disorders of the Neck, Upper Extremity and Low Back. Cincinnati, OH: National Institute for Occupational Safety and Health, 1997.

work would be supported by most physicians. For patients whose degree of impingement falls between the severe and the mild cases described above, there will usually be considerable disagreement among physician evaluators. This is the "How much pain should a person be expected to tolerate?" question, which has no scientific answer.

A temporary period of modified work may be helpful. During this time, shoulder strengthening exercises may be prescribed to improve the impingement, although there is no clear scientific proof of efficacy of this treatment.[13] This is not total cessation of shoulder use, but rather use in a pattern to strengthen specific shoulder muscles. During this time, temporary work guides may be appropriate.

The key is to modify activities but not to have total absence from aggravating activities such as hand use at or above the shoulder. Capacity guides might include limited overhead work (reaching above shoulder) or to shoulder level (90-degree position); reaching above the shoulder limited to less than 15 to 30 times per hour with up to 15 lbs of weight; reaching to shoulder up to 15 to 30 times per hour with up to 25 lbs of weight; holding the arm in abduction or flexion limited to up to 15 to 30 times per hour with up to 15 lbs of weight; pulling and pushing up to 60 lbs 20 to 30 times per hour; lifting and carrying up to 40 lbs 15 to 30 times per hour; and climbing ladders up to 60 rungs per hour. An ergonometric evaluation of the workplace may be helpful. Change in job duties, sharing or alternating tasks, reduced work rate, more frequent rest breaks, and limiting the time and frequency of repetitive activities are important accommodations. Work site modifications can include forearm rests for individuals who use computer keyboards frequently, headsets for those who answer telephones, and changing task performance such that repetitive activities can be done with the arms at a lower level of elevation.

Postoperative instructions might include 0 to 5 days with the arm in a sling or support, with the arm used for assist activities only, 10 lbs or less maximum, frequent use for 5 lbs at waist to chest height, and no arm use at or above shoulder height. At 5 to 28 days after surgery, light-medium to medium work may be permitted (35 to 50 lbs maximum, frequent lift and carry of 20 to 25 lbs with both arms combined, and no use at or above shoulder height). After 4 weeks, gradual increase in weight is permitted but still with limitation of hand over the shoulder. The ability to return to heavy work and very heavy work may be difficult, and permanent restrictions may be appropriate after surgery.

Tolerance is influenced by the individual's age, occupation, dominant or nondominant arm affected, response to treatment, and compliance with treatment recommendations and rehabilitation programs during the recovery (disability) period. Return to work is often linked to the job category. Job categories include sedentary, light, medium, heavy, and very heavy. The data in Table 12-2 reflect the physician's work guides (capacity), the patient's tolerance, and risk of reinjury. Two groups of data are reported. The first set of data is labeled Target, TMinimum, and TMaximum, representing the "best practice guidelines" as reported by The Hand Center.[14] The second set of data is labeled Optimum, Minimum, and Maximum, representing a composite of recommendations by multiple physicians in multiple states as reported by *The Medical Disability Advisor*.[15] The Hand Center data was updated in 2010 for the 2nd edition of this book. *The Medical Disability Advisor* data was updated in 2010 for the MDGuidelines Version 6.1 online version at http://www.mdguidelines.com/. The Hand Center best practice guidelines were developed for The Hand Center by the author (J.M.M.), a physician who enthusiastically educates patients and employers about the advantages of early return to work, assists employers in the development of

Table 12-2 Shoulder Rotator Cuff Impingement Suggested Disability Durations (Days)

Job Classification	ICD-9-CM: 726, 726.2, 840, 840.9					
	ICD-10: M75.4, M75.8, M75.9					
	The Hand Center			The MDGuidelines 2005/2010		
	Target	TMinimum	TMaximum	Optimum	Minimum	Maximum
Nonsurgical Treatment for Shoulder Rotator Cuff Impingement						
Sedentary	0	0	1	3*	0	4
Light	0	0	5	3	0	7
Medium	0	0	7	21	14	42
Heavy	14	0	45	42	28	84
Very Heavy	28	7	56	42	28	84
Arthroscopic Surgery for Shoulder Rotator Cuff Impingement						
Sedentary				10	7	21
Light				10	7	21/42
Medium				42	28	56
Heavy				70	56/42	84/91
Very Heavy				70/84	56	84/112
Open Surgery for Shoulder Rotator Cuff Impingement						
Sedentary	5	0	14	42/10	28/7	70/21
Light	5	0	17	56/21	28/10	84/42
Medium	21	7	35	84/42	42/14	140/56
Heavy	42	14	91	84/70	70/42	140/91
Very Heavy	49	21	105	84	70/56	140/112

* No change between 2005 and 2010 data if only one number in the MDGuidelines section.

Reproduced with permission from Reed. www.mdguidelines.com.

Chapter 12

early return-to-work programs, and promotes return to work through educational venues. To reduce unnecessary disability, physicians are encouraged to aim for the target disability day. The minimum and maximum range is provided with the realization that individuals are unique and many factors contribute to stay at work or early return to work.

The Medical Disability Advisor duration table guidelines outlined in Table 12-2 represent a unique combination of methodologies that have resulted in the development of practical and usable guidelines.[16] Differences may exist between the expected duration tables and the normative graphs. Duration tables provide expected recovery periods based on the type of work performed by the individual. The normative graphs shown in Table 12-3 reflect the actual observed experience of many individuals across the spectrum of physical conditions, in a variety of industries, and with varying levels of case management. Recovery trends (in days) are derived from normative data for cases specifically identified with shoulder rotator cuff syndrome.

Conclusion

For shoulder impingement and rotator cuff syndrome, the decision to stay at work or return to work is primarily based on tolerance. Although the capacity may be limited for a short period after surgery, most individuals can return to previous levels. Capacity may be limited in chronic cases by decreased shoulder motion. Temporary work guides limiting hand-over-shoulder activities may be helpful. Returning to heavy work or very heavy work for extended periods may be difficult after surgery. Believable tolerance of pain in cases of impingement with severe imaging changes may be a basis for physicians to support a patient's decision to choose different work, although the words *work restriction* (based on risk) and *work limitation* (based on capacity) may not apply.

In reviewing the data in the table, it is interesting that the maximum time off work has increased for the "arthroscopic surgery for shoulder rotator cuff impingement" while the days off for "open surgery for shoulder rotator cuff impingement" has decreased. When this data is compared to the medical literature, most "arthroscopic technique" articles describe a shorter recovery time (disability) with their technique.[17–21]

This does not seem to be supported by actual numbers collected, but may illustrate the difference in "tolerance" because most "arthroscopic technique" articles are in "sports medicine" and not "workers' compensation" publications and consider return-to-sports but not return-to-work days.

Table 12-3 Recovery Trends (Days) With Shoulder Rotator Cuff Impingement

Reproduced with permission from Reed. www.mdguidelines.com.

Shoulder: Rotator Cuff Tear

The rotator cuff consists of four muscles that control three basic motions: abduction, internal rotation, and external rotation. The supraspinatus muscle is responsible for initiating abduction, the infraspinatus and teres minor muscles control external rotation, and the subscapularis muscle controls internal rotation. The rotator cuff muscles provide dynamic stabilization to the humeral head on the glenoid fossa, forming a force coupled with the deltoid to allow elevation of the arm. This force couple is responsible for 45% of abduction strength and 90% of external rotation strength. Acromion morphology may contribute to rotator cuff injuries. The risk increases with type 1 flat (17%), type 2 curved (43%), and type 3 anteriorly hooked (40%) acromions.

A rotator cuff injury (ICD-9-CM codes 718.0, 726.1, 726.10, 727.61, 726.19, 840.4 or ICD-10 codes M75.1, M75.8, M75.9) is an injury to one or more of the four tendons attaching muscles to the shoulder. This shoulder injury may come on suddenly and be associated with a specific injury such as a fall (acute), or it may become slowly and progressively worse over time without a specific injury incident. Return to work and outcomes are different for each type. Full-thickness tears are uncommon in individuals younger than 40 years but are present in 25% of individuals older than 60 years. Many of these are asymptomatic.

The Social Security Administration's disability requirements are the same as discussed in the previous section. However, as the size of the tear increases and the age increases, the likelihood of disability increases. Therefore, a shoulder rotator cuff tear may occasionally qualify for one-sided total upper extremity disability.

Risk Assessment

The risk of rotator cuff tear increases with age and is similar to that of shoulder impingement as outlined earlier. In patients with documented tears, repetitive activity that places major force on the cuff does risk extending the tear (increasing in size). Thus, work restrictions (based on risk) against repetitive lifting of heavier objects into positions requiring significant shoulder motion are appropriate. Similarly, after surgical repair of cuff tears, many surgeons impose restrictions on shoulder activity in the hope of preventing recurrent tears.

For surgically repaired rotator cuff tears, surgeons typically consider the effect of occupation on both shoulders. The larger the symptomatic cuff tear, the higher the chance of recurrent tearing after surgical repair.[22-23] Unrepaired partial-thickness and full-thickness cuff tears may worsen, or increase in size, over time.[24-25] Individuals with a symptomatic cuff tear in only one shoulder may have an asymptomatic cuff tear in the contralateral shoulder.[26]

Published epidemiologic studies of risk factors for rotator cuff pathology focus on the incidence or prevalence of rotator cuff tears in the working population and involve those not known to have rotator cuff disease. Those with known symptomatic tears may be genetically predisposed to cuff disease,[27] and thus may have more risk for progression or recurrence than individuals in the general population. This is the traditional justification for postoperative or postrehab physician-imposed activity restrictions based on risk. Unfortunately, other than recognizing that increased risk may be present in these situations, there is no published science to guide physicians in risk assessment, so physicians vary widely in the restrictions they impose in these cases.

Capacity

Capacity may be diminished in patients with rotator cuff tears by decreased motion or decreased strength. The larger the tear, the more it "disconnects" shoulder muscles from their normal bony attachments. Range of motion and strength can be quantified.

In the nonoperative group with small tears, activity modification and functional capacity are similar to those for shoulder impingement. The capacity after surgery is determined by the size of the tear; the quality of the cuff tissue as observed at surgery; whether the cuff could be anatomically repaired; the individual's age, occupation, and overall health; dominant side involvement; and success of rehabilitation. The duration of disability is longer than that for shoulder impingement. The larger the tear, the more likely that permanent weakness will result, and, therefore, heavy or very heavy work may no longer be possible. Additionally, there may be permanent disability regarding certain activities such as hand-over-shoulder movement.

Tolerance

Pain level may limit tolerance. The section on shoulder impingement gives the specifics. Tables 12-4 and 12-5 are provided as guides.

Conclusion

For rotator cuff tears, the decision to stay at work or return to work is primarily based on size of the tear and whether surgery is performed. Outcomes are better for acute rotator cuff tears. This is because the injury usually occurs in a younger patient with better rotator cuff substance. A chronic tear usually represents a wearing out of the cuff substance with age, and therefore repair is more difficult because the remaining tissue is weak. Capacity is further limited for short periods after surgery, and many individuals can return to previous employment levels with permanent work guides

Chapter 12

Table 12-4 Shoulder Rotator Cuff Tear Suggested Disability Durations (Days)

Job Classification	The Hand Center			The MDGuidelines 2005/2010		
	Target	TMinimum	TMaximum	Optimum	Minimum	Maximum
ICD-9-CM: 726.1, 726.10, 726.11, 726.19						
ICD-10: M75.1, M75.8, M75.9						
Nonsurgical Treatment for Shoulder Rotator Cuff Tear						
Sedentary	0	0	1	3*	0	4
Light	0	0	1	3	0	7
Medium	0	0	8	21	14	42
Heavy	14	0	42	42	28	84
Very Heavy	28	7	49	42	28	84
Arthroscopic Surgery for Shoulder Rotator Cuff Tear						
Sedentary				10	7	21
Light				10	7	21/42
Medium				42	28	56/70
Heavy				70/84	56	84/112
Very Heavy				70/112	56	84/140
Open Surgery for Shoulder Rotator Cuff Tear						
Sedentary	5	0	21	42/14	28/7	70
Light	5	0	21	56/21	28/21	84
Medium	21	7	28	84	42/84	140
Heavy	56	14	119	84/98	70/98	140
Very Heavy	70	18	133	84/112	70/112	140

* No change between 2005 and 2010 data if only one number in the MDGuidelines section.

Reproduced with permission from Reed. www.mdguidelines.com.

limiting hand-over-shoulder movement. Some residual long-term discomfort with activities is likely.

In reviewing the data in Table 12-4, it is interesting that, similar to impingement, the maximum time off work has increased for the "arthroscopic surgery for shoulder rotator cuff tear" while the days off for "open surgery for shoulder rotator cuff tear" have decreased for sedentary and light but increased for heavy and very heavy work categories. These data suggest that work demands do have an effect on return-to-work options.

Table 12-5 Duration Trends With Rotator Cuff Tear

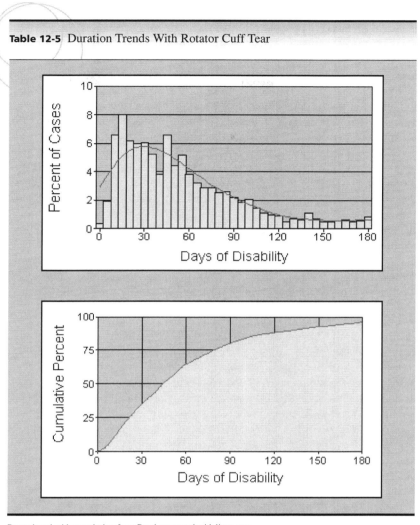

Reproduced with permission from Reed. www.mdguidelines.com.

Elbow: Lateral or Medial Epicondylitis

Epicondylitis (ICD-9-CM codes 726.31, 726.32 or ICD-10 codes M77, M77.0, M77.1) occurs when tendons in the elbow develop microscopic tears, and inflammation occurs at their attachments on the epicondyles, although the point of maximal pain is usually in the tendon substance just distal to the site of origin of the extensor carpi radialis brevis muscle (lateral) or the origin of the flexor/pronator tendons (medial). This process is known as *lateral epicondylitis* ("tennis elbow") if on the outside, or *medial epicondylitis* ("golfer's elbow") if on the inside. The term *epicondylitis* implies inflammation of the epicondyle or tissue adjoining the epicondyle of the humerus. The current opinion is that the early phase is inflammatory and often responds to anti-inflammatory medications and exercises. In the chronic (late) phase, when tissue biopsy is often done, there are no signs of inflammation, only degeneration. The term *angio-fibroblastic degeneration* is consistent with the findings of fibroblastic and vascular response in the tendon at biopsy, which has no evidence of immune cell inflammatory response.

Although the cause is unknown, epicondylitis may be associated with overuse or overexertion of the forearm and wrist muscles. Many tennis players have had symptoms of epicondylitis. Occupations that involve repetitive and/or stressful use of the forearm may be associated with a higher incidence of epicondylitis; affected groups include cooks, utility workers, secretaries (and others spending a great deal of time using a keyboard), assembly line workers, cashiers, carpenters, plumbers, butchers, and politicians. Individuals participating in tennis, golf, baseball, swimming, racquetball, fly-fishing, weight lifting, and track and field sports are at an increased risk of developing epicondylitis. Epicondylitis typically afflicts individuals between the ages of 35 and 50 years. Although men are twice as likely as women to develop medial epicondylitis, lateral epicondylitis afflicts men and women equally. Lateral epicondylitis is common, affecting approximately 2% of the US population, and is eight times more common than medial epicondylitis. The Social Security Administration's disability requirements for epicondylitis are similar and therefore a patient rarely qualifies for one-sided total upper extremity disability.

Risk Assessment

There is no significant risk with epicondylitis. There is no described syndrome of rupture of the involved tendon(s) resulting in disability. One of the surgical options for chronic cases involves removing the already necrotic tendon from its attachment on the epicondyle without reattaching the tendon. Thus, concern that the involved tendon may rupture with continued use is not logical.

The NIOSH review of the factors that may be involved in producing epicondylitis suggests that only jobs that require repetitive performance of high-force movements in awkward postures are epidemiologically linked to this syndrome. (See Table 12-6.) Thus most jobs do not pose a substantial risk, and the common problem is tolerance for symptoms, not risk. A more recent

British systematic review[28] and an American systematic review[29] each have failed to implicate most jobs as causing epicondylitis syndromes, so the vast majority of jobs should not be viewed as "risk factors." Thus, physician-imposed work restrictions are usually not appropriate.

Capacity

Capacity is not usually an issue with epicondylitis. Patients can do things, but they dislike doing what they can do because it hurts (tolerance). If a patient chooses not to use a limb, disuse atrophy may develop, which can be measured. Unlike some other conditions (osteoarthritis of the hip, for example), there is a poor correlation between the severity of imaging findings and the severity of the patient's clinical (pain) problem. Thus, there is not usually "severe objective evidence of pathology" to support physician evaluator agreement.

Tolerance

Tolerance for the pain associated with use of the hand is the issue in epicondylitis. Temporary modification of work activity (work guides) may be helpful while patients are treated with stretching and strengthening exercises, use of a counterforce brace, and perhaps a corticosteroid injection into the area of maximum tenderness.

For chronic cases, temporary work modification is not appropriate. Surgical treatment may decrease the associated pain. Ultimately the patient will need

Table 12-6 Risk Factors for Elbow Musculoskeletal Pain*

Body Part and Risk Factor	Strong Epidemiologic Evidence (+++)	Epidemiologic Evidence (++)	Insufficient Epidemiologic Evidence (+/0)	No Epidemiologic Evidence (−)
Elbow				
Repetition			X	
Force		X		
Posture			X	
Combination	X			

* See Table 12-1 for definitions of levels of evidence.

Source: United States Department of Health and Human Services. Musculoskeletal Disorders and Workplace Factors. A Critical Review of Epidemiologic Evidence for Work-Related Musculoskeletal Disorders of the Neck, Upper Extremity and Low Back. Cincinnati, OH: National Institute for Occupational Safety and Health, 1997.

Chapter 12

to choose to take a different job or to continue to put up with the pain. In many chronic cases the pain ultimately decreases, but this may take years to occur.

Temporary modification of activities includes limiting exposure to precipitating or exacerbating activity, but not total absence of activity. A change in job duties, sharing or alternating tasks, and limiting time and frequency of repetitive activities are important accommodations. Use of vibrating tools such as impact wrenches or jackhammers should be minimized. Increasing or decreasing the size of tool grips so the wrist can be held in the neutral position is also helpful. Use of splints, straps, and casts should be limited, as these can affect dexterity and may temporarily limit the individual's ability to lift and carry heavy or bulky objects, operate equipment, or perform other tasks requiring the use of both hands. An ergonometric evaluation of the workplace may be helpful.

Modified light work may be performed the day after surgery (maximum, 20 lbs or less lift/carry, with frequent lifting at 10 lbs for both arms). Up to 14 days after surgery, a light dressing is applied, no large power or vibratory tools are used, and extremity use on the operated-on side is limited. Work production may initially be decreased in the postoperative period. In general, the individual should gradually increase his or her activities at home and at work.[10]

Tolerance is primarily influenced by pain level and job requirements (use of wrist and forearm with or without power or vibratory tools and intensity of force). Temporary modification of the job on the basis of the following table is appropriate. Because this diagnosis is described as chronic, some persistent chronic pain with activity is likely even with surgical treatment. Table 12-7 includes suggested disability durations in days for elbow conditions.

Conclusion

For epicondylitis, risk and capacity are not the issue, and the decision to stay at work or return to work is primarily based on tolerance. There is thus no basis for permanent physician-imposed work restrictions or physician-described work limitations. Symptoms (pain) tend to be chronic with activities, although often not progressive. Although the capacity may be limited for short periods after surgery, most individuals can return to previous employment levels. Temporary work guides limiting combination activities may be helpful. Returning to very heavy work for expanded periods may be difficult, so the patient must decide whether the rewards of work outweigh the pain involved.

Table 12-7 Elbow Lateral or Medical Epicondylitis Suggested Disability Durations (Days)

Job Classification	The Hand Center			The MDGuidelines 2005/2010		
	Target	TMinimum	TMaximum	Optimum	Minimum	Maximum
Nonsurgical Treatment for Elbow Lateral or Medical Epicondylitis						
Sedentary	0	0	7	7*	0	28
Light	0	0	7	10	1	28
Medium	0	0	14	21	7	56
Heavy	0	0	21	28	14	56
Very Heavy	0	0	28	28	14	56
Open Surgery for Elbow Lateral or Medical Epicondylitis						
Sedentary	0	0	7			
Light	0	0	7			
Medium	7	0	21			
Heavy	14	0	28			
Very Heavy	21	7	32			

ICD-9-CM: 726.31, 726.32
ICD-10: M77, M77.0, M77.1

* No change between 2005 and 2010 data if only one number in the MDGuidelines section.

Reproduced with permission from Reed. www.mdguidelines.com.

Elbow: Ulnar Nerve Entrapment

Ulnar nerve entrapment at the elbow (ICD-9-CM code 354.2, 354.4, 354.8, 354.9 or ICD-10 code G56.2, G56.8, G56.9, S44.0, S54.0, S64.0) is the second most common entrapment neuropathy in the upper extremity (the first being the median nerve at the wrist, ie, carpal tunnel syndrome).

The elbow is the most vulnerable point of the ulnar nerve: here it is superficial and fixed and crosses a joint. Because of the anatomic positioning of the ulnar nerve, it is subject to entrapment and injury. Nerves are fragile and can be damaged by pressure, stretching, or cutting. Because of its superficial position at the elbow, the ulnar nerve may be injured either by sustained excessive pressure or by repetitive contusion (bumping).

Overstretching of the nerve, either from sustained posturing in near-full elbow flexion or from highly repetitive elbow flexion, can also injure the nerve. The nerve loses its ability to conduct, and the small intrinsic muscles of the hand become dysfunctional. Sensory loss may occur, most commonly in the little finger and the ulnar half of the ring finger.

In early cases the symptoms are suggestive, but physical examination and electrodiagnostic tests fail to confirm the diagnosis. Cases that progress to major nerve damage are rare.

The Social Security Administration's disability requirements are the same as discussed earlier in this chapter. Therefore, ulnar nerve entrapment at the elbow rarely qualifies for one-sided total upper extremity disability.

Risk Assessment

Ulnar nerve function can be assessed. Parameters such as two-point sensation testing of the little finger, grip strength, and finger abduction strength can be assessed by physical examination, although these require the cooperation of the patient. Nerve conduction testing can document the conduction velocity of the ulnar nerve in the segment crossing the elbow. No patient cooperation is necessary for this test. These tests can be repeated, permitting assessment of change over time. If repeat nerve conduction testing (electrodiagnostics) is done, only the ulnar nerve studies need to be repeated. If nerve function is documented at multiple office visits, and if it is clearly worsening with continued work activity and subsequently improves with temporary work restrictions, it is reasonable to conclude that this work activity is a risk to this patient's ulnar nerve. Either permanent work restrictions or surgical treatment would be indicated. Generally the weight lifted at work is not a problem. Restrictions should address sustained posturing with the elbow in flexion of greater than 90 degrees, highly repetitive elbow flexion, and repetitive contusion of or sustained pressure on the nerve. Ulnar neuropathy can also cause decreased sensation on the ulnar side of the hand. If "protective" sensation (most easily measured as sharp-dull discrimination) is lost (very unusual), the patient may need restrictions precluding work around hot or sharp objects that would risk cutting or burning skin that lacks its normal protective sensation.

If results of multiple physical examination and nerve conduction tests show that ulnar nerve function is either stable or improving despite continued work activity, the reasonable conclusion is that this work activity does *not* pose a risk to this patient's ulnar nerve. Whether the patient chooses to tolerate symptoms is then the issue.

Two recent systematic reviews have failed to implicate work as a cause of ulnar neuropathy at the elbow,[29–30] so most jobs are unlikely to be a risk for patients with this disorder.

Capacity

Capacity may be affected by ulnar neuropathy. Grip strength (due to weakness in the flexor profundus) and hand dexterity can be affected, and these deficits can be measured. A Jamar dynamometer can quantify grip strength, and tests like the Perdue Peg Board Test (available through physical therapists and/or occupational therapists) can assess hand dexterity. These deficits can affect the ability to do routine factory work and can be described by physicians as work limitations.

Tolerance

Tolerance for symptoms such as pain and paresthesia is the most frequent problem. If tests of nerve function confirm that ulnar neuropathy with significant nerve function impairment is the correct diagnosis, most physicians would feel the symptoms are believable and the condition is at a level of severity that justifies physician support for work modification. This is not work restriction based on risk, but rather guidance and support based on tolerance in the presence of severe, objectively documented pathology. If there is evidence of nerve damage, the nerve may well be at risk, as discussed above.

In the early phases of neuropathy, work activity may be a problem based on tolerance of pain and/or numbness, while in late phases capacity is limited by functional loss. All phases are influenced by the individual's age, occupation, dominant or nondominant arm affected, response to treatment, and compliance with treatment recommendations and rehabilitation programs during the recovery period. Job modification may be helpful. Ergonometric assessment can help with workplace modifications. Suggested disability durations in days for elbow ulnar nerve entrapment are listed in Table 12-8.

Conclusion

For early ulnar nerve elbow entrapment, the decision to stay at work or retur to work is primarily based on tolerance. If the diagnosis and treatment (including surgery) are early, before permanent major nerve damage occurs, residual functional loss should be minimal. However, if muscle atrophy or weakness is present on physical examination, even with surgery, permanent functional loss and residual disability are more likely. Although the capacity may be limited for a short period after surgery, most individuals can return to previous employment levels, especially if permanent modifications, such as task rotation and limitations of power and vibratory tool exposure, can be implemented.

In reviewing the data in Table 12-8, it is interesting that the MDA now provides data for nonsurgical treatment. Additionally, the optimum and

Table 12-8 Elbow Ulnar Nerve Elbow Suggested Disability Durations (Days)

Job Classification	The Hand Center			The MDGuidelines 2005/2010		
	Target	TMinimum	TMaximum	Optimum	Minimum	Maximum
Nonsurgical Treatment for Elbow Ulnar Nerve Elbow						
Sedentary	0	0	7	x/7	x/0	x/28
Light	0	0	7	x/10	x/1	x/28
Medium	0	0	14	x/21	x/7	x/56
Heavy	0	0	21	x/28	x/14	x/56
Very Heavy	0	0	28	x/28	x/14	x/56
Open Surgery for Elbow Ulnar Nerve Elbow						
Sedentary	0	0	7	21/14	7	42/28
Light	0	0	7	28*	7	42
Medium	14	0	28	56/42	28	365/84
Heavy	21	0	47	98/56	28/35	365/112
Very Heavy	28	0	56	98/84	42	365/126

ICD-9-CM: 354.2, 354.4, 354.8, 354.9

ICD-10: G56.2, G56.8, G56.9, S44.0, S54.0, S64.0

* No change between 2005 and 2010 data if only one number in the MDGuidelines section.
x No data for 2005.

Reproduced with permission from Reed. www.mdguidelines.com.

maximum times off work have decreased significantly over the last 5 years (perhaps a result, at least in part, of the efforts to educate physicians regarding the need to reduce unnecessary disabilities days).

Wrist: Carpal Tunnel Syndrome

Considerable controversy continues to surround the cause (etiology), definition, diagnosis, and treatment of persons with carpal tunnel syndrome (CTS) (ICD-9-CM codes 354, 354.0 or ICD-10 codes G56, G56.0, G56.1). CTS is also known as *median nerve compression neuropathy* and is actually a condition (with a known pathophysiology) and not a syndrome, but the name *carpal tunnel syndrome* has become so well known that CTS will be used here rather than median nerve compression neuropathy. It is a condition in which pain, prickling, tingling (paresthesia), or numbness radiates from the wrist into the palm of the hand and then down into the thumb, index finger, middle finger, and the thumb side of the ring finger. It is caused by elevated pressure on the median nerve. The main (median) nerve and its branches enter the hand through an internal opening (the carpal tunnel) formed by the wrist bones (carpal bones) and the tough membrane that holds the bones together (transverse carpal ligament). The median nerve supplies sensation to the palm of the hand, thumb, and radial 3 fingers. Because this passageway is rigid, inflammation, swelling, or increased fluid retention may compress the nerve (nerve entrapment), causing pain and changes in sensation along the pathways where the nerve runs. Pain may eventually extend to the arm, shoulder, or neck.

Carpal tunnel syndrome may be diagnosed clinically, but it is frequently a difficult diagnosis. There is no pathognomonic test on physical examination, and those physical examination findings that exist have a low sensitivity, specificity, and reliability.[31–33] Nerve conduction testing is the only objective test available, and no national organization defines for CTS what is a normal or an abnormal test result, but practice parameters have been attempted.[34] Each physician performing nerve conduction tests must choose his or her own definition of normal.

Most of the literature on causation of CTS is flawed. Most of the studies are cross sectional, which means that they can generate hypotheses for testing by prospective studies, but by themselves they do not prove causation. Many of the studies use a clinical definition of CTS and not nerve conduction testing for diagnosis, so in studies on the relationship of work activity to CTS, many of the individuals labeled as having CTS do not actually have it.[35] Fifty-nine medical conditions (diseases or injuries) have been reported to be associated with CTS.[36] Thus, in a single individual with CTS, it is impossible to reason from the literature whether work activity was part of the cause of the CTS.

Many countries and the state of Virginia do not accept CTS as work related. The debate on causation is critical to a discussion of risk.[37] The unfounded premise that work is a "toxin" to the carpal tunnel and, therefore, physicians should limit exposure to the toxin by having physician-imposed work restrictions, should not be considered to be scientifically proven yet.

The Social Security Administration's disability requirements are the same as discussed earlier in this chapter. Therefore, carpal tunnel syndrome rarely qualifies for one-sided total upper extremity disability.

Risk Assessment
As mentioned earlier, if work activities are considered as a contributor (risk factor) to the development of CTS, physicians should consider limiting

Chapter 12

exposure to the risk factor by providing workplace guides or restrictions. The NIOSH review of studies suggested that only in combination of all the ergonomic factors is there strong evidence of causation. (See Table 12-9.)

The only prospective study published in English that did use nerve conduction studies to diagnose CTS concluded that female sex, greater age at baseline, and obesity predict the later development of CTS. Repetition, force, heavy lifting, and keyboard use were not predictive.[38] Thus, in a single individual with CTS, it is impossible to reason from the literature whether specific work activities contributed to or aggravated a preexisting CTS.[29] The determination of work compensibility is based on a legal definition and is not necessarily based or supported by the medical literature.[40,41]

Similar to the preceding discussion of ulnar neuropathy, median nerve function can be assessed at multiple office visits. Testing of sensation (for example, by two-point discrimination) and testing of motor function (by thenar atrophy and thenar opposition weakness) can be performed during physical examination. Nerve conduction studies on the median nerve can be repeated (the study of all the nerves in the limb does not need to be repeated; only one or some of the median nerve studies need to be repeated).

If nerve function is documented at multiple office visits, and if median nerve function is clearly worse with continued work activity and subsequently improves with temporary work restrictions, it is reasonable to conclude that

Table 12-9 Risk Factors for Carpal Tunnel Syndrome*

Body Part and Risk Factor	Strong Epidemiologic Evidence (+++)	Epidemiologic Evidence (++)	Insufficient Epidemiologic Evidence (+/0)	No Epidemiologic Evidence (−)
Hand/wrist: Carpal Tunnel Syndrome				
Repetition		X		
Force		X		
Posture			X	
Vibration		X		
Combination	X			

* See Table 12-1 for definitions of levels of evidence.

Source: United States Department of Health and Human Services. Musculoskeletal Disorders and Workplace Factors. A Critical Review of Epidemiologic Evidence for Work-Related Musculoskeletal Disorders of the Neck, Upper Extremity and Low Back. Cincinnati, OH: National Institute for Occupational Safety and Health, 1997.

this work activity is a risk to this patient's median nerve. Either permanent work restrictions or surgical treatment would be indicated. Generally the weight lifted at work is not a problem. Restrictions should address sustained posturing with the wrist in flexion or extension of greater than 30 degrees, highly repetitive wrist motion, and sustained pressure on the nerve.

Carpal tunnel syndrome can also cause decreased sensation on the radial side of the hand. If protective sensation (most easily measured as sharp-dull discrimination or two-point discrimination of 15 mm) is lost, the patient may need restrictions precluding work around hot or sharp objects that would risk cutting or burning skin that lacks its normal protective sensation.

If results of multiple physical examination and nerve conduction tests show that median nerve function is either stable or improving despite continued work activity, the reasonable conclusion is that this work activity does *not* pose a risk to this patient's median nerve. Whether the patient chooses to tolerate symptoms is then the issue. In the largest published study of the natural course of untreated CTS, patients were most likely to remain unchanged, but were more likely to improve than to worsen in terms of elec-trodiagnostic study class, symptoms, pain, and function.[41] This suggests that short-term risk is not a major issue in most cases of CTS.

Although the popular media suggests that keyboard activity causes CTS, the science shows otherwise.[29] Nine studies have reviewed this relation-ship. The results show that keyboards are safe to use and do not cause CTS.[35,38,41,43–49] Furthermore, keyboard redesign had no effect on incidence of CTS.[50,51] Symptoms may increase with many activities, including the use of keyboards, but keyboards do not cause CTS.[29]

Capacity

Capacity may be affected by CTS. Grip strength is not usually affected, as the nerve compression occurs distal to the forearm muscles involved in grip. Pain may limit grip, but that is an issue of tolerance. Hand dexterity can be affected, and these deficits can be measured with tests like the Perdue Peg Board Test (available through physical therapists and/or occupational therapists) that can assess hand dexterity. These deficits can affect the abil-ity to do routine factory work and can be described by physicians as work limitations.

Tolerance

Tolerance for symptoms like pain and paresthesia is the most frequent prob-lem. If tests of nerve function confirm that CTS is the correct diagnosis, many physicians would feel the symptoms are believable and the condition is at a level of severity that justifies work restrictions. This is not work restriction based on risk, but rather restriction based on tolerance in the presence of significant, objectively documented pathology. The problem with this position is that there is no uniformly accepted definition of CTS by nerve conduction studies. Many cases diagnosed as "mild CTS" by nerve conduction testing are false-positive cases. These cases explain most of the now-frequent case scenarios of "mild CTS" (false positives) that fail to respond to appropriate treatment. Nonspecific hand and arm pain (ICD-9-CM code 729.5) and numbness (782.0) are common, may be misdiagnosed as CTS, and will fail to respond to carpal tunnel release.

If there is nerve conduction test or physical exam evidence of nerve damage, the nerve may well be at risk, as discussed above. Surgical treatment is logical if there is nerve damage. This is an issue of risk and not of tolerance. Physical exam evidence of nerve damage is a late finding, long after nerve conduction tests become very abnormal.

In the early stages of CTS, work activity may be a problem based on tolerance of pain and numbness, while in late stages capacity is limited by nerve function lost. All phases are influenced by the individual's age, occupation, whether the dominant or nondominant arm is affected, the response to treatment, and the compliance with treatment recommendations and rehabilitation programs during the recovery period. Job modification may be helpful. Ergonometric assessment can help with workplace modifications. Suggested disability durations (in days) for CTS are listed in Table 12-10.

Conclusion

For early cases of CTS, the decision to stay at work or return to work is primarily based on tolerance of symptoms. If diagnosis and treatment (including surgery) are early, residual functional loss is rare. However, if muscle weakness or atrophy or sensory loss is present on physical examination, even with surgery, permanent functional loss and residual disability are more likely. Although the capacity may be limited for a short period after surgery, most individuals can return to previous employment levels, but perhaps with permanent modifications or task rotation and limitations of power and vibratory tool exposure.

In reviewing the data in Table 12-10, it is interesting that the optimum time off work has decreased for light and medium jobs but the maximum time has increased for very heavy jobs. The disability duration days for CTS have decreased some, but not as much as Ulnar Nerve Elbow Entrapment (UNE), also called Cubital Tunnel Syndrome. Why? The disability duration days for UNE were much higher to start with, suggesting that the ability for the physician to modify tolerance through education had a greater window of opportunity.

Table 12-10 Wrist Carpal Tunnel Syndrome Suggested Disability Durations (Days)

	ICD-9-CM: 354. 354.0					
	ICD-10: G56, G56.0, G56.1					
Job Classification	The Hand Center			The MDGuidelines 2005/2010		
	Target	TMinimum	TMaximum	Optimum	Minimum	Maximum
Nonsurgical Treatment for Wrist Carpal Tunnel Syndrome						
Sedentary	0	0	7	7*	0	21
Light	0	0	7	7	0	21
Medium	0	0	12	14	0	28
Heavy	0	0	21	21	0	42
Very Heavy	0	0	28	18/28	0	63
Open Surgery for Wrist Carpal Tunnel Syndrome						
Sedentary	0	0	7	14	1	42
Light	0	0	7	28/21	1/3	42
Medium	14	0	28	42/28	14	56
Heavy	21	0	42	42	28/21	84
Very Heavy	28	3	61	56	28	84/91

* No change between 2005 and 2010 data if only one number in the MDGuidelines section.

Reproduced with permission from Reed. www.mdguidelines.com.

Wrist: De Quervain's Tenosynovitis

Stenosing tenosynovitis of the extensor pollicis brevis and abductor pollicis longus tendons is a condition in which the tendons and their covering tenosynovium, or tendon sheaths, become inflamed. The precise cause of de Quervain's tenosynovitis (ICD-9-CM codes 727.04, 82, 82.0, 82.01 or ICD-10 code M65.4) is unknown. The involved tendons are usually normal, but the tendon covering is inflamed. Because the area within the tunnel for the tendons is confined, any inflammation reduces available space for the tendon-pulley mechanism to function. Pain and increased inflammation are caused when the tendons and their swollen sheaths are pulled through the tighter space. It becomes difficult for the tendons to move, and consequently they begin to catch and rub, producing jerky movements and causing more pain and inflammation.

The Social Security Administration's disability requirements are the same as discussed earlier in this chapter. Therefore, de Quervain's tenosynovitis rarely qualifies for one-sided total upper extremity disability.

Risk Assessment

The NIOSH review of published studies suggests the evidence shown in Table 12-11 that work activities cause de Quervain's tenosynovitis.

It is rare for the involved tendons to rupture, so there is no risk of significant harm that is imminent. It is safe (risk) but painful (tolerance) to do work tasks when afflicted with de Quervain's tenosynovitis. Thus, there is no basis for work restrictions.

Capacity

Work capacity is not usually affected by this condition. Wrist range of motion is preserved. Grip strength and function are normal. Moving the wrist into simultaneous flexion and ulnar deviation provokes the pain of this condition, but patients can do what is painful. Thus, there are no work limitations.

Tolerance

For de Quervain's tenosynovitis, the decision to stay at work or return to work is primarily based on tolerance. Symptoms tend to be chronic with activities, although often not progressive. Temporary work modifications (but not total absence from aggravating tasks) while undergoing treatment may help to minimize symptoms and speed recovery. Surgical treatment is usually successful. Although the capacity for work may be limited for a short period after surgery, most individuals can return to previous employment levels. Work guides limiting combination activities (especially repetitive simultaneous

Table 12-11 Risk Factors for Hand or Wrist Tendinitis*

Body Part and Risk Factor	Strong Epidemiologic Evidence (+++)	Epidemiologic Evidence (++)	Insufficient Epidemiologic Evidence (+/0)	No Epidemiologic Evidence (−)
Hand/Wrist Tendinitis				
Repetition		X		
Force		X		
Posture		X		
Combination	X			

* See Table 12-1 for definitions of levels of evidence.

Source: United States Department of Health and Human Services. Musculoskeletal Disorders and Workplace Factors. A Critical Review of Epidemiologic Evidence for Work-Related Musculoskeletal Disorders of the Neck, Upper Extremity and Low Back. Cincinnati, OH: National Institute for Occupational Safety and Health, 1997.

wrist flexion and ulnar deviation) may be helpful. In general, the individual should gradually increase activities at home and at work.[14]

Returning to very heavy work for expanded periods may be difficult (painful), resulting in the need for career decisions. Table 12-12 includes suggested disability durations (in days) for de Quervain's tenosynovitis.

Conclusion

For de Quervain's tenosynovitis, the decision to stay at work or return to work is primarily based on tolerance. Symptoms may be chronic with activities, although often not progressive. Although the capacity may be limited for a short period after surgery, most individuals can return to previous employment levels. Work guides limiting combination activities may be helpful. Returning to very heavy work for expanded periods may be difficult (painful, an issue of tolerance), resulting in the need for career decisions. Tolerance as the key factor is reflected by little change in the duration days over the last 5 years.

Table 12-12 Wrist de Quervain's Disease Suggested Disability Durations (Days)

Job Classification	The Hand Center			The MDGuidelines 2005/2010		
	Target	TMinimum	TMaximum	Optimum	Minimum	Maximum
ICD-9-CM: 727.04						
ICD-10: M65.4						
CPT: 25000						
Nonsurgical Treatment for Wrist de Quervain's Disease						
Sedentary	0	0	7			
Light	0	0	7			
Medium	0	0	14			
Heavy	0	0	21			
Very Heavy	0	0	28			
Open Surgery for Wrist de Quervain's Disease						
Sedentary	0	0	7	7*	1	21
Light	0	0	7	14	3	21/28
Medium	7	0	14	21	7	42
Heavy	14	0	21	28	21	56
Very Heavy	21	0	35	28	21	56/70

* No change between 2005 and 2010 data if only one number in the MDGuidelines section.

Reproduced with permission from Reed. www.mdguidelines.com.

Chapter 12

Finger or Thumb: Trigger

Trigger finger (ICD-9-CM codes 727.0, 727.03 or ICD-10 codes M65, M65.3) (also known as stenosing tenosynovitis) is the equivalent of de Quervain's tenosynovitis, but affecting a finger or thumb instead of the wrist. *Trigger finger* refers to a sensation in which the fingers or thumb feel stuck or temporarily snagged during efforts to straighten or bend the digit. The condition is caused by swelling often accompanied by inflammation that narrows the hand's tunnels (flexor sheath or A-1 pulley) where tendons glide back and forth to allow movement of the hand and fingers. The tendon itself may develop a knot (nodule) caused by irritation from rubbing against the narrowed tunnel walls of the sheath, similar to a knotted rope repeatedly passing through a constricted area. As the tendon pulls free of any obstacles, a snapping sensation (triggering) accompanied by pain may then be felt. The snapping movement likely will create more damage to the affected area, resulting in even more inflammation and swelling that creates additional narrowing and interference with hand and finger movement. The cycle of damage could result in the finger or thumb becoming stuck or locked, with movement becoming increasingly more painful and difficult. The underlying cause of inflammation creating the condition often is not known, but it can be associated with diseases such as rheumatoid arthritis and diabetes mellitus. Studies indicate that trigger finger is related to certain occupations and repetitive tasks. One Canadian study indicated a 14% prevalence of trigger finger among workers in a meat-packing plant, with the incidence being higher among hand tool users.[52]

The Social Security Administration's disability requirements are the same as discussed earlier in this chapter. Therefore, trigger thumb or finger tenosynovitis rarely qualifies for one-sided total upper extremity disability.

Risk Assessment

The risk for trigger finger or thumb is similar to that of de Quervain's tenosynovitis of the wrist, as outlined above. Even in severe cases it is very rare for the involved tendon to rupture. If the digit becomes locked (unable to flex or unable to extend because the knot in the tendon can no longer pass through the constriction), there is a risk of permanent loss of digit motion. Digits that do not move may become permanently stiff. Thus, for the uncommon locked digit, urgent surgical treatment and work restrictions are appropriate.

Capacity

In the common "triggering" or snapping digit scenario, capacity or grip strength and hand dexterity are minimally affected. Trigger finger thus is not generally an issue of capacity.

Tolerance

For trigger finger or thumb, the decision to stay at work or return to work is primarily based on tolerance. Patients can use the involved digit, but to do so is painful. Nonoperative treatment with a brief period of temporary work modification is frequently successful. Comfortable hand function is compromised enough that patients who fail to respond to nonoperative treatment almost always choose to have surgical treatment. Trigger finger release surgery is almost always successful. Thus, trigger finger is rarely a reason for any permanent work problem. Over time, with continued performance of work tasks, additional digits may become involved, but each usually responds to treatment. Table 12-13 contains suggested disability durations in days for trigger digits, and the duration and trend data is listed in Table 12-14.

Conclusion

For trigger finger or thumb, the decision to stay at work or return to work is primarily based on tolerance. Tolerance is associated with the pain level experienced with movement of the digit. Surgery often results in marked improvement, although the capacity may be limited for a short period after surgery. After surgery, most individuals can return to their previous employment. Temporary work guides limiting combination activities may be helpful. Again, tolerance is the key and therefore little change in the data for the last 5 years is seen.

Chapter 12

Nontraumatic Soft-Tissue Disorder

Nontraumatic soft-tissue disorder, ICD-9-CM code 729.5, (sometimes also considered as 842, 842.1, 842.10, 842.11, 842.12 or ICD-10 codes S63, S63.6, S63.7) is used to describe discomfort affecting any part of an extremity (such as an elbow) or the entire limb (arm or leg). The term is general and could be used to describe pain that arises from various causes. Common synonyms include regional arm pain, musculoskeletal disorders, musculoskeletal pain, cumulative trauma disorder, and repetitive strain injury.

The pain may arise from the skin, nerves, muscles, bones, joints, or even the brain (in psychogenic or phantom pain). Typically, the term *pain in the limb*

Table 12-13 Hand Trigger Finger or Thumb Suggested Disability Durations (Days)

	ICD-9-CM: 727.0, 727.03					
	ICD-10: M65, M65.3					
Job Classification	The Hand Center			The MDGuidelines 2005/2010		
	Target	TMinimum	TMaximum	Optimum	Minimum	Maximum
Nonsurgical Treatment for Hand Trigger Finger or Thumb						
Sedentary	0	0	7	7*	1	21/14
Light	0	0	7	7	1	21
Medium	0	0	7	7	3	28
Heavy	0	0	14	7	5	35
Very Heavy	0	0	14	7	5	42
Open Surgery for Hand Trigger Finger or Thumb						
Sedentary	0	0	7	14	1	28
Light	0	0	7	14	3	28
Medium	7	0	28	21	7	35
Heavy	21	3	35	28	21	42
Very Heavy	21	7	35	28	21	42

* No change between 2005 and 2010 data if only one number in the MDGuidelines section.

Reproduced with permission from Reed. www.mdguidelines.com.

would be used to describe a person's symptoms until a definitive diagnosis is made (such as a broken arm, tendinitis, peripheral neuropathy, etc). In many of these cases, no specific diagnosis is ever possible.

The Social Security Administration's disability requirements are the same as discussed earlier in this chapter. Therefore, nontraumatic soft-tissue disorder or musculoskeletal disorder rarely qualifies for one-sided total upper extremity disability.

Risk Assessment

Although the pain may be associated with physical activities, it is often difficult to establish a reasonable cause and effect: *post hoc ergo propter hoc* (after the fact, therefore because of the fact).[53] Arguments based only on temporal relationships for workers' compensation causation or impairments are logic fallacies, especially in degenerative conditions, as the normal progression of degeneration will lead to worsening in and of itself over time.[54]

Table 12-14 Real-world Disability Case Data

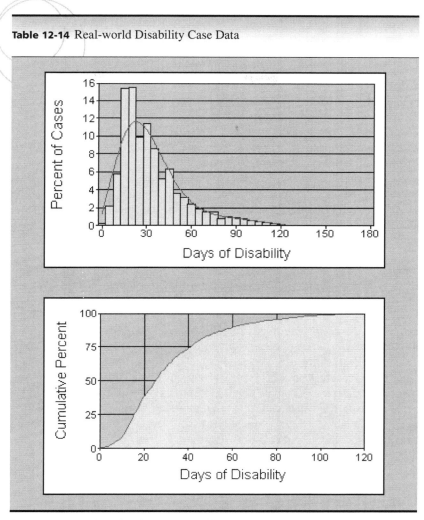

Reproduced with permission from Reed. www.mdguidelines.com.

In the absence of a specific objectively verifiable diagnosis, there is no risk, and thus no basis for physician-imposed work restrictions.

Capacity

Because the individual often lacks a specific musculoskeletal diagnosis, unless limited capacity is currently present on the basis of deconditioning, nonspecific hand and/or arm pain does not affect capacity. In general, the goal is to encourage maximum function and limit dysfunction.

Tolerance

Pain is the limiting factor for tolerance of work activities. Pain is a fluid concept and cannot be proved or disproved by a physician.[55] The International Association for the Study of Pain defines *pain* as an unpleasant sensory and emotional experience associated with actual or potential tissue damage, or described in terms of such damage.[56] At its most basic level, pain is both a physical phenomenon (presence of activity in discrete neural pathways) and a psychological or emotional experience ("it hurts"). Theoretically, pain serves the useful function of prevention of tissue damage. Pain is actually a homeostatic mechanism.[57] It is only when pain becomes chronic, and no longer predictive of possible tissue damage, that it serves no useful function.[58]

Tolerance for pain is the limiting factor for the patient's decision to stay at work or return to work in nonspecific hand and/or arm pain. Symptoms tend to be chronic with activities, although often not progressive. Although work modifications for short periods may be recommended, physicians should encourage increasing tolerance through education and communication and through progressive increases in activity. This can be difficult when the individual reports that any and all activities make the pain worse. Discussions regarding musculoskeletal pain and its relationship to the individual and workplace risk factors may be helpful.[57] General physical conditioning, appropriate diet and sleep habits, and limitation of caffeine and nicotine are helpful.[59] Ergonometric assessment and modification of the workplace may be considered. Suggested disability durations in days for nontraumatic soft-tissue disorders are listed in Table 12-15.

Conclusion

Patients with nontraumatic soft-tissue disorders or work-related nonspecific musculoskeletal pain are often the most frustrating for the health care provider. The response to treatment is often intermittent and inconsistent. Symptoms can remain disproportional to the clinical findings despite appropriate conservative medical care and reasonable modifications to the workplace. Because pain is a plural concept with biological, psychological, and social components, and because its perception is influenced by cognitive, behavioral, environmental, and cultural factors, successful management requires the health care provider to go beyond the traditional medical model.[60] Treatment must also address these nonmedical issues to obtain better outcomes.[61–64] Prevention has been the most successful management for this group of patients.[65]

Table 12-15 Nontraumatic Soft-Tissue Disorders Suggested Disability Durations (Days)

Job Classification	The Hand Center			The MDGuidelines 2005/2010		
	Target	TMinimum	TMaximum	Optimum	Minimum	Maximum
MDGuidelines 2010 as sprains and strains hand or fingers interphalangeal joint						
ICD-9-CM: 842, 842.1, 842.10, 842.11, 842.12						
ICD-10: S63, S63.6, S63.7						
Nonsurgical Treatment for Nontraumatic Soft-Tissue Disorders						
Sedentary	0	0	4	0/7	3/1	7/14
Light	0	0	5	0/7	3/1	7/21
Medium	0	0	7	1/14	3/1	7/42
Heavy	0	0	14	1/21	3/2	7/56
Very Heavy	0	0	14	1/21	3/2	7/70

* No change between 2005 and 2010 data if only one number in the MDGuidelines section.

Reproduced with permission from Reed. www.mdguidelines.com.

In reviewing the data in Table 12-16, it is interesting that the maximum time off work has increased for the "nontraumatic soft-tissue disorders" while the minimum has decreased. This reflects an understanding by some physicians that tolerance is the issue with which doctors, employers, employees, and insurers struggle. Tolerance is the ability to put up with the symptoms (like pain or fatigue) that accompany doing work tasks in order to gain the rewards of work (income, self-esteem, health benefits, etc). Tolerance means the ability to tolerate the symptoms produced by doing an activity the individual clearly can do. Tolerance is not a scientific concept, and tolerance is not scientifically measurable. Early after major injury or surgery, physicians have fair agreement on work guidelines based in tolerance issues, but for chronic problems studies have shown physicians cannot agree on work guidelines based on tolerance issues. Patients consider factors like income and finances, job satisfaction, need for employer-provided health insurance benefits, availability of disability or workers' compensation insurance to maintain income, ability to switch to physically easier careers, etc when deciding whether the rewards of working are to them worth the "cost" of working.

Additional diagnosis-specific reviews have been added at the request of readers to provide additional insight to suggested disability durations. Readers are encouraged to contact Dr. Melhorn by email at Melhorn@CtdMAP.com with additional upper limb diagnoses they would like to see added to future editions of this book.

Chapter 12

Table 12-16 Wrist Ulnar Nerve Wrist Suggested Disability Durations (Days)

Job Classification	The Hand Center			The MDGuidelines 2005/2010		
	Target	TMinimum	TMaximum	Optimum	Minimum	Maximum
Nonsurgical Treatment for Wrist Ulnar Nerve Wrist						
Sedentary	a/0	a/0	a/7	x/7	x/0	x/21
Light	a/0	a/0	a/7	x/7	x/0	x/21
Medium	a/0	a/0	a/14	x/14	x/0	x/28
Heavy	a/0	a/0	a/14	x/21	x/0	x/42
Very Heavy	a/0	a/0	a/21	x/28	x/0	x/63
Open Surgery for Wrist Ulnar Nerve Wrist						
Sedentary	0 b	0	7			
Light	0	0	7			
Medium	14	0	21			
Heavy	21	0	28			
Very Heavy	28	3	35			

ICD-9-CM: 354.2, 354.4, 354.8, 354.9

ICD-10: G56.2, G56.8, G56.9, S44.0, S54.0. S64.0

* No change between 2005 and 2010 data if only one number in the MDGuidelines section.
x No data for 2005.
a Data available in 2005 but not published.
b Very small numbers available for this diagnosis.

Reproduced with permission from Reed. www.mdguidelines.com.

Ulnar Neuropathy at the Wrist

Ulnar nerve entrapment at the wrist (ICD-9-CM codes 354.2, 354.4, 354.8, 354.9 or ICD-10 codes G56.2, G56.8. G56.9, S44.0, S54.0, S64.0) can occur where the ulnar nerve and artery pass through a very small tunnel called Guyon's canal. Entrapment of the ulnar nerve at the wrist is uncommon and is usually a result of a direct blow over this area, on the palm, or near the wrist that can cause inflammation and compression of the nerve. An example is fracture of the hook of the hamate, which is next to the ulnar nerve. Even less common is compression or inflammation from repetitive trauma such as using a hammer. A cyst (ganglion) or an aneurysm in the ulnar artery in the canal also can put pressure on the nerve.

The Social Security Administration's disability requirements are the same as discussed earlier in this chapter. Therefore, ulnar nerve entrapment at the wrist rarely qualifies for one-sided total upper extremity disability.

Risk Assessment

Studies for association with activities for ulnar nerve wrist entrapment are limited. Therefore, the consensus suggestion would be to use the NIOSH CTS data that suggests only in combination of all the ergonomic factors is there strong evidence of causation. (See Table 12-9.)

Capacity

Capacity can be affected by ulnar nerve wrist entrapment, depending on the cause of the entrapment. For example, a cyst (mass) may swell and be painful with gripping. An aneurysm may enlarge and be painful with activities. Gripping power tools may be difficult.

Tolerance

Each individual's tolerance for symptoms like pain and paresthesia is different. Nerve testing is sometimes helpful to gauge tolerance and confirm diagnosis. Believable symptoms often result in work restrictions. These work restrictions may not be based on risk, but rather on tolerance in the absence of objectively documented pathology. Tolerance is influenced by the individual's age, occupation, whether the dominant or nondominant arm is affected, the response to treatment, and the compliance with treatment recommendations and rehabilitation programs during the recovery period. Job modification may be helpful. Ergonometric assessment can help with workplace modifications. Suggested disability durations (in days) for ulnar nerve wrist are listed in Table 12-16, and the duration trend is listed in Table 12-17.

Conclusion

For early cases of ulnar nerve wrist entrapment, the decision to stay at work or return to work is primarily based on tolerance of symptoms. If diagnosis and treatment (including surgery) are early, residual functional loss is rare. However, if muscle weakness or atrophy or sensory loss is present on physical examination, even with surgery, permanent functional loss and residual disability are more likely. Although the capacity may be limited for a short period after surgery, most individuals can return to previous employment levels, but perhaps with permanent modifications or task rotation and limitations of power and vibratory tool exposure.

Synovial Cyst

A synovial cyst or ganglion (ICD-9-CM codes 727.4, 727.40, 727.41, 727.42, 727.43, 727.51 or ICD-10 codes M67.4, M71.2, M71.3) is a small, fluid-filled sac or pouch that can develop over a tendon or joint. As the cyst

Chapter 12

Table 12-17 Duration Trend From Normative Data for Cases Specifically Identified With Carpal Tunnel Syndrome

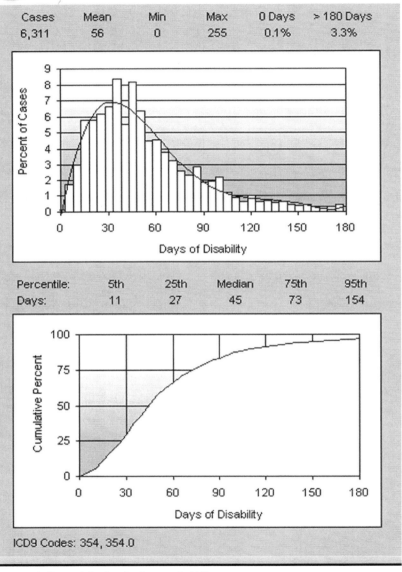

Cases	Mean	Min	Max	0 Days	> 180 Days
6,311	56	0	255	0.1%	3.3%

Percentile:	5th	25th	Median	75th	95th
Days:	11	27	45	73	154

ICD9 Codes: 354, 354.0

Reproduced with permission from Reed. www.mdguidelines.com.

Chapter 12

enlarges, the "mass" creates a swelling visible and palpable through the skin that can be soft to firm, depending on the amount of fluid in the sac and the length of time the cyst has been present. A synovial cyst may or may not be painful, depending on its size and location. The cause for most synovial cysts is unknown or idiopathic, although there is some evidence that trauma may be a risk factor. The size of the sac or cyst can change with activity and may disappear for some time, only to recur.

Ganglionic cysts are the most common cysts found on the hands and feet. A mucus (myxoid) cyst is a synovial cyst of the last joint, the distal inter-phalangeal (DIP) of a finger or the interphalangeal (IP) of a thumb. Myxoid cysts are thought to be caused by leakage of synovial fluid from the joint, usually associated with underlying degenerative joint disease.

Risk factors for developing synovial cysts are osteoarthritis, rheumatoid arthritis, acute or chronic trauma, joint instability, or overuse injuries from repetitive movement, and cysts are most common in women ages 20 to 30. If these cysts are caused by repetitive trauma, they should be increasingly more common with age, instead of having a peak incidence in the young. Ganglion cysts of the wrist and hand comprise 50% to 70% of all masses found in the hand with 80% of such cysts located on the back of the hand (dorsal surface).[66]

The Social Security Administration's disability requirements are the same as discussed earlier in this chapter. Therefore, synovial cysts and ganglions would not qualify for one-sided total upper extremity disability.

Risk Assessment
Most risk factors are felt to be nonoccupational with the incidence increased with female gender and arthritides.[67]

Capacity
Capacity is usually not limited by the cyst, ganglion, or mass. However, sometimes the cyst, ganglion, or mass may be painful with activities, or spontaneously rupture (leak fluid), which will result in a temporary reduction in activity.

Tolerance
The individual's tolerance for symptoms like pain and appearance varies. Aspiration of the fluid can sometimes help, but recurrence is high. Believable symptoms may result in inappropriate work "restrictions" that are based solely on tolerance rather than pathology. Tolerance is influenced by the individual's age, occupation, whether the dominant or nondominant

arm is affected, and the response to treatment. Job modification to avoid contact of hard objects with the mass may be helpful. Suggested disability durations (in days) for synovial cysts are listed in Table 12-18, and the duration trend is listed in Table 12-19.

Conclusion

Most individuals will not require time off work. Treatment is based on symptoms. Although the capacity may be limited for a short period after surgery, most individuals can return to previous employment levels.

Table 12-18 Synovial Cyst Suggested Disability Durations (Days)

	ICD-9-CM: 727.4, 727.40, 727.41, 727.42, 727.43, 727.51					
	ICD-10: M67.4, M71.2, M71.3					
Job Classification	The Hand Center			The MDGuidelines 2005/2010		
	Target	TMinimum	TMaximum	Optimum	Minimum	Maximum
Nonsurgical Treatment for Synovial Cyst						
Sedentary	a/0	0	1	x/1	x/1	x/7
Light	0	0	5	x/1	x/1	x/14
Medium	0	0	7	x/1	x/1	x/28
Heavy	0	0	7	x/1	x/1	x/35
Very Heavy	0	0	14	x/1	x/1	x/42
Aspiration for Synovial Cyst						
Sedentary	a/0	0	1	x/1	x/1	x/7
Light	0	0	5	x/1	x/1	x/14
Medium	0	0	7	x/4	x/3	x/28
Heavy	0	0	14	x/6	x/3	x/35
Very Heavy	0	0	21	x/9	x/3	x/42
Open Surgery for Synovial Cyst						
Sedentary	a/0	a/0	a/3	x/3	x/1	x/14
Light	a/0	a/0	a/5	x/3	x/1	x/21
Medium	a/5	a/0	a/7	x/14	x/7	x/28
Heavy	a/7	a/0	a/14	x/21	x/14	x/42
Very Heavy	a/14	a/7	a/21	x/28	x/14	x/54

* No change between 2005 and 2010 data if only one number in the MDGuidelines section.

x No data for 2005.

a Data available in 2005 but not published.

Reproduced with permission from Reed. www.mdguidelines.com.

Chapter 12

Table 12-19 Synovial Cyst Trend

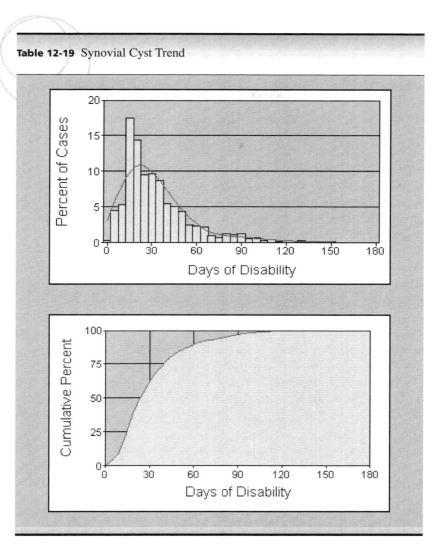

Reproduced with permission from Reed. www.mdguidelines.com.

Amputation: Finger or Thumb

Amputations (ICD-9-CM codes 84.01, 84.02, 885.0, 885.1, 886.0, 886.1 or ICD-10 code T14.7) are performed when blood supply is irreversibly compromised by disease or severe injury to an extremity. In workers' compensation, the surgical approach is the same: determine the appropriate amputation level (adequate blood supply), wound closure, rehabilitation, and use of artificial limbs (prosthetics) if appropriate. The goal is to remove diseased or damaged tissue, relieve pain, and to prepare a site for a possible prosthesis, helping the individual return to the most comfortable and functional life. The Social Security Administration's disability requirements are the same as discussed earlier in this chapter. Therefore, single or limited finger or thumb amputation rarely qualifies for one-sided total upper extremity disability. Bilateral hand amputations would clearly qualify.

Risk Assessment
This is a return-to-work risk assessment, not progression of disease risk. Function of the upper limb is affected by which digit (thumb or finger) is injured and therefore amputated, along with the length of loss for each amputated digit and the number of digits amputated. The risk can also be complicated by functional loss of other digits (stiffness, loss of feeling, etc) but not completely amputated.

Capacity
Capacity is affected by the same items outlined in risk assessment, but must also consider job tasks. If a concert pianist has a little finger amputation, his or her functional capacity is the same as a surgeon, but his or her ability to return to his or her previous level of employment is unlikely.

Tolerance
If a specific requirement of a job is not a limiting factor, then tolerance becomes the key. A self-employed farmer may return to work the same day ("If I don't feed the cows, who will?"), where a receptionist may be off for several days. Suggested disability durations (in days) for amputations are listed in Table 12-20.

Conclusion
The length of disability depends on the type and level of amputation, the number of digits involved, comorbidities, the option of possible prosthesis use, job requirements, and tolerance.

Miscellaneous

Can I Drive With A Cast?
A study was presented to the American Society for Surgery of the Hand to address this issue. Thirty police officers participated in the study. The participants were variously managed with splinting on the right and left sides,

Table 12-20 Amputation Finger or Thumb Suggested Disability Durations (Days)

Job Classification	The Hand Center			The MDGuidelines 2005/2010		
	ICD-9-CM: 84.01, 84.02, 886.0, 886.1, 885.0, 885.1					
	ICD-10: T14.7					
	CPT: 26910, 26951, 26592					
	Target	TMinimum	TMaximum	Optimum	Minimum	Maximum
Open Surgery for Amputation Finger or Thumb						
Sedentary	a/0	a/0	a/7	x/14	x/7	x/42
Light	a/0	a/0	a/14	x/14	x/7	x/42
Medium	a/7	a/0	a/21	x/28	x/14	x/49
Heavy	a/14	a/5	a/28	x/42	x/14	x/63
Very Heavy	a/21	a/7	a/35	x/42	x/21	x/91

* No change between 2005 and 2010 data if only one number in the MDGuidelines section.

x No data for 2005.

a Data available in 2005 but not published.

Reproduced with permission from Reed. www.mdguidelines.com.

proximal and distal to the elbow, and with or without the thumb included in the cast (spica) and were asked to complete a standard driving skills test on a cone-marked course. Regardless of hand dominance, splints on the left arm resulted in the worst driving scores, with the participants with above-the-elbow splints doing worse than those with below-the-elbow splints. The reasons for this effect were not determined but might be related to the left-sided driver position in the United States, with the left arm having less freedom to maneuver because of the fixed constraint of the driver-side door. It would be interesting to see if a right-hand cast is associated with worse driving performance in cars in which the driver sits on the right side. However, in countries in which the driver sits on the left side, patients wearing left-arm casts should probably be advised that their driving ability may be impaired as a result of the cast.[68] A Medline search returned only one other article in 2002. The right Colles' cast was found to have no effect on ability to drive. Scaphoid and Bennett's casts were found to have an effect on driving ability.[69] A call to the Kansas Department of Transportation Highway Patrol returned the following: "It is not illegal to drive your car while wearing a cast. A police officer generally cannot pull you over or give you a citation simply for driving with a cast on. However, if you are involved in an accident, the officer may determine that the cast impaired your ability to drive safely." Therefore, the physician should caution the patient in the above context regarding driving.

Chapter 12

What's New?

As databases become more sophisticated, their size increases, the ability to analyze data improves, and the Internet allows this data to be shared with the end user. Disability durations are entering a new era. Two commercial products have become available. This is not an endorsement for either but an effort to provide insight. My disclaimer: I have been and continue to be a paid medical consultant for both organizations. Commercial products in alphabetical order:

MDGuidelines Predictive Model™ benchmarks against the predicted duration at www.MDguidelines.com, and the ODG (Official Disability Guidelines) Comorbidity Calculator™ at www.disabilitydurations.com. The two products take slightly different approaches. I will highlight their similarities and differences.

Database content

MDGuidelines is obtained from large employers and disability insurance companies. ODG is obtained from guidelines from the BLS (Bureau of Labor and Statistics), CDC (Center for Disease Control), and OSHA (Occupational Safety and Health Administration), and from phone surveys.

Disability Duration Content

MDGuidelines: Select key ICD-9-CM code, age, gender, job class (DOT, as used in this chapter), co-existing conditions (up to 3 additional ICD-9-CM codes), workers' comp (yes or no), region by zip code, and year injury incurred.

ODG: Select key ICD-9-CM code, one co-existing condition, and age. ODG states that DOL job class is not predictive of disability duration and provides additional information to support this position on its Web site.

After entering the information above, a disability duration is provided.

Disability Duration Results

MDGuidelines: The report provides the median disability duration for the primary diagnosis and shows the additional days for each of the above reference items, followed with total disability duration in days.

ODG: Provides the total disability duration in days.

Comparing the Results

First, the two products are not identical and therefore this is not an apples-to-apples comparison but rather a discussion of what can we learn about disability duration days using these additional tools. Our first comparison will be by using a few common diagnosis patterns. Table 12-21 is used to compare the primary diagnosis/ICD-9-CM of carpal tunnel syndrome (CTS)/354.0 and secondary diagnosis/ICD-9-CM of ulnar nerve elbow (UNE)/354.2. Table 12-22 CTS and secondary diagnosis/ICD-9-CM of diabetes mellitus/250. Table 12-23 CTS and secondary diagnosis/ICD-9-CM of de Quervain's disease/727.04.

Table 12-21 Median Disability in Days – CTS UNE

	Primary ICD-9-CM code: 354.0 (carpal tunnel syndrome)	
	Secondary ICD-9-CM code: 354.2 (ulnar nerve elbow entrapment)	
	MDGuidelines Predictor using 45 female, light work, and zip 67208	
Age	**MDGuidelines Predictor**	**ODG Comorbidity Calculator**
35	97.6	116
45	101.6	119
55	105.5	146
65	109.4	177

Reproduced with permission from Reed. www.mdguidelines.com.
Reproduced with permission from Work Loss Data Institute, publisher of ODG (www.disabilitydurations.com).

Table 12-22 Median Disability in Days – CTS Diabetes

	Primary ICD-9-CM code: 354.0 (carpal tunnel syndrome)	
	Secondary ICD-9-CM code: 250 (diabetes mellitus)	
	MDGuidelines Predictor using 45 female, light work, and zip 67208	
Age	**MDGuidelines Predictor**	**ODG Comorbidity Calculator**
35	115	55
45	118.9	56
55	122.8	69
65	126.8	84

Reproduced with permission from Reed. www.mdguidelines.com.
Reproduced with permission from Work Loss Data Institute, publisher of ODG (www.disabilitydurations.com).

Chapter 12

Table 12-23 Median Disability in Days – Quervain's

Primary ICD-9-CM code: 354.0 (carpal tunnel syndrome)		
Secondary ICD-9-CM code: 727.04 (de Quervain's or radial styloid tenosynovitis)		
MDGuidelines Predictor using 45 female, light work, and zip 67208		
Age	MDGuidelines Predictor	ODG Comorbidity Calculator
35	105.8	94
45	109.7	97
55	113.7	119
65	117	144

Reproduced with permission from Reed. www.mdguidelines.com.
Reproduced with permission from Work Loss Data Institute, publisher of ODG (www.disabilitydurations.com).

1. Days reported in decimal point does not imply a higher level of statistical significance.

2. The results vary depending on the source of the data, and therefore the two products provide similar ranges for disability duration by diagnosis, but they are not the same.

Second, the MDGuidelines provides an opportunity to see just how job class affects disability durations. In Table 12-24, I selected a 45-year-old female

Table 12-24 Median Disability in Days by Job

Primary ICD-9-CM code: 354.0 (carpal tunnel syndrome)				
Secondary ICD-9-CM code: none				
MDGuidelines Predictor using 45 female by job class for zip 67208				
Job Class	No WC	No WC	WC	WC
	Total days	Days for job class	Total days	Days for job class
Sedentary	86.2	+3.3	101.4	+4.0
Light	92.6	+7.3	108.2	+8.6
Medium	99.6	+11.9	114.9*	+10.2
Heavy	106.3	+16.9	121.6	+18.6
Very Heavy	113	+22.2	128.3	+24.0

No WC = No workers' compensation
WC = Workers' compensation
Days for job class are included in the total days.

Reproduced with permission from Reed. www.mdguidelines.com.

with ICD-9-CM of CTS/354.0 in the zip code of 67208 as my standard. I then change the job class for sedentary, light, medium, heavy, and very heavy for "No WC" (data based on nonworkers' compensation patients). With the same standard, I repeated the process for "WC" (data based on workers' compensation patients). In Table 12-25, I selected a 45-year-old female with ICD-9-CM of CTS / 354.0 as my standard and repeated the job classes but for two different zip codes (67208 Wichita, KS and 90017 Los Angeles, CA).

1. Job Class does seem to affect disability duration. As the job class increased (becomes heavier), the disability duration days linked to the job class increased.

Table 12-25 Median Disability in Days by Zip Code

Primary ICD-9-CM code: 354.0 (carpal tunnel syndrome)				
Secondary ICD-9-CM code: none				
MDGuidelines Predictor using 45 female by job class				
Zip	**67208**			
City	**Wichita, KS**			
	No WC	**No WC**	**WC**	**WC**
Job Class	**Total days**	**Days for job class**	**Total days**	**Days for job class**
Sedentary	86.2	+3.3	101.4	+4.0
Light	92.6	+7.3	108.2	+8.6
Medium	99.6	+11.9	114.9	+10.2
Heavy	106.3	+16.9	121.6	+18.6
Very Heavy	113	+22.2	128.3	+24.0
Zip	**90017**			
City	**Los Angeles, CA**			
	No WC	**No WC**	**WC**	**WC**
Job Class	**Total days**	**Days for job class**	**Total days**	**Days for job class**
Sedentary	62.6	+2.7	77.9	+3.7
Light	69.3	+6.5	54.6	+8.0
Medium	76.0	+10.9	91.3	+12.8
Heavy	82.7	+15.8	98.0	+17.9
Very Heavy	89.4	+21.0	104.7	+23.2

No WC = No workers' compensation
WC = Workers' compensation
Days for job class are included in the total days.

Reproduced with permission from Reed. www.mdguidelines.com.

Chapter 12

2. Workers' compensation also seems to affect disability duration. All disability durations were higher in the "WC" compared to the "No WC" groups for each of the job classes. Additionally as the job class increased in the "WC" group, so did the additional duration disability days.

Physical Therapy Visits

Unfortunately, the medical literature provides little evidence-based medicine for the ideal number of physical therapy visits per specific diagnosis. Therapy can be used to enhance the ability to stay at work or return to work. Both of the commercial products now include recommendations for a reasonable number of visits per diagnosis primarily based on consensus opinion. For most conditions of the upper limb that require therapy, 6 or fewer visits appear to be appropriate (MDGuidelines and ODG). The most successful programs include a "home education program" commonly labeled as HEP. Most studies demonstrate that having the patient take responsibility for his or her therapy results in better outcomes, shorter periods of disability or lost work time, and a reduction in the number of formal therapy visits[70] or legislatively imposed limits.[71]

Functional Capacity Evaluation

Functional capacity evaluations (FCEs) are commonly used to help determine return-to-work readiness and workplace guides or restrictions following work-related injury. Most reports suggesting benefit of FCEs are at a case report level of quality with little evidence-based medicine to confirm their validity. In a study by Gross and Battie, the authors examined the performance on the Isernhagen Work Systems' FCE as a predictor of timely and sustained recovery in workers' compensation claimants with upper extremity disorders. A secondary objective was to determine whether FCE is more predictive in claimants with specific injuries (like a fracture) when compared to less-specific, pain-mediated disorders (like myofascial pain). The longitudinal study reviewed 336 claimants with upper extremity disorders undergoing FCE. FCE indicators were maximum performance during handgrip and lift testing, and the number of tasks in which performance was rated below required job demands. Outcomes investigated were days receiving time-lost benefits (a surrogate of return to work or work readiness) in the year following FCE, days until claim closure, and future recurrence defined as whether benefits restarted, the claim reopened, or a new upper extremity claim was filed. Cox and logistic regression were used to determine the prognostic effect of FCE crudely and after controlling for potential confounders. Analysis was performed separately on claimants with specific and pain-mediated disorders. The authors found that most subjects (95%) experienced time-loss benefit suspension within one year following FCE. The one-year recurrence rate was 39%. Higher lifting performance was associated with faster benefit suspension and claim closure, but explained little variation in these outcomes (r2 = 1.2–11%). No FCE indicators were associated with future recurrence after controlling for confounders. Results were similar between the specific injury group and the less-specific injury group. The authors conclude that better FCE performance was a weak predictor of faster benefit suspension and was unrelated to sustained recovery. Therefore, FCE was no more predictive in claimants with specific pathology and injury than in those with more ambiguous, pain-mediated conditions.[72] These authors also found that FCEs did not predict sustained employment in patients with chronic low back pain.[73] In a similar unpublished study, Melhorn found the same to be true, FCE did not predict sustained employment, for upper limb conditions.[74]

Coworkers' Effect on Return to Work

Tjulin et al. concluded that workplace-based return-to-work interventions need to take social relations among workplace participants into consideration. They highlight the importance and relevance of the varied roles of different workplace participants during two relatively appreciated areas of the return-to-work process: the prereturn and the postreturn sustainability phase. Attention to these "invisible phases" can facilitate a successful return to work.[75]

Summary

Musculoskeletal pain may affect any body location. Converting the subjective complaints to a specific pathoanatomic diagnosis can often be challenging. The first step is the traditional medical history and examination. Most individuals can be placed into one of five categories for insight into treatment and outcomes: (1) at risk but without injury or current symptoms, (2) acute traumatic injuries, (3) acute onset of nontraumatic symptoms, (4) chronic symptoms with return to work likely, and (5) chronic symptoms with return to work unlikely (based on severe pathology or psychosocial factors).[76]

When patients are disabled (unable to work), everyone loses. As a patient advocate, the physician has the best opportunity to encourage staying at work or early return to work. Benefits for the individual include better self-image, improved ability to cope, improved work survivability, and improved ability to be self-sufficient. (See Chapter 1.) Conversely, prolonged time away from work makes recovery and return to work progressively less likely. Benefits

Chapter 12

for the employer and insurer are financial, while the workers' compensation system lives up to its goal of intended fairness. Severe conditions require the consideration of risk (work restrictions) and capacity (work limitations). Most often, the factor hindering return to work is tolerance.

Returning the individual to work requires a balance between the demands of the job and the capability of the patient, while limiting the risk of additional injury. Communication and education are key to addressing tolerance concerns. Temporary workplace guides must include an understanding for individual tolerance, which varies to allow for an appropriate early return to work, while considering the patient's desires and concerns. This approach provides treating physicians with a unique opportunity and obligation to provide reasonable work guides in an effort to reduce work disability, improve the outcome for work-related injuries, and advance the quality of life for their patients.

In addition to their medical outcome, the physicians of the future will be measured by their ability to return patients to work within the "appropriate" disability durations.

References

1. US Bureau of Labor Statistics. Nonfatal occupational illness data by category of illness. Washington, DC:US Department of Labor, 1995.

2. Kaufman LR, Green A, Haas NS, Hoffman H, Melhorn JM, Michener LA, Saechao K, Watson, Jr. RR , Zuckerman, JD. Shoulder disorders. In: Hegmann KT, ed. *Occupational Medicine Practice Guidelines*. Elk Grove Village, IL: American College of Occupational and Environment Medicine; 2008:549–572.

3. US Bureau of Labor Statistics. Lost-worktime injuries and illnesses: characteristics and resulting time away from work, 2005. Washington, DC: 2006.

4. Silverstein B, Welp E, Nelson N, and Kalat J. Claims incidence of work-related disorders of the upper extremities: Washington state, 1987 through 1995. *Am J Public Health*. 1998;88(12):1827–1833.

5. US Bureau of Labor Statistics. *Survey of Occupational Injuries and Illnesses, 1996*. Washington, DC: US Government Printing Office; 1998:1–58.

6. US Bureau of Labor Statistics. BLS issues 1996 lost-worktime injuries and illnesses survey. *Am Coll Occup Environ Med Rep*. 1998;98:6–7.

7. Brady W, Bass J, Royce M, et al. Defining total corporate health and safety costs: significance and impact. *J Occup Environ Med*. 1997;39:224–231.

8. Feuerstein M, Miller VL, Burrell LM, Berger R. Occupational upper extremity disorders in the federal workforce. *J Occup Environ Med*. 1998;40:546–555.

9. Webster BS, Snook SH. The cost of compensable upper extremity cumulative trauma disorders. *J Occup Environ Med*. 1994;7:713–718.

Chapter 12

10. Social Security Administration. *Social Security Determination Book for Muscular Skeletal*. Washington, DC: Social Security Administration; 2004:1–45.

11. US Department of Health and Human Services. *Musculoskeletal Disorders and Workplace Factors: A Critical Review of Epidemiologic Evidence for Work-Related Musculoskeletal Disorders of the Neck, Upper Extremity, and Low Back*. Cincinnati, Ohio: National Institute for Occupational Safety and Health; 1997.

12. Melhorn JM. Epidemiology of musculoskeletal disorders and workplace factors. In: Mayer TG, Gatchel RJ, Polatin PB, eds. *Occupational Musculoskeletal Disorders Function, Outcomes, and Evidence*. Philadelphia, PA: Lippincott Williams & Wilkins; 1999:225–266.

13. Albright J, Allman R, Bonfiglio RP, Conill A, Dobkin B, Guccione AA, Hasson S, Russo R, Shekelle P, Susman JL, Brosseau L, Tugwell P, Wells GA. Philadelphia Panel evidence-based clinical practice guidelines on selected rehabilitation interventions for shoulder pain. *Phys Ther*. 2001;81:1719–1730.

14. Melhorn JM. *Work Guides, Functional Capacity, Work Restrictions Used by the Hand Center*. Wichita, KS: Hand Center; 2003.

15. Reed P. *The Medical Disability Advisor*. Boulder, CO: Reed Group Ltd; 2001.

16. Reed P. *The Medical Disability Advisor: Workplace Guidelines for Disability Duration*. 5th ed. Westminster, CO: Reed Group, Ltd; 2005.

17. Baker CL, Liu SH. Comparison of open and arthroscopically assisted rotator cuff repairs. *Am J Sports Med*. 1995;23:99–104.

18. Ramsey ML, Getz CL, Parsons BO. What's new in shoulder and elbow surgery. *J Bone Joint Surg Am*. 2007;89:220–230.

19. Henn RF, Kang L, Tashjian RZ, Green A. Patients' preoperative expectations predict the outcome of rotator cuff repair. *J Bone Joint Surg Am*. 2007;89: 1913–1919.

20. Kang L, Henn RF, Tashjian RZ, Green A. Early outcome of arthroscopic rotator cuff repair: a matched comparison with mini-open rotator cuff repair. *Arthroscopy*. 2007;23:573–82, 582.

21. Henn RF, Kang L, Tashjian RZ, Green A. Patients with workers' compensation claims have worse outcomes after rotator cuff repair. *J Bone Joint Surg Am*. 2008;90:2105–2113.

22. Mellado JM, J. Calmet J, Olona M, et al. Surgically repaired massive rotator cuff tears: MRI of tendon integrity, muscle fatty degeneration, and muscle atrophy correlated with intraoperative and clinical findings. *AJR*. 2005;184:1456–1463.

23. Galatz LM, Ball CM, Teefey SA, et al. The outcome and repair integrity of completely arthroscopically repaired large and massive rotator cuff tears. *J Bone Joint Surg Am*. 2004;86:219–224.

24. Sher JS, Uribe JW, Posada A, Murphy BJ, Zlatkin MB. Abnormal findings on magnetic resonance images of asymptomatic shoulders. *J Bone Joint Surg Am*. 1995;77:10–15.

25. Yamanaka K, Matsumoto T. The joint side tear of the rotator cuff: a followup study by arthrography. *Clin Orthop Relat Res*. 1994;304:68–73.

26. Yamaguchi K, Ditsios K, Middleton WD. The demographic and morphological features of rotator cuff disease. A comparison of asymptomatic and symptomatic shoulders. *J Bone Joint Surg Am*. 2006;88:1699–1704.

Chapter 12

27. Tashjian RZ, Farnham JM, Albright FS, et al. Evidence for an inherited predisposition contributing to the risk for rotator cuff disease. *J Bone Joint Surg Am.* 2009;91:1136–1142.

28. Palmer KT, Harris EC, David CE. Compensating occupationally related tenosynovitis and epicondylitis: a literature review. *Occupational Medicine.* 2007;57:67–74.

29. Melhorn JM, Martin D, Brooks CN, Seaman S. Upper limb. In: Melhorn JM, Ackerman JM, eds. *Guides to the Evaluation of Disease and Injury Causation.* Chicago, IL: AMA Press; 2008:141–202.

30. Katz RT. Ulnar neuropathy at the elbow due to repetition: myth or reality? *The Guides Newsletter*, Sep/Oct 2006. American Medical Association.

31. D'Arcy CA, McGee S. The rational clinical examination: does this patient have carpal tunnel syndrome? *JAMA.* 2000;283:3110–3117.

32. Marx RG, Hudak PL, Bombardier C, et al. The reliability of physical examination for carpal tunnel syndrome. *J Hand Surg.* 1998;23B:499–502.

33. Salerno DF, Franzblau A, Werner RA, et al. Reliability of physical examination of the upper extremity among keyboard operators. *Am J Ind Med.* 2000;37: 423–430.

34. American Academy of Neurology. Practice parameter for electrodiagnostic studies in carpal tunnel syndrome (summary statement). *Neurology.* 1993;43: 2404–2405.

35. Hadler NM. *Occupational Musculoskeletal Disorders.* Philadelphia, PA: Lippincott Williams & Wilkins; 1999.

36. Michelson H, Posner MA. Medical history of carpal tunnel syndrome. *Hand Clin.* 2002;18:257–268.

37. Carrico HL. Virginia declares carpal tunnel not a job injury. *Occup Health Manage.* July 1996:79–80.

38. Nathan PA, Meadows KD, Istvan JA. Predictors of carpal tunnel syndrome: an 11-year study of industrial workers. *J Hand Surg.* 2002;27A:644–651.

39. Hegmann KT, Oostema SJ. Causal associations and determination of work-relatedness. In: Melhorn JM, Ackerman WE. *Guides to the Evaluation of Disease and Injury Causation*, Chicago, IL: AMA Press; 2008:33–46.

40. Melhorn JM, and Hegmann KT. Methodology. In: Melhorn JM, Ackerman WE. *Guides to the Evaluation of Disease and Injury Causation.* Chicago, IL:AMA Press; 2008:47–60.

41. Padua L, Padua R, Aprile I, Pasqualetti P, Tonali P. Multiperspective follow-up of untreated carpal tunnel syndrome: a multicenter study. *Neurology.* 2001;56:1459–1466.

42. Andersen JH, Thomsen JF, Overgaard E, et al. Computer use and carpal tunnel syndrome: a 1-year follow-up study. *JAMA.* 2003;289:2963–2969.

43. Stevens CJ, Witt JC, Smith BE, Weaver AL. The frequency of carpal tunnel syndrome in computer users at a medical facility. *Neurology.* 2001;56:1568–1570.

44. Nordstrom DL, Vierkant RA, DeStefano F, Layde PM. Risk factors for carpal tunnel syndrome in a general population. *Occup Environ Med.* 1997;54:734–740.

45. Hadler NM. A keyboard for "Daubert." *J Occup Environ Med*. 1996;38:469–476.

46. Egilman D, Punnett L, Hjelm EW, Welch L. Evidence for work-related musculo-skeletal disorders. *J Occup Environ Med*. 1996;38:1079–1080.

47. Garland FC, Garland CF, Doyle EJ, et al. Carpal tunnel syndrome and occupation in U.S. Navy enlisted personnel. *Arch Environ Health*. 1996;51:395–407.

48. Lo SL, Raskin K, Lester H, Lester B. Carpal tunnel syndrome: a historical perspective. *Hand Clin*. 2002;18:211–217.

49. Kryger AI, Andersen JH, Lassen CF, et al. Does computer use pose an occupational hazard for forearm pain; from the NUDATA study. *Occup Environ Med*. 2003;60:14.

50. Rempel D, Tittiranonda P, Burastero S, Hudes M, So Y. Effect of keyboard key-switch design on hand pain. *J Occup Environ Med*. 1999;41:111–119.

51. Lincoln AE, Vernick JS, Ogaitis S, et al. Interventions for the primary prevention of work-related carpal tunnel syndrome. *Am J Prev Med*. 2000;18:37–50.

52. Gorsche R, Wiley JP, Renger R, et al. Prevalence and incidence of stenosing flexor tenosynovitis (trigger finger) in a meat-packing plant. *J Occup Environ Med*. 1998;40:556–560.

53. Melhorn JM. Work-related upper extremity musculoskeletal pain: successful disability prevention. In: Genovese E, ed. *First Do No Harm: Medical and Ethical Issues in Disability Management*. Philadelphia, PA: IMX Medical Management Services Inc; 2004.

54. Melhorn JM. The top 10 most medically controversial or dubious treatments in workers comp. In: International Association of Industrial Accident Boards and Commissions, *IAIABC 31st International Workers Compensation College*. Madison, Wis: 2004.

55. Melhorn JM. *Employer's Modified Work Program Agreement*. Wichita, KS: Hand Center; 2003.

56. International Association for the Study of Pain. *Pain Definitions*. Seattle, WA: International Association for the Study of Pain; 2002. Available at: www.iasp-pain.org/defsopen.html. Accessed January 26, 2011.

57. Melhorn JM. Understanding and managing chronic non-malignant pain for the occupational orthopaedists. In: Melhorn JM, Strain RE Jr, eds. *Occupational Orthopaedics and Workers' Compensation: A Multidisciplinary Perspective*. Rosemont, IL: American Academy of Orthopaedic Surgeons; 2002.

58. Melhorn JM. Return to work: negotiation strategies. In: Melhorn JM, Strain RE Jr, eds. *Occupational Orthopaedics and Workers' Compensation: A Multidisciplinary Perspective*. Rosemont, IL: American Academy of Orthopaedic Surgeons; 2002.

59. Melhorn JM. Return to work issues: arm pain. In: Melhorn JM, Strain RE Jr, eds. *Occupational Orthopaedics and Workers' Compensation: A Multidisciplinary Perspective*. Rosemont, IL: American Academy of Orthopaedic Surgeons; 2002.

60. Melhorn JM, Gardner P. How we prevent prevention of musculoskeletal disorders in the workplace. *Clin Orthop*. 2004;419:285–296.

61. Melhorn JM, Kennedy EM. Musculoskeletal disorders, disability, and return-to-work (repetitive strain): the quest for objectivity. In: Gatchel RJ, Schultz IZ, eds.

At Risk Claims: Predication of Occupational Disability Using a Biopsychosocial Approach. New York, NY: Kluwer Academic/Plenium; 2004.

62. Melhorn JM. Upper extremities: return to work issues. In: Melhorn JM, Spengler DM, eds. *Occupational Orthopaedics and Workers' Compensation: A Multidisciplinary Perspective.* Rosemont, IL: American Academy of Orthopaedic Surgeons; 2003:256–285.

63. Melhorn JM. Occupational orthopaedics: evidence-based medicine, HIPAA privacy compliance, and functional capacity evaluations. In: Melhorn JM, Spengler DM, eds. *Occupational Orthopaedics and Workers' Compensation: A Multidisciplinary Perspective.* Rosemont, IL: American Academy of Orthopaedic Surgeons; 2003:41–80.

64. Talmage JB. Injury healing and maximum medical improvement (MMI): the basic sciences. In: Melhorn JM, Strain RE Jr, eds. *Occupational Orthopaedics and Workers Compensation: A Multidisciplinary Perspective.* Rosemont, IL: American Academy of Orthopaedic Surgeons; 2002:453–474.

65. Melhorn JM, Wilkinson LK, O'Malley MD. Successful management of musculoskeletal disorders. *J Hum Ecol Risk Assessment.* 2001;7:1801–1810.

66. Cassidy, C., and V. Chung. Hand and wrist ganglia. In: Frontera WR, Silver JK, Rizzo TD, eds. *Essentials of Physical Medicine and Rehabilitation.* 2nd ed. W.B. Saunders; 2008:149–154.

67. STanaka S, Seligman PJ, Halperin W. Use of worker's compensation claims data for surveillance of cumulative trauma disorders. *J Occup Environ Med.* 1988;30:488–492.

68. Amadio PC. What's new in hand surgery. *J Bone Joint Surg Am.* 2010;92(3): 783–789.

69. Blair S, Chaudhri O, Gregori A. Doctor, can I drive with this plaster? An evidence based response. *Injury.* 2002;33(1):55–56.

70. Jamieson, J. An evaluation of the effectiveness of using a prospective peer review process to control excessive physical therapy visits. *IAIABC Journal.* 2009;46(1):143–154.

71. Barrett S. *New California Law Limits Workers' Compensation Visits to Chiropractors,* Cambridge, MA: Workers Compensation Research Institute, 2005.

72. Gross DP, Battie MC. Does functional capacity evaluation predict recovery in workers' compensation claimants with upper extremity disorders? *Occup Environ Med.* 2006;63(6):404–410.

73. Gross DP, Battie MC. Functional capacity evaluation performance does not predict sustained return to work in claimants with chronic back pain. *J Occup Rehabil.* 2005;15(3):285–294.

74. Melhorn JM. *Functional Capacity Evaluations in Patients with Upper Limb Conditions Do Not Predict Future Employment,* Wichita, KS: Hand Center, 2008.

75. Tjulin A, Maceachen E, Ekberg K. Exploring workplace actors experiences of the social organization of return-to-work. *J Occup Rehabil.* 2009;20(3): 311–321.

76. Melhorn JM. The advantages of early return to work. *IAIABC J.* 2003;41:128–147.

Chapter 13

Working With Common Lower Extremity Problems

Randy Lea, MD

Lower extremity injuries commonly occur in the workplace and result in significant time away from work. According to the Bureau of Labor and Statistics (2008), the number of nonfatal work-related lower extremity injuries involving days away from work was comparable to those involving the back and upper extremities. Furthermore, the reported median days away from work in lower and upper extremity injuries were within a similar range (1 to 23 days vs 7 to 18.6 days).[1]

In spite of the prevalence of lower extremity injuries, there remains a relative paucity of published research on work-related lower extremity problems in contrast to occupational lower back and upper extremity disorders. Furthermore, scientific studies regarding activity restrictions and limitations due to sports-related lower extremity injuries are much more prevalent than those for work-related lower extremity injuries and illnesses. Finally, what information is available tends to be more consensus or opinion based rather than evidence based. Even though these research limitations exist, there is some data available to facilitate well-reasoned decisions by an examiner in the context of the risk-capacity-tolerance model.

Risk

Assessment of risk in the context of returning to work means estimating whether a worker can return to work without a significant risk of reinjury, injuring another body part, slowing the healing process, or causing an outcome that is less satisfactory than would have occurred if the patient had not returned to work. Nearly all lower extremity injuries have some potential risk for activity-related reinjury during the time required for healing. This necessitates that the examiner have knowledge about the science regarding the time required for healing of specific injuries. Some lower extremity injuries even carry some degree of risk for reinjury and/or persistence of symptoms long after healing has occurred. Lower extremity disease processes such as arthritis can also be worsened or aggravated with certain activities. These risks have been described in detail in other texts in this series.[2] However this chapter will focus on risk assessment for activity-related reinjury in lower extremity injuries commonly encountered in the workplace rather than specific diseases. It will address some of the early risks associated with healing as well as risks for reinjury or additional injury that may exist even after healing is complete.

Capacity

Lower extremity injuries or conditions may result in permanent abnormal physical findings and symptoms regardless of how appropriate the treatment may have been. Depending on an individual's accommodative capabilities, these physical findings and symptoms may even result in permanent functional restrictions or limitations.

Therefore the examiner needs to have some idea as to the type of physical findings and complaints that commonly occur as a result of a specific injury or clinical condition. The examiner then needs to have knowledge about what type of functional limitations are associated with various physical findings and complaints. For example, postoperative joint contractures, joint deformities from a fracture malunion, and arthritis can all lead to diminished motion in the knee. The limited motion can, in turn, prevent the individual from satisfactorily performing certain activities of daily living (ADLs) (see Table 13-1).

In the early postinjury or postoperative healing period, activity restrictions (things the patient can do, but should not do) and limitations (things the patient cannot physically do) may be indicated in order to minimize the risk for reinjury or additional injury. Once the patient reaches maximal medical improvement (MMI), then permanent modification of the initial capacity recommendations is usually required. The examiner's opinion regarding capacity should be formulated by first considering what is medically reasonable or scientifically valid based on current research and evidence-based literature. When necessary, a validity-based functional capacity evaluation (FCE) may be helpful when differences regarding an individual's ability to return to work exist among the various players in the compensation system (employer, insurer, physician, patient). In those situations, a formal functional job analysis is also needed in order to know the specific physical requirements of an occupation. The examiner can then compare the job

Table 13-1 Lower Limb Considerations

Injury/Condition	Physical Finding/ Symptom	Functional Implication
Joint contracture (postoperative or postfracture) Degenerative Joint Disease (DJD) Bony deformity (malunion with articular incongruity)	Decreased ROM	Gait Postures* Balance Sitting Standing
Ligamentous insufficiency Malaligned or loose joint prosthesis Bucket handle meniscus tear Patellofemoral instability	Laxity/instability	Gait Postures* Balance
Direct muscle injury Prolonged immobilization with atrophy Ligament/tendon injury Bony deformity (malunion with shaft shortening, rotation, or angulation)	Decreased strength	

Postures = squat, stoop, kneel, climb

requirements with the patient's measured functional capacity and then determine whether the individual can perform a certain activity or job.

This chapter discusses the physical residuals and associated capacity alterations that are seen in some of the more commonly encountered lower extremity injuries.

Tolerance

Once adequate healing has occurred, most people sustaining noncatastrophic lower extremity injuries are usually able to return to their preinjury activity level, as there are rarely "risk" or "capacity" factors present that would preclude them from doing so. Resumption of these activities is often possible even though the injury may result in residual discomfort and/or physical abnormalities. Many individuals are willing to resume preinjury activities even though they may have to tolerate some level of discomfort when doing so. Research regarding tolerance limits after lower extremity injuries is sparse given the fact that there are both medical (quantifiable) and nonmedical (nonquantifiable) factors that play a role in an individual's willingness to return to work. This chapter will focus on some of the medically acceptable reasons that an individual may have decreased tolerance to certain activities using several lower extremity injuries as examples. It will also review some

Chapter 13

of the trends reported regarding the effect that nonmedical factors have on individuals returning to work or sports after various lower extremity injuries or procedures.

Presumed Disability

Under the guidelines set forth in the musculoskeletal section of *Disability Evaluation under Social Security*,[3] a lower extremity disorder that produces total disability must result in "a loss of function." The term *loss of function* in the context of lower extremity impairment is based on the rather broad categories of ineffective ambulation and pain. The Social Security guides specifically define what is meant by ineffective ambulation and pain.

Functional loss is considered present if there is an inability to ambulate effectively on a sustained basis for any reason, including pain associated with the underlying musculoskeletal impairment. The Social Security Administration's Blue Book defines the inability to ambulate effectively as:

"… an extreme limitation of the ability to walk; i.e., an impairment(s) that interferes very seriously with the individual's ability to independently initiate, sustain, or complete activities. Ineffective ambulation is defined generally as having insufficient lower extremity functioning (see 1.00J) to permit independent ambulation without the use of a hand-held assistive device(s) that limits the functioning of both upper extremities. To ambulate effectively, individuals must be capable of sustaining a reasonable walking pace over a sufficient distance to be able to carry out activities of daily living. They must have the ability to travel without companion assistance to and from a place of employment or school. Therefore, examples of ineffective ambulation include, but are not limited to, the inability to walk without the use of a walker, two crutches or two canes, the inability to walk a block at a reasonable pace on rough or uneven surfaces, the inability to use standard public transportation, the inability to carry out routine ambulatory activities, such as shopping and banking, and the inability to climb a few steps at a reasonable pace with the use of a single hand rail. The ability to walk independently about one's home without the use of assistive devices does not, in and of itself, constitute effective ambulation."

Under the Social Security system, pain or other symptoms can be considered an important factor contributing to lower extremity functional loss. "In order for pain or other symptoms to be found to affect an individual's ability to perform basic work activities, medical signs or laboratory findings must show the existence of a medically determinable impairment(s) that can reasonably be expected to produce the pain or other symptoms." The presumed diagnosis that is causing the pain or loss of ambulatory function

Chapter 13

should be based on observable or measurable physical findings in addition to objective diagnostic testing, rather than subjective complaints alone.

In addition to ineffective ambulation and pain, the Blue Book also lists five impairment categories that could potentially involve lower extremity disorders:

> Section 1.02 Major dysfunction of a joint(s) (due to any cause): Characterized by gross anatomical deformity (e.g., subluxation, contracture, bony or fibrous ankylosis, instability) and chronic joint pain and stiffness with signs of limitation of motion or other abnormal motion of the affected joint(s), and findings on appropriate medically acceptable imaging of joint space narrowing, bony destruction, or ankylosis of the affected joint(s). With: A. Involvement of one major peripheral weightbearing joint (i.e., hip, knee, or ankle), resulting in inability to ambulate effectively, as defined in 1.00B2b; **example: Osteomyelitis**

> Section 1.03 Reconstructive surgery or surgical arthrodesis of a major weight-bearing joint, with inability to ambulate effectively, as defined in 1.00B2b, and return to effective ambulation did not occur, or is not expected to occur, within 12 months of onset. **Example: Dislocating or loose hip or knee prosthesis; knee or hip arthrodesis**

> Section 1.05 Amputation (due to any cause); One or both lower extremities at or above the tarsal region, with stump complications resulting in medical inability to use a prosthetic device to ambulate effectively, as defined in 1.00B2b, which have lasted or are expected to last for at least 12 months; or Hemipelvectomy or hip disarticulation

> Section 1.06 Fracture of the femur, tibia, pelvis, or one or more of the tarsal bones. With:

> A. Solid union not evident on appropriate medically acceptable imaging and not clinically solid; and B. Inability to ambulate effectively, as defined in 1.00B2b, and return to effective ambulation did not occur or is not expected to occur within 12 months of onset. **Example: Nonunion of tibia or femur; nonunion femoral neck fracture**

> Section 1.08 Soft tissue injury (e.g., burns) of an upper or lower extremity, trunk, or face and head, under continuing surgical management, as defined in 1.00M, directed toward the salvage or restoration of major function, and such major function was not restored or expected to be restored within 12 months of onset. **Example: Complex open wound with or without compound fracture necessitating reconstructive procedures such as flap or grafting.**

Chapter 13

The more commonly seen and noncatastrophic occupational lower extremity injuries rarely meet the Social Security defined criteria for disability. Therefore the risk, capacity, and tolerance model will be used to illustrate how the examiner can approach return to work issues for these injuries.

Sprains

Ligament stretch/disruption injuries are called *sprains* and can be divided into three grade classifications based on physical findings (area of tenderness, amount of joint laxity, or joint specific provocative tests) and/or diagnostic studies (stress X rays and MRI). A grade I sprain indicates that there has been a stretch injury of the ligament itself, but no actual disruption of the ligament has occurred nor has there been any change in ligament strength. A grade II sprain means there has been a partial ligament disruption and the length and/or strength of the ligament has been altered to some degree. Grade III sprains represent complete disruption of the ligament. In general, grade I and II injuries require some level of protection/immobilization while selected grade II anterior cruciate ligament (ACL) injuries and other grade III ligament injuries may even require operative repair or reconstruction. Grade is only one indicator of severity as healing may also be dependent on the joint-specific ligament involved, the location of the ligament injury (midsubstance or directly off bone), and whether there is more than one ligament involved. Sprains of the knee and ankle are two of the most common lower extremity sprains encountered in the workplace.

Risk

When a knee or ankle ligament is injured, the primary risk concern is how long the functional stability of the affected joint or extremity will be compromised during the healing process and even after the ligament has healed.

Knee injuries of the medial collateral ligament (MCL): Isolated grade I and grade II medial collateral ligament injuries of the knee are generally treated nonoperatively, sometimes with functional bracing in combination with early range of motion (ROM) and progressive weight bearing as tolerated. Quadriceps and hamstring strengthening is also instituted once the initial pain and swelling have subsided.

Healing usually occurs spontaneously with near-complete healing seen within 10 to 20 days for grade I and grade II MCL injuries.[4] Almost all MCL injuries have healed within 6 to 12 weeks. Some grade III MCL injuries may require a year or more for complete healing to occur.[5] Nonetheless, these individuals are still allowed to return to full preinjury activity levels fairly soon after the initial postinjury symptoms have abated and prescribed rehabilitative goals have been met.

<u>Knee ACL:</u> Injuries of the anterior cruciate ligament most often occur within the ligament and not at the bone-ligament interface. Due to this fact, and their intra-articular location bathed in synovial fluid, they do not heal spontaneously.

Older individuals who sustain an ACL tear and have concomitant degenerative changes in the knee are usually treated nonoperatively. Younger individuals who do not do heavy work and who are not active in recreational sports or activity on uneven ground are sometimes also treated nonoperatively. A variety of nonoperative protocols have been proposed that are goal oriented and include some form of initial protected motion/bracing and weight bearing; limited modalities to decrease swelling; restoration of ROM; hamstring and quadriceps strengthening; and proprioceptive training. Individuals are considered to be at risk for further injury until the predetermined functional goals are met or it becomes clear that symptomatic functional instability is going to persist in spite of the rehabilitation given.

Surgery is considered appropriate for younger people functioning at high activity levels without any type of degenerative comorbidities. However, protocols exist for identifying younger individuals who may be able to functional well without surgery.[6] When surgery is the preferred treatment, the current operative standard is arthroscopic-assisted reconstruction utilizing autogenous grafting (patellar tendon or hamstring) or allograft materials. Although there have been recent advances in surgical technique and tissue engineering, osseointegration of the graft within the bone tunnels does not occur until 6 to 12 weeks post operatively[7] with revascularization of graft taking 3 to 6 months.[8] Full maturation of the graft may not occur until 12 months postoperatively. This means that there is a potential risk for graft disruption and the development of persistent knee instability during this time frame. Due to this concern, most of the postoperative protocols initially developed were very conservative and included immobilization, limited weight bearing, and gradual restoration of motion. However, recent research favors the use of accelerated protocols without bracing that focus on reducing pain, swelling, and inflammation as well as restoring ROM, strength, and neuromuscular control.[9] This more aggressive rehabilitation has not resulted in an increased incidence of graft disruption or instability problems.

An increased incidence of graft rupture has been reported with higher activity levels[10] and competitive side-stepping, pivoting, and jumping sports.[11] However, there are factors other than activity level alone that may be important in determining whether an individual will have a retear or

Chapter 13

not. One investigation regarding the increased incidence of ACL retears in female jumping athletes found that those individuals having retears also had weaker quadriceps and hamstring strength prior to retear[12] than those athletes who did not have retears. This suggests that the adequacy of initial rehabilitation may be as important as activity level when evaluating the risk for possible retear.

Even though there is a risk for graft rupture for the first 12 months, most protocols allow for full return to work activities within 4 to 6 months post-injury provided the rehabilitative goals have been met.

Ankle: Grade I lateral ankle sprains have traditionally been thought to be relatively minor, requiring minimal treatment and associated with early return to preinjury activities. A more rapid return to work and sports activities has been found in those patients treated with functional protocols instead of immobilization.[13] Even though accelerated functional programs have resulted in early return to preinjury activities, a high incidence of persistent physical findings and symptoms indicative of chronic ankle instability have been reported at one year postinjury.[14] A variety of reasons for chronic ankle instability after a sprain have been proposed, including the possibility that acute injuries may be undertreated.[15] This underlines the fact that treatment programs should be based on sound basic science and research. Specifically, ligament injuries generally require 6 to 12 weeks for healing and therefore may require some form of protective bracing during that time frame.[16] Additionally, functional treatment programs incorporating physical therapy should address any deficits in strength, ROM, proprioception/postural control, and neuromuscular control.[15,17]

Capacity

Knee MCL: There are rarely long-term risk, capacity, or medically based tolerance concerns that prevent patients with healed MCL injuries from returning to work, as most are able to return to preinjury activity levels.[18] Grades I and II MCL injuries have been found to have the ability to return to preinjury activities fairly early, with one study reporting that 95% of the study subjects returned to work no later than 3 months postinjury.[20] However there are those individuals who complain of persistent pain or instability beyond the normal healing time. In those situations the examiner should ensure that there are no associated knee injuries (meniscus tear or ACL tear) that could serve as a legitimate basis for ongoing symptoms resulting in functional limitations. Some patients who have sustained a medial collateral ligament injury may demonstrate persistent mild medial joint line opening on valgus stressing of the knee after they have healed. This finding should not be the sole basis for ongoing activity restrictions.

Although this may be suggestive of instability, many times no actual functional instability exists. Accommodative devices such as injury-specific bracing can be offered in such situations; however, studies regarding the effectiveness of prophylactic knee bracing for the prevention of medial collateral ligament injuries in sports are still inconclusive.[20]

Knee ACL: Many individuals with nonoperatively treated ACL injuries have been reported to have relatively good knee function and capacity when treated by early activity modifications combined with rehabilitation.[21] However, achieving a functional status compatible with higher activity levels may take up to 6 to 12 months.[22] Those patients having both persistent clinical and functional instability after that time frame may necessitate permanent activity modifications (capacity limitations) or surgical treatment.

With the exception of individuals requiring exceptionally high levels of knee function (vigorous sports or heavy work), most surgically treated ACL injuries are allowed to return to preinjury activities as soon as an adequate healing period has transpired and predetermined functional goals indicative of adequate knee stability have been obtained. This usually takes at least 4 to 6 months after surgery. Sedentary and lighter activities can be resumed as soon as the surgical wounds are healed as long as appropriate accommodative devices (bracing or limited crutch usage) are allowed as needed.

If clinical and functional instability persist after an individual reaches maximal medical improvement (MMI) from operative or nonoperative treatment, then a functional performance evaluation may be indicated in order to qualify any potential deficits or alterations in balance, gait, or posture.

Ankle: Uncomplicated lateral ankle sprains may result in decreased work ability for the first few days until the initial swelling and pain have diminished. Sedentary work done sitting should not be affected 1 to 3 days after injury, but sedentary work done standing could be difficult and thus limited for a slightly longer period. However, most individuals are able to return to work within 8 to 10 days.[13] Those patients having more complex sprains or chronic instability may take as long as 6 to 12 weeks before returning to very heavy activities. Even so, most of these patients are able to ultimately resume preinjury activity levels. In some cases, a variety of supportive braces or splints may be recommended in order to expedite an individual's safe and early return to work.

Tolerance

Knee MCL: Most grades I and II MCL injuries heal fairly well with minimal residuals. However, if an individual continues to have symptoms after an appropriate healing time, some consideration should be given to the possibility that there may be concomitant injuries such as an ACL tear, meniscus tear, or chondral injury. If an adequate diagnostic workup has been completed and no additional abnormalities are found, then it may be that nonmedical factors are contributing to the individual's ongoing complaint profile.

Knee ACL: There is research suggesting that nonmedical issues play a definite role in determining whether an individual will return to work after an ACL injury. Wexler analyzed patients with work-related ACL injuries and found that they all returned to work.[23] However, other studies strongly suggest that there are nonmedical factors influencing an individual's willingness to return to work after an ACL injury. Barrett's and Noyes' research have shown that work-related ACL injuries are associated with longer disability durations and higher subjective complaints than those that were nonwork related.[24,25] Furthermore, the number of mean days of lost employment in the workers' compensation group could not be accounted for from factors that normally affect ACL reconstruction results.[25]

Ankle: Although there are no recent studies specifically focusing on return to work after a work-related ankle sprain, tolerance issues may play a role in an individual's willingness to return to work given the fact that a fairly high number of ankle sprains result in persistence of pain and symptoms. However, most individuals return to work even if they have persistence of symptoms, suggesting that there are rarely permanent risk or capacity issues that would preclude successful activity resumption.

Strains: Strains are injuries of the muscle or muscle-tendon unit such as those occurring in the hamstrings or medial gastrocnemius. Most patients with these types of injuries are managed conservatively with symptomatic

Table 13-2 Surgical Treatment, Arthroscopic Reconstruction of Anterior Cruciate Ligament

Job Classification	Duration in Days		
	Minimum	Optimum	Maximum
Sedentary	3	10	35
Light	7	42	49
Medium	21	56	70
Heavy	84	91	112
Very Heavy	91	112	140

Reproduced with permission from Reed. www.mdguidelines.com.

Table 13-3 Supportive treatment, ankle sprain or strain (first or second degree)

Job Classification	Duration in Days		
	Minimum	Optimum	Maximum
Sedentary	0	3	7
Light	1	3	7
Medium	3	7	14
Heavy	7	14	28
Very Heavy	7	14	28

Reproduced with permission from Reed. www.mdguidelines.com.

Table 13-4 Supportive treatment, ankle sprain or strain (third degree)

Job Classification	Duration in Days		
	Minimum	Optimum	Maximum
Sedentary	1	3	7
Light	1	7	28
Medium	7	14	42
Heavy	14	21	70
Very Heavy	14	21	84

Reproduced with permission from Reed. www.mdguidelines.com.

treatment and functional rehabilitation. Furthermore, these patients typically heal well and are able to return to their preinjury activity level. Healing to this extent can occur even when there has been a complete tear that leaves a permanent void in the muscle that can be seen and felt on physical exam.

Risk

Even though strains rarely result in permanent impairment, they can still be a cause for seemingly prolonged temporary activity restrictions. Such restrictions can be considered appropriate if the specific strain has a varied or prolonged healing time or is associated with a high risk of reinjury. For example, medial gastrocnemius strains have a wide range of reported healing times starting as early as 2 weeks postinjury for minimal strains and extending up to 4 months postinjury for more severe injuries.[26] Hamstring injuries have a recurrence rate of 30% for the first year post-injury with some researchers suggesting that this high reinjury rate could be due to inadequate rehabilitation prior to returning to the preinjury activities.[27] These data suggest that activity modifications can be considered reasonable until an adequate healing time has transpired and the appropriate rehabilitation completed.

Unlike most muscle strains, Achilles tendon ruptures may require surgery depending on the patient's age, activity level, and comorbid conditions. Operatively treated patients have been found to have a lower incidence of retears when compared to those injuries treated nonoperatively.[28] However, surgically treated patients have a higher incidence of wound and skin complications than Achilles injuries treated by casting or bracing alone. Healing time is variable with one study reporting a mean return-to-work time of 8 to 16 weeks postinjury.[29]

Capacity

Strains are usually associated with pain-related strength loss until the musculotendinous unit heals. Furthermore, residual strength loss after a strain heals is also common. Nonetheless most people sustaining a strain are able to accommodate to the extent that they can return to their preinjury activity level. In other words, there are rarely long-term capacity issues involved with common strains of the lower extremity.

Tolerance

The inability to tolerate preinjury activities in the early poststrain time frame is medically understandable. Although unusual, when complaints continue after an adequate healing time period has occurred, consideration needs to be given to the possibility that there are some additional medical or nonmedical problems affecting an individual's ability to tolerate activity.

Table 13-5 Surgical Treatment, Ruptured Achilles Tendon Repair

Job Classification	Duration in Days		
	Minimum	Optimum	Maximum
Sedentary	1	3	7
Light	7	14	28
Medium	28	56	84
Heavy	42	84	156
Very Heavy	56	112	180

Reproduced with permission from Reed. www.mdguidelines.com.

For example, undiagnosed avulsion injuries of the hamstring origin can be a cause of chronic pain and disability.[30] If there are no recognizable physical explanations, poor activity tolerance due to psychosocial issues may be the problem.

Fractures

Risk

The treatment of lower extremity fractures involves the use of operative or nonoperative measures in order to achieve the best alignment and stability of the fracture that is possible. However, there is still some risk for displacement due to muscular activity or varying degrees of axial loading that can occur while the fracture is healing. Healing times for lower extremity fractures are variable (Table 13-6), and a number of factors exist that potentially effect fracture healing.

Multipart fractures (comminuted) can present more treatment and healing difficulties than those that are simple (two pieces) and nondisplaced. Open fractures with associated soft tissue damage are generally more complex and require longer healing times than closed fractures. Comorbid medical conditions such as advanced age, diabetes, rheumatoid arthritis, and osteoporosis are associated with prolonged healing times. Tobacco and alcohol use can delay fracture healing. Various medications such as cytotoxic drugs, coritcosteroids, and NSAIDs can result in delayed healing. Regional and fracture-specific variations in complexity also exist. For example, femoral neck fractures can disrupt the blood supply to the femoral head resulting in *delayed unions* (fractures that extend beyond the healing time frame but show some evidence of healing), *nonunions* (fractures with healing times that extend beyond the accepted consolidation time and show evidence of incomplete healing), or avascular necrosis. However, intertrochanteric femur fractures do not affect the femoral head fragment blood supply and thus do not present the same treatment and healing problems.

Once most lower extremity fractures have completely healed, refractures due to specific activities are not that common. The incidence of femoral shaft refracture varies from 2% to 10%, with most refractures occurring in patients who have been treated with plate fixation.[31] Femoral fractures treated with IM rodding that heal satisfactorily can refracture after removal of the rod if protected weight bearing is not utilized for 6 to 8 weeks after rod removal. The incidence of tibial shaft refractures after plating is variable as well, with one study reporting an 11% refracture rate,[32] but a later study had no refractures reported.[33] When refracture occurs it is almost always

Table 13-6 Lower Limb Fracture Considerations

Fracture	Healing Time	Potential Complication(s)	Physical Residuals	Functional Implications
Femoral neck	3–12 months	Nonunion DJD AVN	Articular Collapse Loss of motion	Gait and standing limitations due to pain Lifting limitations
Intertrochanteric femur	3–4 months	Nonunion Malunion	Rotational deformity Shortening	Gait and standing
Femoral shaft	3–6 months	Delayed Union Malunion Nonunion	Angulation Rotation Shortening	Gait and standing
Tibial plateau	3–6 months	Arthritis Malunion Ligament injury	Motion Loss Joint depression/ angulation Joint instability	Balance Gait Postures*
Tibial shaft	Low energy 10–13 weeks High energy 13–20 weeks Open 16–26 weeks	Nonunion Delayed Union Malunion	Angulation Rotation Shortening	Gait
Tibial plafond	2–4 months	DJD Nonunion Malunion	Loss of motion Angulation	Gait Balance Postures*
Ankle-Malleolar	8–14 weeks	Arthritis	Loss of motion	Gait and standing Postures*
Talus (head, neck, body)	3–4 months	Osteonecrosis Arthritis Nonunion/ malunion	Joint collapse Loss of motion (ankle and subtalar)	Gait and standing Postures*
Calcaneus	3–4 months	Malunion-heel deformity Subtalar arthritis Peroneal impingement		Gait and standing Postures*
Metatarsal shaft	6–12 weeks	Malunion	Excessive plantar-dorsiflexion of metatarsal	Gait and standing Postures*

Postures = squat, stoop, kneel, climb

Reproduced with permission from Reed. www.mdguidelines.com.

caused by a second injury and not an activity the individual is accustomed to doing repetitively.

Gait and/or balance impairments may pose a risk to activities that risk a fall from a height, like structural steel work in which workers walk on narrow steel beams as buildings are being constructed.

There are other fractures, such as those seen in the femoral and talar neck regions that may heal in satisfactory alignment but develop complications such as avascular necrosis (AVN). Furthermore, those individuals with AVN of the hip can be at risk for worsening (collapse of the bone of the femoral head) if they are involved in heavy lifting.

Capacity

Even when an individual has the best treatment for a lower extremity fracture, some residual impairment or symptoms that could potentially limit function may be unavoidable (see Table 13-6). Some fractures may heal, but with an unacceptable degree of angulation, rotation, or shortening and are classified as a *malunion*. Angular deformities of a tibial plateau fracture can lead to functional instability of the knee and subsequent balance and gait abnormalities. Angular deformities of the distal femur can lead to arthritis in the knee, and those of the tibial shaft can contribute to the development of ankle degenerative joint disease. Rotational deformities of the femur or tibia can result in significant gait or balance disturbances. Kootstra found that 35% of patients with femoral external rotation deformities of 20 degrees or more were symptomatic.[34] Bråten reported the patients having femoral rotational differences less than 15 degrees did not have any significant complaints, but those with more than 15 degrees of malrotation did have difficulties.[35] Shortening due to bone loss or fracture comminution can also occur after a lower extremity long bone fracture. Most individuals are able to tolerate up to 2 cm of shortening. Some individuals can compensate for a limb length discrepancy of 3 cm while others complain of abnormal body posture, non-physiologic gait patterns, and pain.[36] Articular fractures involving the hip, knee, or ankle can lead to the development of significant osteoarthritis, which can cause joint stiffness and loss of motion. Certain activities of daily living (ADLs) may be limited if the motion loss is severe enough (see Table 13-7).

Tolerance

Even though lower extremity fractures can be associated with prolonged healing times and residual impairment, not all of the individuals sustaining significant lower extremity fractures have significant persisting pain. One prospective study on patients with lower extremity fractures found major

Chapter 13

Table 13-7 Range of Motion (ROM) Needed for Activities of Daily Living (ADLs)

Activity	Knee[37]	Knee[38]	Knee[36]	Ankle[39]
Walking	0–67	Less than 90		10 degrees dorsiflexion 20 degrees Plantar flexion
Ascending stairs	0–83	90–120	100–109	
Descending stairs	0–90	90–120	100–109	
Sitting	0–93	90–120	100–109	
Bathing	—	135		
Lifting	0–117	—		
Tying a shoe	0–106	—	110–124	
Squatting	—	—	125	

deficits in ROM as well as loss of thigh and calf strength in up to 1/4 of the study subjects. However, there were low levels of residual pain reported.[40] Bednar's research on femoral shaft fractures reported that 80% of his injured subjects returned to work within 4 months.[41] Hardy reported that 70% of his subjects with femoral shaft fractures returned to work within 6 to 7 months.[42] Christiansen's study of tibial shaft fractures treated surgically revealed that 90% of the patient's returned to work within 6 months.[33] However another study done by Ferguson found that 47% of the patients reported work-related disability with 40% experiencing persistent pain one year after fracture of the tibial shaft.[43]

Investigations have been performed regarding the effect of nonmedical factors affecting outcome and disability after various lower extremity fractures. Mock and MacKenzie found that the degree of physical impairment accounted for only a small amount of the variance in disability seen after a lower extremity fracture.[44] However, factors such as age, socioeconomic status, preinjury health, and social support account for more than half the variance in long-term disability.[44] A later study by MacKenzie reported poorer outcomes in older individuals, females, nonwhite race, lower educational levels, living in a poor household, smoking, and involvement in the legal system in an effort to obtain disability payments.[45] An investigation of four independent measures affecting the outcome of tibial plafond fractures emphasized the importance of socioeconomic factors on an individual's outcome and also found poorer outcomes in work-related injuries.[46] Calder's study on Lisfranc fractures reported poorer outcomes in those patients who had delayed diagnoses or a compensation claim, but found no association between poor outcomes and age, gender, or previous occupation.[47]

Total Joint Arthroplasty (Hip and Knee)

End-stage and severe arthritic conditions of the hip and knee are often treated with joint arthroplasty (replacement). The replacement may be total (complete) or partial, depending on the patient's age, activity level, and extent of disease. The prosthetic components may be held in place by being cemented into proper position, uncemented/press-fit, or some combination of the two. The decision as to whether the component should be cemented or uncemented is based on the patient's age, lifestyle, bone architecture, and comorbid conditions.

Risk

A total hip arthroplasty requires that some of the stabilizing soft tissues about the joint be cut then repaired. Healing of these tissues usually takes at least 12 weeks to occur. The primary risk concern in the early postoperative period is dislocation of the replaced joint. Specific activity restrictions should be mandated during this time frame and are dependent on whether an anterior, posterior, or anterolateral approach is utilized. If an anterior approach is performed, the patient should minimize extremes of hip flexion, abduction, and external rotation. If the posterior approach has been selected, then the patient should avoid extreme hip flexion, adduction, and internal rotation. Late instability of hip replacements occurs less frequently than early postoperative dislocation and is usually associated with malpositioned components, a new trauma, deterioration in muscle mass or mental status, and polyethylene wear.[48]

Hip instability could also occur if the prosthesis becomes dislodged from the bone into which it has been implanted. Those patients having cemented replacements usually have immediate bony stability and are allowed to put full weight on the operated extremity in the early postoperative period. Patients receiving uncemented or press-fit femoral stems have traditionally been limited to partial weight bearing for the first 6 to 12 weeks in order to facilitate osseointegration of the prosthesis. However, a recent review reported that there was no subsidence or lack of osseous integration found in individuals receiving uncemented femoral stems that were allowed to have immediate and unrestricted postoperative weight bearing.[49]

Chapter 13

Knee arthroplasty also requires a period of about 3 months in order for the surgically manipulated soft tissue to heal. Even though late instability can occur due to ligamentous imbalance or incompetence, malalignment of the prosthesis, a deficient extensor mechanism, an inadequate prosthetic design, or surgical error,[50] early instability or dislocation is not that common.

Most surgeons suggest permanent restrictions against high-impact activity (contact sports, jumping, etc) after joint replacement because of the risk of wear and subsequent implant loosening.

Capacity

Many individuals undergoing technically successful joint replacements still experience some activity-modifying discomfort.[51] However, unless there are problems with ROM or stability, they are able to perform their ADLs better than they did preoperatively and perform at least sedentary-to-light activities. Nonetheless, research regarding the assignment of specific activity restrictions following a joint arthroplasty is incomplete and based more on consensus than evidence-based data.[52,53] Design differences between total hip and knee replacements are such that hip replacement patients are allowed to do heavier activities than patients who have undergone knee replacement.[54] Furthermore, arthroplasty patients may have the actual capacity to pursue heavy occupational or sports activities but traditionally have been limited to lighter activities due to the concern for increased wear and subsequent loosening with vigorous activity (risk).[55] However, one recent study showed that higher-impact sports had no significant effect on the survivorship of total knee arthroplasties.[56] Researchers are also hopeful that hip resurfacing procedures instead of traditional hip replacement will allow patients to participate in heavier activities without increased wear.[57] Naal recently reported that patients who had hip resurfacing procedures instead of traditional total joint replacement returned to a higher level of sports after surgery, but further follow up is necessary in order to assess the influence of high activity level on loosening and revision.[58]

The effect of arthroplasty on employment status has been studied. Bohm found that 86% of the patients who were working prior to total hip replacement returned to work after recovery from the surgery.[59] He also concluded that total hip arthroplasty has positive effects on work capacity in those individuals who return to work. Another investigation demonstrated that hip arthroplasty was effective in keeping patients under the age of 60 employed.[60] This same study found hip replacement to be effective in allowing those patients already off work due to hip pain to return to work, although there was a greater delay noted. Research regarding return to work after total or unicompartmental knee arthroplasty in patients under the age of 60 found that 82% of the study subjects were able to return to work after the surgery within 3 months following surgery.[61] Moreover, Lyall et al. reported that 97.5% of their patient population under age 60 who were working prior to their knee replacement were able to return to their previous work.[62] However, those patients not working prior to their knee arthroplasty continued to be unemployed after their procedure.[62]

Tolerance

Chronic pain, functional disability, and generalized patient dissatisfaction after knee arthroplasty are not uncommon. Certainly surgical technique and implant factors can contribute to poor outcomes. However, much of the pain and disability after knee arthroplasty has been described by one researcher as "medically unexplained."[63]

Table 13-8 Knee Replacement: Consensus Criteria

| | Duration, days | | |
Job Classification	Minimum	Optimum	Maximum
Sedentary	14	28	42
Light	21	42	84
Medium	84	112	Indefinite
Heavy	Indefinite	Indefinite	Indefinite
Very Heavy	Indefinite	Indefinite	Indefinite

Reproduced with permission from Reed. www.mdguidelines.com.

Table 13-9 Surgical Treatment, Total Hip Replacement

| | Duration in Days | | |
Job Classification	Minimum	Optimum	Maximum
Sedentary	7	28	56
Light	42	98	140
Medium	84	112	182
Heavy	Indefinite	Indefinite	Indefinite
Very Heavy	Indefinite	Indefinite	Indefinite

Reproduced with permission from Reed. www.mdguidelines.com.

Chapter 13

Most of the studies evaluating total knee arthroplasty in workers' compensation and non–workers' compensation patients have found inferior outcomes in the workers' compensation population. Mont did not find any major differences in the objective measurements performed on patients with work-related knee versus nonwork-related knee replacements.[64] He did however note much lower Knee Society scores in those individuals with work-related knee problems and advised surgeons that workers' compensation was one of several variables that could have an untoward effect on the outcome of a total knee replacement. De Beer compared patients with work- and nonwork-related knee replacements and concluded that the outcomes of primary knee replacement in patients with work-related injuries were poorer; with higher pain scores, poorer self-perceived outcomes, and lower range of knee flexion.[65] Another study involving work- and nonwork-related knee replacements did not identify any significant differences between the two groups as far as objective measurements such as ROM, strength, instability, deformity, or radiographic criteria.[66] Brinker noted higher pain and disability complaints in the work-related replacements and concluded that suboptimal outcomes could be anticipated in workers' compensation patients. Additionally they found this to be associated with claims that had not been settled at the time of surgery. Saleh's research found that whether the individual's knee replacement was considered to be work related or not, high satisfaction levels were reported. Nonetheless, only 20% of the patients with work-related knee replacements returned to their previous occupation.[67] Thus medical factors do not explain the poorer results in joint replacement patients with workers' compensation–funded surgery, and psychosocial factors must account for the difference.

Although the data regarding outcomes after total knee arthroplasty in the workers' compensation population is somewhat negative, one optimistic report has been published in workers' compensation patients undergoing total hip replacement. Specifically, Hostin et al. found that workers' compensation did not negatively affect the outcome of total hip arthroplasty.[68]

Arthroscopic Meniscectomy

Arthroscopic meniscectomy is one of the most common orthopedic procedures performed. If the location of the tear is such that there is sufficient vascularity in the meniscus and there is an absence of degenerative changes within the meniscus, then repair can be performed. Otherwise, the most conservative meniscal resection is indicated. The methods for the repair or removal of an isolated torn meniscus have evolved over the years to the extent that nearly all procedures to address this problem are done arthroscopically as an outpatient. These procedural improvements have resulted in a significant decrease in the recovery time.[69,70]

Risk

If a technically appropriate meniscectomy has been performed for a torn meniscus, the risk for retear or additional tear within the same meniscus is not a commonly seen complication during the early postoperative time frame. Therefore, the only risk for additional injury involves unrestricted or unprotected use of the extremity during the time required for the postoperative soft tissue inflammation to resolve. This generally takes 1 to 6 weeks, depending on the extent of the tear and any comorbid conditions. High-profile athletes typically return to contact sports within 3 to 6 weeks of arthroscopic partial meniscectomy.

The healing time for meniscal repairs is variable, taking anywhere from 3 to 12 months for complete healing. Some modification or restriction of higher-level activities may be indicated during that time frame.

Capacity

Arthroscopic meniscectomy has been touted as a near-perfect procedure, yet a significant number of patients undergoing arthroscopic meniscectomy may have residual symptoms or clinical findings.[71] A recent study has found that some degree of quadriceps weakness may exist up to 6 months postoperatively.[72] Long-term studies confirm that osteoarthritis can still be a complication of meniscectomy.[73] Nonetheless, most of these individuals are able to return to their previous activity level and do so fairly soon after an uncomplicated procedure. Umar reported that sedentary workers returned to work within 3 weeks and heavy laborers returned to their occupation within a mean time of 5 weeks.[74] Lubowitz's research found that most patients who underwent an uncomplicated arthroscopy had no knee-related activity restrictions 4 weeks after their arthroscopy.[75] However, patients with workers' compensation claims were not included as study subjects.

Table 13-10 Arthroscopic Meniscectomy: Consensus Criteria

	Duration, days		
Job Classification	**Minimum**	**Optimum**	**Maximum**
Sedentary	7	14	28
Light	7	14	35
Medium	14	21	56
Heavy	21	42	84
Very Heavy	28	42	112

Reproduced with permission from Reed. www.mdguidelines.com.

Chapter 13

Tolerance

When a patient has persistence of pain after an uncomplicated arthroscopy, some consideration should be given to the possibility that there is additional pathology present, such as osteoarthritis, an associated ligament injury, or unrecognized hip pathology referring pain into the knee region. If no additional pathology is found, then nonmedical factors could be contributing to the unexpected duration and extent of reported pain.

References

1. US Bureau of Labor Statistics, US Department of Labor. TABLE R68. Number and percent distribution of nonfatal occupational injuries and illnesses involving days away from work by part of body affected by injury or illness and number of days away from work, 2008. http://www.bls.gov/iif/oshwc/case/ostb 2150.pdf. Accessed March 19, 2010.

2. Melhorn JM, Ackerman WE. *Guides to the Evaluation of Disease and Injury Causation.* Chicago, IL: AMA; 2008.

3. Blue Book – September 20081.00 Musculoskeletal System – Adult. http://www.socialsecurity.gov/disability/professionals/bluebook/1.00-Musculo skeletal-Adult.htm (1of 17). Accessed March 15, 2010.

4. Derscheid GL, Garrick JG. Medial collateral ligament injuries in football: nonoperative management of grade I and grade II sprains. *Am J Sports Med.* 1981;9:365–368.

5. Woo SLY, Vogrin TM, Abramowitch SD. Healing and repair of ligament injuries. *J Am Acad Orthop Surg.* 2000;8:364–372.

6. Mosknes H, Snyder-Mackler L, Risberg MA. Individuals with an anterior cruciate ligament-deficient knee classified as noncopers may be candidates for non-surgical rehabilitation. *J Orthop Sports Ther.* 2008;38(10):586–595.

7. Chen CH. Graft healing in anterior cruciate ligament reconstruction. *Sports Medicine, Arthroscopy, Rehabilitation, Therapy, and Technology.* 2009;1:21.

8. West RV, Harner CD. Graft selection in anterior cruciate ligament reconstruction. *J Am Acad Orthop Surg.* 2005;(13)197–207.

9. van Grinsven S, van Cingel RE, Holla CJ, van Loon CJ. Evidence-based rehabilitation following anterior cruciate ligament reconstruction. *Knee Surg Sports Traumatol Arthrosc.* 2010;18(8):1128–1144.

10. Borchens JR, Pedroza A, Kaeding C. Activity level and graft type as risk factors for anterior cruciate ligament graft failure: a case-control study. *Am J Sports Med.* 2009;37(12):2362–2367. Epub 2009 Aug 14.

11. Salmon L, Russell V, Musgrove T, Pinczewski L, Refshauge K. Incidence and risk factors for graft rupture and contralateral rupture after anterior cruciate ligament reconstruction. *Arthroscopy.* 2005;21(8):948–957.

12. Tanaka Y, Yonetani Y, Shiozaki Y, Kitaguchi T, Sato N, Takeshita S, Horibe S. Re-tear of anterior cruciate ligament grafts in female basketball players: a case

series. *Sports Med Arthrosc Rehabil Ther Technol.* 2010;2(1):7. {Epub ahead of print}

13. Kerkoffs GM, Rowe BH, Assendelft WJ, Kelly K, Struijs PA, van Dijk CN. *Cochrane Database Syst Rev.* 2002;(3):CD003762.

14. van Rij RM, van Os AG, Bernsen RM, Luijsterburg PA, Koes BW, Bierma-Zeinstra SM. What is the clinical course of acute ankle sprains? a systematic literature review. *Am J Med.* 2008;121(4):324–331.

15. Maffulli N, Ferran NA. Management of acute and chronic ankle instability. *J Am Acad Orthop Surg.* 2008;16(10):608–615.

16. Hubbard TJ, Hicks-Little CA. Ankle ligament healing after an acute ankle sprain: an evidence-based approach. *J Athl Train.* 2008;43(5):523–529.

17. Holmes A, Delahunt E. Treatment of common deficits associated with chronic ankle instability. *Sports Med.* 2009;39(3):207–224.

18. Chen L, Ahmad CS, Levine WN. Medial collateral ligament injuries of the knee: current treatment concepts. *Curr Rev Musculoskeletal Med.* 2008;1(2):108–113.

19. Lundberg M, Messner K. Long-term prognosis of isolated partial medial collateral ligament ruptures: a ten-year clinical and radiographic evaluation of a prospectively observed group of patients. *Am J Sports Med.* 1996;24:160–163.

20. Pietrosimone BG, Grindstaff TL, Linens SW, Uczekaj E, Hertel J. A systematic review of prophylactic braces in the prevention of knee ligament injuries in collegiate football players. *J Ath Train.* 2008;43(4):409–415.

21. Kostogiannis I, Ageberg E, Neuman P, Dahlberg L, Friden T, Roos H. Activity level and subjective knee function 15 years after anterior cruciate ligament injury: a prospective, longitudinal study of nonreconstructed patients. *Am J Sports Med.* 2007;35(7):1135–1143.

22. Hartigan EH, Axe MJ. Time line for noncopers to pass return-to-sports criteria after anterior cruciate ligament reconstruction. *J Orthop Sports Phys Ther.* 2010;40(3):141–154.

23. Wexler G, Bach BR, Bush-Joseph CA, Smink D, Ferrari JD, Bojchuk J. Outcomes of anterior cruciate ligament reconstruction in patients with worker's compensation claims. *Arthroscopy.* 2000;16(1):49–58.

24. Barrett GR, Rook RT, Nash CR, Coggin MR. The effect of worker's compensation on clinical outcomes of arthroscopic assisted autogenous patellar tendon anterior cruciate ligament reconstruction in an acute population. *Arthroscopy.* 2001;17(2):132–137.

25. Noyes FR, Barber-Westin SD. A comparison of results of arthroscopic-assisted anterior cruciate ligament reconstruction between worker's compensation and noncompensation patients. *Arthroscopy.* 1997;13(4):474–484.

26. Kivi P, Aho H, Jarvinen M. "Tennis Leg"—calf muscle rupture of the middle-aged tennis aficionado. *Duodecim.* 2009;125(16):1441–1443.

27. Heiderscheit BC, Sherry MA, Silder A, Chumanov ES, Thelen DG. Hamstring strain injuries: recommendations for diagnosis, rehabilitation, and injury prevention. *J Orthop Sports Phys Ther.* 2010;40(2):67–81.

Chapter 13

28. Khan RJ, Fick D, Keogh A, Crawford J, Brammar T, Parker M. Treatment of Achilles tendon ruptures. A meta-analysis of randomized, controlled trials. *J Bone Joint Surg Am*. 2005;87(10):2202–2210.

29. Metz R, Verleisdonk EJ, van der Heijden GJ, Clevers GJ, Hammacher ER, Verhofstad MH, van der Werken C. Acute Achilles tendon rupture: minimally invasive surgery versus nonoperative treatment with immediate full weightbearing—a randomized controlled trial. *Am J Sports Med*. 2008;36(9): 1688–1694.

30. Gidwani S, Bircher MD. Avulsion injuries of the hamstring origin—a series of 12 patients and management algorithm. *Ann R Coll Surg Engl*. 2007;89(4): 394–399.

31. Breederveld RS, Patka P, van Mourik JC. Refractures of the femoral shaft. *Neth J Surg*. 1985;37(4):114–116.

32. Jensen JS, Hansen FW, Johansen J. Tibial shaft fracture. A comparison of conservative treatment and internal fixation with conventional plates or AO compression plates. *Acta Orthop Scand*. 1977;48(2):204–212.

33. Christensen J, Greiff J, Rosendahi S. Fractures of the tibia treated with AO compression osteosynthesis. *Injury*. 1982;13(4):307–314.

34. Kootstra G. Femoral shaft fractures in adults. A study of 329 consecutive cases with a statistical analysis of different methods of treatment. Thesis. University of Groningen. Van Gorcum & Comp. B.V. Assen 1973.

35. Bråten M, Terjesen T, and Rossvoll I. Femoral shaft fractures treated by intramedullary nailing. A follow-up study focusing on problems related to the method. *Injury*. 1995;26(6):379–383.

36. FemoralShaftFractures.http://www.rcsed.ac.uk/fellows/Ivanrensburg/Femoral. htm. Accessed May 4, 2010.

37. Laubenthal KN, Smidt GL, Kettelkamp DB. A quantitative analysis of knee motion during activities of daily living. *PhysicalTherapy*. 1972;52(1):34–45.

38. Rowe PJ, Myles CM, Walker C, Nutton R. Knee joint kinematics in gait and other functional activities measured using flexible electrogoniometry: how much knee motion is sufficient for normal daily life? *Gait and Posture*. 2000;12: 143–155.

39. McPoil TG, Knecht HG. Biomechanics of the foot in walking: a functional approach. *J Orthop Sports Phys Ther*. 1985;7(2):69–72.

40. Faergemann C, Frandsen PA, Rock ND. Residual impairment after lower extremity fracture. *J Trauma*. 1998;45(1):123–126.

41. Bednar DA, Ali P. Intramedullary nailing of femoral shaft fractures; reoperation and return to work. *Can J Surg*. 1993;36(5):464–466.

42. Hardy AE. The treatment of femoral fractures by cast-brace application and early ambulation. A prospective review of one hundred and six patients. *J Bone Joint Surg Am*. 1983;65(1):56–65.

43. Ferguson M, Brand C, Lowe A, et al. Outcomes of isolated tibial shaft fractures treated at level one trauma centers. *Injury*. 2008;39(2):187–95.

44. Mock C, MacKenzie E, Jurkobich G, et al. Determinants of disability after lower extremity fracture. *J Trauma.* 2000;49(6):1002–1011.

45. MacKenzie E, Bosse MJ, Pollak AN, et al. Long term persistence of disability following lower limb trauma. Results of seven-year follow up. *J Bone Joint Surg Am.* 2005;87(8):1801–1809.

46. Williams TM, Nepola DV, DeCoster TA, Hurwit SR, Dirschi DR, Marsh JL. Factors affecting outcome in tibial plafond fractures. *Clin Orthop Relat Res.* 2004;(423):93–98.

47. Calder JD, Whitehouse ST, Saxby TS. Results of isolated Lisfranc injuries and the effect of compensation claims. *J Bone Joint Surg Br.* 2004;86(4):527–530.

48. Pulido L, Restrepo C, Parvizi J. Late instability following total hip arthroplasty. *Clin Med Res.* 2007; 5(2):139–142.

49. Hol AM, van Grinsven S, Lucas C, van Susante JL, van Loon CJ. Partial versus unrestricted weight bearing after an uncemented femoral stem in total hip arthroplasty: recommendation of concise rehabilitation protocol from a systematic review of the literature. *Arch Orthop Trauma Surg.* 2010;130(4):547–555.

50. Fehring TK, Valadie AL. Knee instability after total knee arthroplasty. *Clin Orthop Relat Res.* 1994;(299):157–162.

51. Weller IM, Kunz M. Physical activity and pain following total hip arthroplasty. http://www.sciencedirect.com/science?_ob=ArticleURL&_udi=B7CVK-4M7 CMH5-1&_u. Accessed March 13, 2010.

52. Swanson EA, Schmalzried TP, Dorey FJ. Activity recommendations after total hip and knee arthroplasty: a survey of the American Association for Hip and Knee Surgeons. *J. Arthroplasty.* 2009;24(6 Suppl):120–126.

53. Healy WL, Sharma S, Schwartz B, Iorio R. Athletic activity after total joint arthroplasty. *J. Bone Joint Surg Am.* 2008;90(10):2245–2252.

54. Kuster MS. Exercise recommendations after total joint replacement: a review of the current literature and proposal of scientifically based guidelines. *Sports Med.* 2002;32(7):433–445.

55. Seyler TM, Mont MA, Ragland PS, Kachwala MM, Delanois RE. Sports activity after total hip and knee arthroplasty: specific recommendations concerning tennis. *Sports Med.* 2006;36(7):571–583.

56. Parratte S. Dahm DL, Syuart MJ. Paper #507. Presented at the 2010 annual meeting of the American Academy of Orthopedic Surgeons. March 9–13. New Orleans. http://wwworthosupersite.com/print.aspx?rid=61919. Accessed March 15, 2010.

57. Fowble VA, dela Rosa MA, Schmalzried TP. A comparison of total hip resurfacing and total hip arthroplasty—patients and outcomes. *Bull NYUHosp Jt Dis.* 2009;67(2):108–112.

58. Naal FD, Maffiuletti NA, Munzinger U, Hersche O. Sports after hip resurfacing arthroplasty. *Am J Sports Med.* 2007;35(5):705–711.

59. Bohm ER. The effect of total hip arthroplasty on employment. *J Arthroplasty.* 2010;25(1):15–18.

Chapter 13

60. Mobasheri R, Gidwani S, Rosson JW. The effect of total hip replacement on the employment status of patients under the age of 60. *Ann R Coll Surg.* 2006;88(2): 131–133.

61. Foote JA, Smith HK, Jonas SC, Greenwood R, Weale AE. Return to work following knee arthroplasty. *Knee.* 2010;17(1):19–22.

62. Lyall H, Ireland J, El-Zebdeh MY. The effect of total knee replacement on employment in patients under 60 years of age. *Ann R Coll Surg.* 2009;91(5): 410–413.

63. Wylde V, Dieppe P, Hewlett S, Learmonth ID. The total knee replacement: is it really an effective procedure for all? *Knee.* 2007;14(6):417–423.

64. Mont MA, Mayerson JA, Krackow KA, Hungerford DS. Total knee arthro-plasty in patients receiving workers' compensation. *J Bone Joint Surg Am.* 1998;80(9):1285–1290.

65. de Beer J, Petruccelli D, Gandhi R, Winemaker M. Primary total knee arthro-plasty in patients receiving workers' compensation benefits. *Can J Surg.* 2005;48(2):100–105.

66. Brinker MR, Savory CG, Weeden SH, Aucoin HC, Curd DT. The results of total knee arthroplasty in workers' compensation patients. *Bull Hosp Jt Dis.* 1998; 57(2):80–83.

67. Saleh K, Nelson C, Kassim R, Yoon P, Haas S. Total knee arthroplasty in patients on workers' compensation: a matched cohort study with an average follow up of 4.5 years. *J Arthroplasty.* 2004;19(3):310–312.

68. Hostin E, Mont MA, Mayerson JA, Jones LC, Hungerford DS. Total hip arthro-plasty in patients receiving workers' compensation. *Clin Orthop Relat Res.* 2000;(379):161–168.

69. St. Pierre DM. Rehabilitation following arthroscopic meniscectomy. *Sports Med.* 1995;20:338–347.

70. Pettrone FA. Meniscectomy: arthrotomy versus arthroscopy. *AM J Sports Med.* 1982;10:355–359.

71. Roos EM, Ostenberg A, Roos H, Ekdahi C, Lohmander LS. Long-term outcome of meniscectomy: symptoms, function, and performance tests in patients with or without radiographic osteoarthritis compared to matched controls. *Osteoarthritis Cartilage.* 2001;9(4):316–324.

72. Glatthorn JF, Berendts AM, Bizzini M, Munzinger U, Maffuletti NA. Neuromuscular function after arthroscopic partial meniscectomy. *Clin Orthop Relat Res.* 2010;468(5):1336–1343.

73. Fabricant PD, Joki P. Surgical outcomes after arthroscopic partial meniscectomy. *J Am Acad Orthop Surg.* 2007;15(11):647–653.

74. Umar M. Ambulatory arthroscopic knee surgery results of partial meniscectomy. *J Pak Med Assoc.* 1997;47(8):210–213.

75. Lubowitz JH, Ayala M, Appleby D. Return to activity after knee arthroscopy. *Arthroscopy.* 2008;24(1):58–61.

Chapter 14

Working With Common Cardiovascular Problems

**Mark H. Hyman, MD, Jawali Jaranilla, MD, MPH
and Thomas E. Kottke, MD, MSPH**

This chapter explores the common cardiovascular problems encountered in clinical return-to-work evaluations. Heart disease and associated vascular conditions continue to dominate Western society as the number-one cause of death and medical expenditures.[1] As industrialized nations continue to experience an aging workforce, physicians are certain to be confronted with disability determinations in patients with these cardiovascular conditions that accompany aging.

General Considerations in Cardiovascular Assessment

The key to cardiovascular evaluations is understanding the use of objective testing. Appropriate testing may include exercise treadmill, echocardiography, Holter monitoring, serial blood pressure testing, or measuring ankle-brachial indices. A brief explanation here of these procedures will allow a better understanding of the illnesses discussed in this chapter. More comprehensive reviews, summaries, and studies are available.[2–6]

In treadmill testing, exercise (or work) capacity is measured. There are different treadmill testing protocols, including the Bruce, Balke, Naughton, and Ellestad tests. These tests vary in how fast patients walk and how steep an incline the patient must work against. The most common protocol is the Bruce, which changes these parameters every three minutes.

Adequate testing usually means a patient achieved at least 85% of his or her maximum predicted heart rate (MPHR). There are normal tables of target heart rate based on patient age, an example of which is shown in Table 14-1.[7] There are also tables of the expected duration of exercise capacity for individuals of varying ages, as shown in Table 14-2.[8]

An important concept in treadmill testing is the metabolic equivalent (MET) system. One MET equals the oxygen cost of, or the oxygen consumed in, sitting at rest in a room of normal temperature and humidity. The numerical value of 1 MET is 3.5 mL of oxygen per kilogram per minute. Each activity to be performed requires a unique or specific amount of energy (or oxygen). Physicians can estimate the maximum exercise ability of patients as the maximum number of METs expended on a treadmill (Tables 14-3 and 14-4). The number of METs an individual should be capable of achieving on the basis of age and sex is shown in Table 14-5. The objective test outlined in Table 14-6 may be used to identify an individual's functional capacity.

Several factors must be considered when exercise performance is interpreted. The most important is effort. This can be assessed subjectively by a physician watching the patient's performance during testing. If the testing was previously monitored by someone else and no comment on patient effort during testing was recorded, the decision to accept the previous test

Table 14-1 Maximal Predicted Heart Rate Averages for Exercise

| Age, y | Maximum | Maximal Predicted Heart Rate, beats/min | | | | | | | |
		95%	90%	85%	80%	75%	70%	65%	60%
25	190	180	171	162	152	143	133	124	114
30	186	177	167	158	149	140	130	121	112
35	182	173	164	155	146	137	127	118	109
40	181	172	163	154	145	136	127	118	109
45	179	170	161	152	143	134	125	116	107
50	175	166	158	149	140	131	123	114	105
55	171	162	154	145	137	128	120	111	103
60	168	160	151	143	134	126	118	109	101
65	164	156	148	139	131	123	115	107	98
70	160	152	144	135	128	120	112	104	96
75	156	148	140	131	125	117	109	101	94
80	152	144	137	130	122	114	106	99	91
85	148	140	133	126	118	111	104	96	89

Adapted from Sheffield.[7]

Table 14-2 Cardiorespiratory Fitness Classification for Bruce Protocol

Age, y	Classification by Expected Duration of Exercise Capacity, min				
	Low	Fair	Average	Good	High
Males					
20–29	<6	8	11	14	>15
30–39	<5	7	10	13	>14
40–49	<4	6	9	12	>13
50–59	<3	4	8	11	>12
60–69	<3	4	8	10	>12
Females					
20–29	<6	7	9	11	>13
30–39	<4	5	8	10	>12
40–49	<3	4	7	9	>11
50–59	<3	3	5	8	>10
60–69	<2	3	4	7	>9

Adapted from Bruce et al.[8]

result or to repeat treadmill testing can be difficult. If the patient's condition seems "too good" for the reported exercise ability on a previous treadmill test, retesting may be indicated.

A patient who achieves 85% of his or her MPHR but at an early stage of testing (low work load) is probably deconditioned. Deconditioning means that the individual is usually sedentary and thus currently has a low exercise capacity, but this capacity may be increased with an activity program. This activity program may mean cardiac rehabilitation (supervised, medically safe progressive exercise) or progressive home-based exercise like walking, or it may mean return to work with work limitations that progressively decrease over time as work assignments become progressively more strenuous.

If a patient terminates treadmill testing because of nonspecific symptoms such as fatigue at a low workload with a heart rate far below the MPHR and without any worrisome ischemic, hemodynamic, or arrhythmic changes, then a poor tolerance for exercise exists despite adequate capacity. If a patient terminates treadmill testing because of nonspecific symptoms at a very low workload and by history that patient routinely performs activities of daily living (ADLs) that require exertion to higher work loads, either malingering or unconscious symptom magnification should be suspected.

Chapter 14

Table 14-3 Relationship of METs and Functional Class According to Five Treadmill Protocols*

METs	1.6	2	3	4	5	6	7	8	9	10	11	12	13	14	15	16
Treadmill tests																
Ellestad																
Miles per hour					1.7	3.0			4.0						5.0	
% grade					10	10			10						10	
Bruce																
Miles per hour					1.7		2.5		3.4					4.2	5.0	
% grade					10		12		14					16	18	
Balke																
Miles per hour				3.4	3.4	3.4	3.4	3.4	3.4	3.4	3.4	3.4	3.4	3.4	3.4	3.4
% grade				2	4	6	8	10	12	14	16	18	20	22	24	26
Balke																
Miles per hour			3.0	3.0	3.0	3.0	3.0	3.0	3.0	3.0	3.0	3.0				
% grade			0	2.5	5	7.5	10	12.5	15	17.5	20	22.5				
Naughton																
Miles per hour	1.0	2.0	2.0	2.0	2.0	2.0	2.0									
% grade	0	0	3.5	7	10.5	14	17.5									

METs	1.6	2	3	4	5	6	7	8	9	10	11	12	13	14	15	16
Clinical status																
Symptomatic patients		←—	——	——	——	——	—→									
Diseased, recovered		←—	——	——	——	——	—→									
Sedentary healthy					←—	——	——	——	——	—→						
Physically active							←—	——	——	——	—→					
Functional class*	IV	←III→			←II→		←——	——	——	——	—I and Normal	——	——	——	——	—→

Adapted from: Fox et al.[9]

Table 14-4 Energy Expenditure in METs During Bicycle Ergometry

Body Weight		Work Rate on Bicycle Ergometer, kg m⁻¹ min⁻¹ (Watts)												
kg	(lb)	75 (50)	150 (75)	300 (100)	450 (125)	600 (150)	750 (175)	900 (200)	1050 (225)	1200 (250)	1350 (275)	1500 (300)	1650	1800
20	(44)	4.0	6.0	10.0	14.0	18.0	22.0							
30	(66)	3.4	4.7	7.3	10.0	12.7	15.3	17.9	20.7	23.3				
40	(88)	3.0	4.0	6.0	8.0	10.0	12.0	14.0	16.0	18.0	20.0	22.0		
50	(110)	2.8	3.6	5.2	6.8	8.4	10.0	11.5	13.2	14.8	16.3	18.0	19.6	21.1
60	(132)	2.7	3.3	4.7	6.0	7.3	8.7	10.0	11.3	12.7	14.0	15.3	16.7	18.0
70	(154)	2.6	3.1	4.3	5.4	6.6	7.7	8.8	10.0	11.1	12.2	13.4	14.0	15.7
80	(176)	2.5	3.0	4.0	5.0	6.0	7.0	8.0	9.0	10.0	11.0	12.0	13.0	14.0
90	(198)	2.4	2.9	3.8	4.7	5.6	6.4	7.3	8.2	9.1	10.0	10.9	11.8	12.6
100	(220)	2.4	2.8	3.6	4.4	5.2	6.0	6.8	7.6	8.4	9.2	10.0	10.8	11.6
110	(242)	2.4	2.7	3.4	4.2	4.9	5.6	6.3	7.1	7.8	8.5	9.3	10.0	10.7
120	(264)	2.3	2.7	3.3	4.0	4.7	5.3	6.0	6.7	7.3	8.0	8.7	9.3	10.0

Adapted from American College of Sports Medicine.[10]

Table 14-5 Normal MET Values for Men and Women

Age, y	Men			Women		
	10th Percentile	Mean	90th Percentile	10th Percentile	Mean	90th Percentile
20–29	9.0	11.0	13.5	6.2	8.6	10.8
30–39	8.6	10.5	13.2	6.2	8.6	10.2
40–49	7.8	10.0	12.8	6.0	7.6	10.0
50–59	7.0	9.4	12.4	5.0	7.0	9.4
60+	5.7	8.2	11.7	4.5	6.2	8.6

Adapted from Pollock et al.[11]

Cardiopulmonary (metabolic) testing can help differentiate among cardiac, pulmonary, and low tolerance for a patient expressing limitation on treadmill testing.[14]

Studies and guidelines suggest that a person has the capacity to perform sustained work, ie, an 8-hour workday with typical breaks, to at least 40% of his or her maximal MET level. He or she could also be expected to perform for 15-minute intervals, once or twice a day, at 80% of the maximal MET level.[13,15,16] Certain occupations, while generally having low demands, could at times be associated with a sudden increase in either physical or psychological demands. Examples include police officer, firefighter, airline pilot, air traffic controller, and commercial vehicle driver.[16] Estimates of the oxygen cost of many jobs and activities (in METs) have been published.[16,17]

For example, if a patient can exercise to 10 METs safely on the treadmill and the job in question requires sustained exertion of 2.5 METs and brief periods of exertion to 5 METs, then the patient should be safe in this job. (A level of 2.5 METs is less than 40% of 10 METs, and 5 METs is less than 80% of 10 METs.)

The US Social Security Administration (SSA) considers inability to exercise during treadmill testing to 5.0 METs due to symptoms or physiologic observations that terminate testing (arrhythmia, hypotension, ischemia, etc) as a criterion for total disability.[18]

Another important measure of cardiovascular disability estimation comes from the ejection fraction.[2] This measure of systolic heart function appears to be a more reliable indicator of disability than diastolic dysfunction, the latter being harder to measure and interpret.[19] The gold standard of systolic function is angiographic left ventriculography, and the gold standard of

Table 14-6 Physical Demand, Energy Requirements, and Activities

Demand Level	Energy Required (METs)	Work Lifting Demand, lbs			Sample Occupations	Home Activity	Recreational Activity	Physical Conditioning
		Occasional (0%–33% of Workday)	Frequent (34%–66% of Workday)	Constant (67%–100% of Workday)				
Sedentary	1.5–2.1	10	None	None	Clerical, store clerk, bartender, truck driver, crane operator	Washing, shaving, dressing, writing, washing dishes, driving car	Shuffleboard, horseshoes, billiards, archery, golf with cart	Walking 2 mph, stationary bicycle, very light calisthenics
Light	2.2–3.5	20	10	None and/ or operating controls while seated	Light welding, carpentry, auto repair, machine assembly	Raking leaves, weeding, painting, cleaning windows, waxing floor	Dancing, golf walking, sailing, horseback riding, doubles tennis	Walking 3–4 mph, cycling 6–8 mph, light calisthenics
Medium or Moderate	3.6–6.3	20–50	10–25	10	Carpentry, shoveling, pneumatic tools	Gardening, lawn mowing, slow climbing of stairs	Badminton, singles tennis, skiing downhill, basketball, football, ice skating, light backpacking	Walking 4–5 mph, cycling 9–10 mph, swimming breast-stroke
Heavy	6.4–7.5	50–100	25–50	10–20	Ditch digging, pick and shovel	Sawing wood, heavy shoveling	Canoeing, mountain climbing, fencing, paddleball	Jogging 5 mph, cycling 12 mph, swimming crawl, rowing
Very Heavy	>7.5	>100	>50	>20	Lumberjack, heavy labor	Heavy snow shoveling, fast stairs	Handball, squash, cross-country skiing	Running $\geq$ 6 mph, cycling $\geq$ 13 mph, jumping rope

Adapted from Haskell[12] and Astrand.[13]

Chapter 14

diastolic function is the left ventricule end diastolic pressure measurement. For disability investigation, radionuclide angiography can be used to measure the ejection fraction, although transthoracic echocardiography with Doppler is noninvasive, less expensive, useful with associated valvular disease, and equally acceptable.[20,21] An ejection fraction greater than 50% is considered normal, 40% to 50% is considered a mild or slight impairment or dysfunction, 30% to 40% is a moderate impairment or dysfunction, and less than 30% is considered a severe or total impairment or dysfunction. While ejection fraction, ventricular arrhythmias, and peak oxygen uptake are all independent predictors of all-cause mortality in patients with reduced physical work capacity, they are poorly correlated.[22] The implication of this observation is that cardiopulmonary exercise testing is a better tool than ejection fraction to determine physical work capacity.

The SSA considers an ejection fraction of 30% or less to be evidence of total disability if there is a history of episodes of clinical congestive heart failure. Congestive heart failure, also called heart failure, is a constellation of symptoms secondary to the inability of the heart to pump blood to meet the needs of the body. An alternative criterion is a left ventricular end diastolic dimension of greater than 6.0 cm. The criteria for total disability for diastolic dysfunction include a left ventricular posterior wall and septal thickness sum of 2.5 cm or more, and a left atrial size of greater than 4.5 cm.

Risk in Cardiovascular Disease

Later sections of this chapter briefly explore what little is known about the *risk of working* with a condition. When discussing cardiovascular disease *risk*, it is often helpful to consider the known risk factors that may have contributed to the disease formation in the first place. For patients with heart disease, treatment of risk factors can slow the progression of disease and markedly reduce clinical events. Many reviews stress the importance of both primary and secondary prevention in risk/causative factor treatment.[23] A more detailed discussion of disease risk and causation can be found in the companion book *Guides to the Evaluation of Disease and Injury Causation.*[24]

Coronary Artery Disease

Presumed Disability
The SSA estimates that, in general, if a patient has a treadmill study with an exercise capacity of at most 5 METs of work, *or* an ejection fraction of at most 30%, *or* significant angiographic coronary artery disease, then total

disability is presumed to exist.[25] The treadmill would be limited on the basis of at least 1mm (mV) ST segment change, failure to increase systolic blood pressure by 10 mm Hg, or significant reversible ischemic defect on imaging. The angiographic disease must be associated with typical angina or dyspnea limitations (Tables 14-7) and must meet or exceed criteria for significant narrowing (Table 14-8). Some individuals with sedentary jobs work despite meeting these criteria.

Table 14-7 New York Heart Association Functional Classification of Cardiac Disease

Class	Description
I	Individual has cardiac disease but no resulting limitation of physical activity; ordinary physical activity does not cause undue fatigue, palpitation, dyspnea, or anginal pain.
II	Individual has cardiac disease resulting in slight limitation of physical activity; is comfortable at rest and in the performance of ordinary, light, daily activities; greater-than-ordinary physical activity, such as heavy physical exertion, results in fatigue, palpitation, dyspnea, or anginal pain.
III	Individual has cardiac disease resulting in marked limitation of physical activity; is comfortable at rest; ordinary physical activity results in fatigue, palpitation, dyspnea, or anginal pain.
IV	Individual has cardiac disease resulting in inability to carry on any physical activity without discomfort; symptoms of inadequate cardiac output, pulmonary congestion, systemic congestion, or anginal syndrome may be present, even at rest; if any physical activity is undertaken, discomfort is increased.

Adapted from Criteria Committee of the New York Heart Association.[26]

Table 14-8 SSA Listing for Significant Angiographic Disease

Percent Narrowing	Involved Coronary Vessel
50	Left main
70	Any vessel
50	Any vessel where narrowing is >1 cm in length
50	Any 2 vessels
100	Any previously bypassed graft vessel

Adapted from the US Social Security Administration.[25]

Risk Assessment

There is little information about workers with documented ischemic heart disease and specific occupations they cannot perform. Certain occupations that place a worker at risk of developing cardiovascular morbidity and mortality have been identified. Depending on the study, examples of these can include workers in metal processing, paper, chemicals, plastics, air traffic control, bus operation, assembly, firefighters, nursing, and waiting tables.[27–30] If chemical exposure at work is thought to play a role in the development of an individual's heart disease, a physician should prevent further potentially harmful exposure to that substance by work restrictions. (Restrictions are based on risk.) When work ability is assessed in patients with coronary artery disease, the risks to consider are angina, myocardial infarction, and hemodynamically significant arrhythmias.

Angina

Angina is the chest pain syndrome associated with reversible myocardial ischemia. With angina of short duration (eg, less than 15 to 30 minutes), there is generally no significant heart muscle damage; thus, no change in impairment has occurred. The frequency and severity of angina can identify a patient who's chest pain or anginal equivalent is truly cardiac in origin, then the symptom of angina can be used as a gauge to restrict a work activity. This should be supported by an evaluation of exercise capacity as discussed below. If there is doubt about whether or not angina is occurring at work, the patient can wear a Holter monitor during a workday This permits the evaluation of heart rate and pattern of ECG changes such as ST segment change at the times when chest pain occurred at work.

For a patient who is off work, a trial of return to work is reasonable if the job demands of potential employment are below the exercise level that provokes angina on treadmill testing.

Myocardial Infarction

A second risk concern is myocardial infarction (or acute unstable angina). Exercise capacity is predictive of the risk of death in normal subjects, as well as in patients with coronary artery disease and noncardiac conditions that include chronic lung disease, diabetes, hypertension, elevated body mass index, hypercholesterolemia, and cigarette smoking.[31,32] Physical exertion becomes a stronger predictor of myocardial infarction when patients are inactive, male, hyperlipidemic, and cigarette smokers.[33] If patients and physicians are concerned that the work environment will precipitate an acute coronary syndrome, an exercise test can be performed, and if the heart rate expected at work (or ideally observed on ambulatory monitoring during work) is less than the heart rate at the ischemic threshold on the exercise test, the patient should

Chapter 14

be able to safely perform work-related tasks. While depression has been associated with development of and poor outcomes in cardiovascular conditions, treatment with medication has not brought great benefit.[34] This may be that the depression affects physical activity and does not have a direct independent influence.[35] As with leisure-time physical activity, the exercise experienced at work may be protective against future coronary events.

While there are many well-known risk factors that predict who will ultimately develop coronary artery disease,[2,3,36–45] these risk factors do *not* predict who will experience problems on returning to work. Perhaps the best study on the risk of returning to work after myocardial infarction was done in Israel.[46] Two hundred sixteen patients were evaluated for return-to-work ability after myocardial infarction. Of the 168 who attempted to return to work, 150 successfully did so and were followed up for 2 years. Six sustained a second infarction, but only two of these occurred while the patient happened to be at work. Thus, returning to work did not pose a significant risk to these patients.

Because the medical literature contains few studies on the risk of working despite known heart disease, following consensus guidelines may be rational and may provide some medicolegal protection for physician opinion. One excellent source of consensus guidelines for activity is to use those developed for athletes. Studies have been done on athletic competition requirements and the risks of competition-induced cardiovascular complications for athletes. A good summary of presumably safe exercise levels for various cardiovascular conditions, known as the 26th Bethesda Conference, has been published by the American College of Cardiology. One section discusses the risk of competitive athletics for athletes with known coronary artery disease.[47] Updated information on this area also exists.[48] The approach promulgated is to assess each sport's activity in terms of its dynamic/isotonic endurance requirement along with its static/isometric lifting requirements. Parallels can be drawn between a worker's Bethesda static requirement and the work demands estimate listed in Table 14-6.

Capacity

Measuring current capacity in cardiovascular conditions has been described above. In general, if a patient has simple chronic stable angina, a normal stress treadmill study, and normal ejection fraction, there has been no change in his or her work capacity. If one or more measures of heart function are altered, then Table 14-6 offers parameters for work limitation. If the measured safe exercise capacity is less than the job demands (sustained exertion exceeds 40% of treadmill-determined maximum ability or infrequent exertion exceeds 80% of capacity), then the individual is not currently

Chapter 14

safely capable of performing the job in question, and there is a medically determined work limitation. (Limitations are based on capacity.)

A useful analogy may be the Department of Transportation criteria for commercial drivers.[49] The criteria are adequate cardiac function despite coronary artery disease to permit commercial driving, which is most often light work with occasional periods of heavy work. The criteria are an ejection fraction of at least 40%, exercise capacity of 6 METs or better (finish stage II on the Bruce protocol, achieving at least 85% of MPHR without evidence of ischemia while systolic blood pressure increases at least 20 mm Hg from its resting level), and tolerance of medications without orthostatic symptoms (systolic blood pressure of 95 mm Hg or greater with less than a 20 mm Hg drop in blood pressure when the patient arises to a standing position).

Cardiac rehabilitation is an important intervention for the management of ischemic heart disease. Both individual trials and meta-analyses have shown that cardiac rehabilitation will reduce mortality and increase a patient's physical capacity and survival but not necessarily translate into return to work.[50–54] Among Medicare beneficiaries, the number of cardiac rehabilitation sessions attended is positively associated with good outcomes.[55] Cardiac rehabilitation improves psychosocial outcomes.[56] There is also information on patients returning to work who have undergone cardiac transplantation.[57] The fact that improved work capacity does not often result in return to work raises the issue of tolerance.

Tolerance

Many factors explain why a patient with ischemic heart disease may not want to tolerate his or her job when work capacity appears more than adequate. Risk factors for refusal to work due to tolerance despite adequate capacity include lower socioeconomic class, poor social network, high psychosocial stressors, shift work, low job satisfaction, anger, hostility, and excessive fatigue. These components of a job and personal psychosocial factors are helpful to consider when patients are looking at returning to work. As an example, one study found that while angioplasty returned patients to work sooner than coronary artery bypass grafting, nonmedical factors predominated in determining long-term employment.[58] Many studies from various countries and across medical disciplines have concurred that these nonmedical findings are predictive, and different models have been developed to explain these findings.[59–64] A good summary of this area is available.[65] Unfortunately, attempts at treating the more well-recognized psychosocial factors have not translated into a reduction in future cardiovascular events.[66] The American College of Cardiology has advocated that patients should undergo psychological assessment when their capacity seems sufficient for their job yet they claim intolerance. This is especially true when the claim is primarily stress related. However, screening and treating for depression may improve depressive symptoms, it may not improve cardiac outcomes.[67,68] Thus the perception of stress may influence the underlying ischemic symptoms, but rarely to a degree that changes capacity or places the patient at significant risk.[16,69]

Disability Duration

Expected disability durations for patients with more commonly used International Classification of Diseases, Ninth Revision, Clinical Modification (ICD-9-CM) codes for ischemic heart disease are shown in Table 14-9. In comparing an individual patient with these normative data, variances can be explained by the factors outlined in this section. In particular, effort on objective testing, identified risk factors or comorbid conditions, and psychosocial factors would be the areas to pursue in a patient falling below these expected outcomes.

Hypertension and Hypertensive Heart Disease

Screening and treatment benefits for high blood pressure are one of the strongest societal recommendations.[71,72] The most important first step in hypertension evaluation is a correct diagnostic method. Many resources have advocated proper methods for measuring blood pressure.[73,74] A growing trend, supported by the literature, is using 24-hour ambulatory blood pressure monitoring to permit more accurate diagnosis and prognosis and to measure the response to intervention.[75–78] The cornerstone of all studies and recommendations is that blood pressure must be measured with good technique in the office and, ideally, supplemented with measures taken in the home and work environments.

Presumed Disability

The presumed criteria for disability from hypertension or hypertensive heart disease are the same as outlined earlier for coronary artery disease. Complications of hypertension (eg, stroke, renal failure) may be severe enough to constitute evidence of presumed disability by SSA criteria.

Risk Assessment

The complications of long-standing untreated or poorly treated hypertension include retinopathy, nephropathy, peripheral vascular disease, coronary

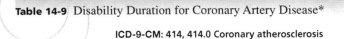

Table 14-9 Disability Duration for Coronary Artery Disease*

ICD-9-CM: 414, 414.0 Coronary atherosclerosis

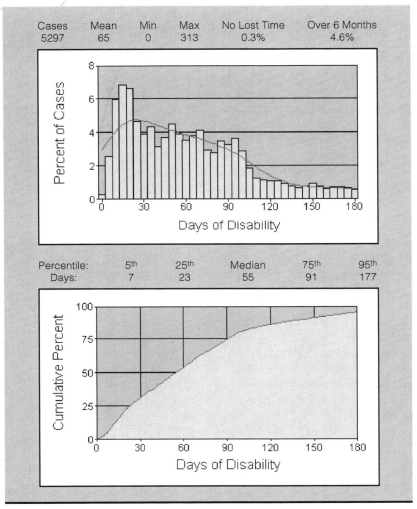

Cases	Mean	Min	Max	No Lost Time	Over 6 Months
5297	65	0	313	0.3%	4.6%

Percentile:	5th	25th	Median	75th	95th
Days:	7	23	55	91	177

* Recovery trends (in days) from normative data for cases specifically identified with
    ICD-9-CM codes 414.0, 414.8, and 414.9.
† Differences may exist between the expected duration tables and the normative graphs. Duration tables
    provide expected recovery periods based on the type of work performed by the individual. The normative
    graphs reflect the actual observed experience of many individuals across the spectrum of physical
    conditions, in a variety of industries, and with varying levels of case management.

Reproduced with permission from Reed. www.mdguidelines.com.

artery disease, cerebrovascular disease, and left ventricular hypertrophy. The presence of these complications might influence the risk of a particular occupation independent of blood pressure measures.

Blood pressure is easily measured, and the consequences of hypertension are rarely immediate. Thus, a trial of return to work with blood pressure monitoring at work is almost always indicated. A most important focus for long-term risk is left ventricular hypertrophy. Left ventricular hypertrophy observed before adulthood is primarily genetic. Among adults, the most frequent causes of left ventricular hypertrophy are hypertension and obesity. The presence of left ventricular hypertrophy increases cardiovascular morbidity and mortality.[79] This argument parallels other known risk factors, their time to cause secondary effects, and stabilization or regression of end-organ damage with treatment.[80] Lifestyle, particularly a diet high in sodium and the development of obesity, are the most common causes of hypertension. The benefits of nonpharmacologic as well as more standard medication interventions have been clearly documented.[81–86]

Psychological stress can influence blood pressure and left ventricular mass.[87] However, stress would need to be present on a fairly constant basis for many months to years to produce left ventricular hypertrophy through hypertension. There is no job that has been described in the medical literature as "free of stress," and there is no case report in the medical literature of an individual whose personal life has always been free of stress.

Blood pressure that is acceptable at rest but that increases to unacceptable levels with exercise represents undertreatment of hypertension. Exercise to the level of severe hypertension is contraindicated only until a change in treatment brings the blood pressure with exercise under control. Exercise is recommended as treatment because sustained endurance exercise leads to increasing aerobic fitness, resulting in decreased blood pressure. Similarly, blood pressure that increases to unacceptable levels at work does not usually mean that work is contraindicated. Rather, it reflects the need for better treatment of the blood pressure. When a change in blood pressure treatment has occurred, two or three weeks may be required for blood pressure stabilization. Patients most commonly can continue to work during this period, except if there is accelerating or severe elevation in their reading. Adequate blood pressure treatment permits exercise or work and can be determined by measuring blood pressure at work intermittently, by ambulatory blood pressure monitors, or by treadmill testing. Decreasing blood pressure translates to increased measures of cardiovascular function as well as diminished secondary complications and would be associated with greater job capacity.

Chapter 14

The risks of commercial driving despite hypertension have been extensively reviewed by the US Department of Transportation (DOT).[49] The DOT criteria for commercial drivers permit continued work (1-year medical certification) for drivers with a resting blood pressure of 140 to 159 mm Hg systolic and 90 to 99 mm Hg diastolic. The DOT criteria still permit continued work but with only a 3-month certification for drivers with blood pressures of 160 to 179 mm Hg systolic and 100 to 109 mm Hg diastolic. In both of these scenarios, the examining physician is to refer the driver for treatment so that the blood pressure is lowered during the certification interval. A blood pressure of greater than 180 mm Hg systolic or greater than 110 mm Hg diastolic is considered disqualifying for commercial drivers, but only until treatment results in lower blood pressure. These criteria are expected to protect the general public from risk, while the stated treatment goal of a resting blood pressure of less than or equal to 140/90 mm Hg is expected to protect the driver from long-term personal health risk. By analogy, even in safety-sensitive jobs, the above consensus criteria can be applied, and individuals can be considered safe to work while treatment is begun or modified. Physicians may modify the goal of treatment to less than 130/80 mm Hg if the patient has concomitant diabetes or kidney disease.

When treadmill testing is performed, most protocols demand that the test be stopped before target work loads are achieved if the blood pressure exceeds 250 mm Hg systolic (220 mm Hg if there has been a prior infarction) or 120 mm Hg diastolic. If work activity results in blood pressures near these levels, such work should not be performed. This would be a basis for physician-imposed work restrictions until a change in therapy results in improved blood pressure control.

Capacity

For purposes of capacity, hypertension is viewed as being associated with hypertensive heart disease. In other words, the tests for capacity center on not just the absolute blood pressure reading but also whether there is any effect on cardiopulmonary function. Cardiopulmonary evaluation is pursued by means of the methods outlined in the introduction to this chapter. If the individual has adequate capacity for work at acceptable risk by treadmill testing, work should be recommended. Many studies show the benefits of lifestyle intervention to increase capacity, similar to a cardiac rehabilitation program used in ischemic heart disease.[88]

Tolerance

Hypertension does not usually cause symptoms. Few individuals are able to predict their own blood pressure measurements. The fear that one's blood pressure may be elevated with work activity can be addressed by arranging for self-monitoring or professional monitoring of blood pressure during work activities.

Disability Duration

Table 14-10 shows the expected duration of disability from this condition. The area of discrepancy between objective capacity measures and ability to return to work in hypertensive disease parallels the findings in coronary artery disease. In particular, stress may influence both conditions as discussed previously. Literature from different studies suggests that stress predicts hypertension.[89–91] Long-standing efforts at using psychotherapy and alternative medicine to control hypertension have had mixed results with data on the effects of treatment being based on traditional medical pharmacology (Table 14-11).[92]

Cardiomyopathy/Heart Failure

Presumed Disability

SSA criteria are normally applied to congestive heart failure and include cardiac enlargement with a cardiothoracic ratio of greater than 0.5 on a postero-anterior (PA) view on chest x-ray with good inspiratory effort, *or* left ventricular diastolic diameter of greater than 5.5 cm, both with significant symptom limitation. An alternative criterion would be the same evidence of cardiac enlargement with an ejection fraction less than 30% or a treadmill limitation to less than 5 METs. Here the treadmill limitation would be symptoms and 3 or more consecutive ventricular premature beats, 3 or more multiform beats, failure to increase systolic blood pressure by 10 mm Hg, or signs of inadequate cerebral perfusion. Finally, disability is presumed in the presence of Cor pulmonale associated with the same limitations in treadmill and ejection fraction.

Risk Assessment

Heart failure, traditionally viewed as the domain of elderly patients, has been estimated to occur in 14% of middle to elderly aged patients[92] and is responsible for nearly 1 million hospital discharges in the United States each year.[93] The cardiomyopathies are classified by different schemes.[94] This may include right side versus left side, high output versus low output, forward versus backward, acute versus chronic, systolic versus diastolic, dilated/congestive versus hypertrophic versus restrictive/obliterative. Both right- and left-sided disease can be due to multiple causes, whereas right-sided failure most commonly results from left-sided failure or associated lung disease. The most common type referred to is usually congestive heart failure, though

Chapter 14

Table 14-10 Disability Duration for Hypertension or Hypertensive Heart Disease

DURATION TRENDS

ICD-9-CM: 401

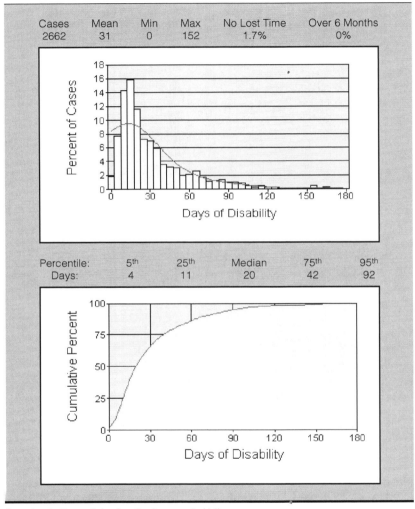

Cases	Mean	Min	Max	No Lost Time	Over 6 Months
2662	31	0	152	1.7%	0%

Percentile:	5th	25th	Median	75th	95th
Days:	4	11	20	42	92

Reproduced with permission from Reed. www.mdguidelines.com.

the current preferred term is *heart failure*. Thus, an understanding of the cause of an individual's heart failure is needed in risk assessment. For example, if the underlying cause is ischemia and, as noted above, risk factors are not addressed, then symptoms and risk will progress. Recurrent cardiac events have a direct effect on heart failure mortality.[95] Reviews of

Table 14-11 Medical Treatment, Hypertensive Heart Disease[124]

DURATION TRENDS

ICD-9-CM: 401.1, 401.9

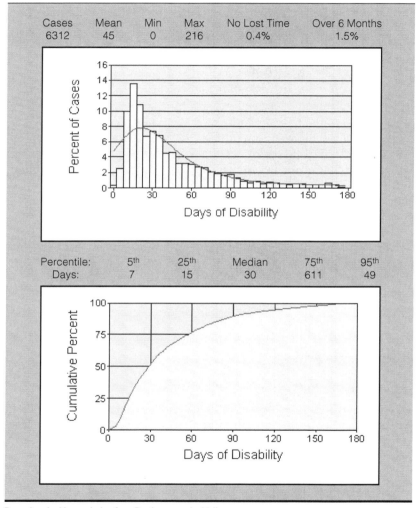

Cases	Mean	Min	Max	No Lost Time	Over 6 Months
6312	45	0	216	0.4%	1.5%

Percentile:	5th	25th	Median	75th	95th
Days:	7	15	30	611	49

Reproduced with permission from Reed. www.mdguidelines.com.

the underlying pathophysiology are available to aid in determination of risk as well as medication optimization.[96] Especially in injured workers, concurrent use of nonsteroidal anti-inflammatory medication can increase heart failure risk.[97] If primary pulmonary disease is at issue, then concurrent consideration of pulmonary status will be mandated.

Chapter 14

Capacity

Symptoms of heart failure include orthopnea, paroxysmal nocturnal dyspnea, edema, fatigue, palpitations, shortness of breath, and chest pain. These can also be functionally classified in heart disease (see Table15-7). The cardiovascular evaluation is pursued using the methods outlined in the introduction to this chapter. As seen in coronary artery disease, there are studies showing the safety and efficacy of cardiac rehabilitation for heart failure patients.[98,99] Capacity can also be altered when there is treatment of concurrent cardiac dysynchrony.[100] Diastolic heart failure due to obesity may be reversed with significant weight loss.[101]

Tolerance

Heart failure, as a marker of the most common cardiomyopathy, displays broad disability duration data (see Table 14-12). The tolerance for symptoms of heart failure can be difficult for patients. In particular, the feelings of breathlessness are alarming for any patient. Yet, patients can do surprisingly well. Even the elderly, who are the most common group of heart failure patients, can regain good short-term ADLs function after hospitalization.[102] Psychosocial factors described above would again be important to consider in this cardiovascular problem. In addition, if the heart failure is of a more acute or recent onset, the patient may not have developed a tolerance for understanding the significance of his or her symptoms. The other important factor in the literature is that much of heart failure is undertreated and needs to be aggressively managed.[96,103–104] This will minimize symptoms, enhance capacity, and improve survival.

Arrhythmias

Presumed Disability

SSA listing for disability requires uncontrolled repeated episodes of cardiac syncope (or near syncope) and arrhythmia despite prescribed treatment. The arrhythmia must be objectively documented coincident with the episode of syncope or near syncope.

Risk Assessment

When assessing arrhythmias, diagnostic evaluation and treatment considerations are critical. In general, the first step is to identify the patient's type of arrhythmia. The second step is determining whether the irregular heartbeat is due to underlying structural or organic cause. The third step is determining whether the arrhythmia correlates with the patient's symptoms. The fourth step is determining whether a treatment is available for the arrhythmia. The final step is determining whether the patient has been given

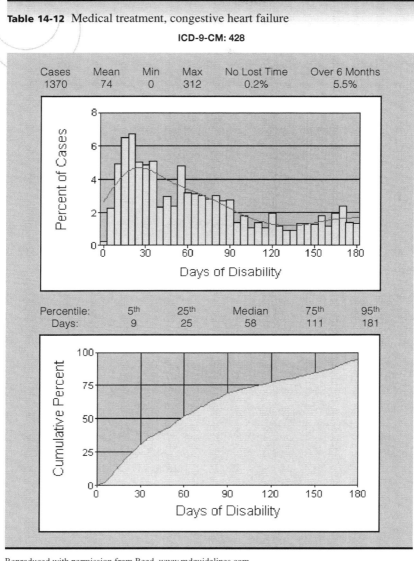

Table 14-12 Medical treatment, congestive heart failure

ICD-9-CM: 428

Cases	Mean	Min	Max	No Lost Time	Over 6 Months
1370	74	0	312	0.2%	5.5%

Percentile:	5th	25th	Median	75th	95th
Days:	9	25	58	111	181

Reproduced with permission from Reed. www.mdguidelines.com.

optimal therapy and explanation as to the nature of the condition. There is no information in the literature on specific jobs causing arrhythmias.

Because there are numerous arrhythmias, a full discussion is beyond the scope of this chapter. The risk of a particular rhythm is influenced by the degree of underlying heart disease, particularly the patient's ejection

Chapter 14

fraction.[105] Thus if a patient has known ischemia, or structural or congenital changes to their conduction system, he or she would be at risk for recurrent arrhythmias. Sick sinus syndrome is an example of the many causes of brady/tachy arrhythmias that at times require pacemaker implantation.[106] The indication for implantation of a permanent pacemaker is symptomatic bradycardia due to sinus node dysfunction or abnormalities of atrio-ventricular node function.[107] Patients with left atrial enlargement are at risk of persistent atrial fibrillation, and those with cardiomyopathy and left ventricular dysfunction are at risk for persistent ventricular arrhythmias.[108] Treatment of atrial fibrillation, while difficult,[109] should focus on elimination of causal agents, heart rate control, and prevention of stroke. Common causal agents include the use of alcohol, stimulants, and herbal supplements. Clinical trials demonstrate that most patients have similar outcomes with strategies to simply control ventricular rate compared to restoring sinus rhythm.[110] Strong evidence exists that warfarin reduces risk of stroke. The evidence that aspirin reduces the risk of stroke is suggestive. Use of the CHADS2 score (an acronym of congestive heart failure, hypertension, age >75, diabetes mellitus, and prior stroke or transient ischemic attack) can help distinguish between patients who are at relatively low risk of stroke and can be treated with aspirin and patients who are at higher risk of stroke and would benefit more from warfarin.[111] Comparison studies between medication and invasive treatment for the management of atrial fibrillation are also available.[112]

Risk factors or behaviors the patient is pursuing that caused the arrhythmia should be addressed. These would include cigarette smoking, obesity, physical inactivity, alcohol or caffeine consumption, stress, and the use of illicit drugs, cold preparations that contain decongestants, weight loss products, or herbal products. Cigarette smoking, poor diet, alcohol consumption, and physical inactivity are modifiable behavioral risk factors implicated as the true, underlying, most-common reasons for death in the United States; with sudden cardiac death due to arrhythmia as a final common pathway.[113–115] The correlation of symptoms with rhythm disturbance is not straightforward and will be described under tolerance.

Optimal treatment requires consideration of reassurance, medications, and procedures such as ablation or revascularization or the introduction of implantable devices. Implantable cardioverter defibrillators (ICDs) and biventricular pacemakers are indicated for patients who have a left ventricular ejection fraction that is persistently less than 30% to 40%. Implantable devices are the only therapies that reduce mortality in this group of patients.[116] The indications for implantable devices have been published.[117] Treatment with antiarrythmic agents other than amiodarone has been documented to increase mortality.[118–119] While implanted defibrillators do usually convert potential lethal arrhythmias (like ventricular fibrillation) to sinus rhythm, the time required for the device to verify the arrhythmia and deliver a series of increasing powerful shocks until the rhythm converts may exceed the 10 to 15 seconds of cerebral hypoperfusion that results in unconsciousness (syncope). Thus the patient may well have syncopal episodes even though the ICD functions successfully and as intended. Due to this risk, patients with implanted ICDs should not perform safety-sensitive work in which unexpected loss of consciousness can result in injury to themselves or others (eg, commercial driver, pilot, nuclear power plant operator, heavy equipment operator, etc). Similarly they should not perform nonsafety-sensitive jobs in which syncope would result in personal injury (eg, climbing to heights, operating unguarded factory presses or sawmill saws, being the only guard in an isolated area, etc).[120]

Capacity

The cardiovascular evaluation is pursued using the methods outlined in the introduction to this chapter. However, additional testing is usually required in rhythm disturbance. This is necessary to document the abnormal rhythm and attempt to correlate the findings with the patient's symptoms. These methods may include Holter monitoring, internal loop recording, event monitors, tilt-table testing, signal averaged ECG, body surface mapping, esophageal electrophysiology, or invasive electrophysiology.[121] Again, it can be useful to use research done about athletes.[122] Once a diagnosis has been made and a therapeutic program initiated, only arrhythmias that are associated with syncope or presyncope preclude work abilities, and that is usually based on risk, not capacity. Because arrhythmias occur during activities one can do, capacity is not usually the issue.

Tolerance

The expected disability duration depends greatly on the type of rhythm disturbance (Tables 14-13 and 14-14). Cardiovascular psychosocial factors, described previously, must be explored when objective testing fails to reveal a significant cause for a patient's symptoms. In particular, patients should not require work limitations if they have only isolated premature ventricular contractions (PVC) or premature atrial contractions (PAC) with a normal left ventricular ejection fraction. Antiarrhythmic therapy, other than beta blockers, is contraindicated. While some patients may feel better taking a beta blocker, others may develop fatigue and depression from the drug. A brief course of cognitive-behavioral therapy may benefit patients who have persistent symptoms that are interfering with their day-to-day functioning. Patient reports of palpitations correlate very poorly with objective abnormal rhythm findings.[123]

Chapter 14

Table 14-13 Medical Treatment, Atrial Fibrillation

DURATION TRENDS

ICD-9-CM: 427.3, 427.31

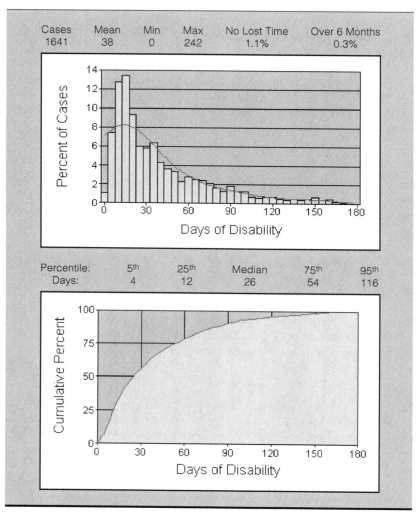

Cases	Mean	Min	Max	No Lost Time	Over 6 Months
1641	38	0	242	1.1%	0.3%

Percentile:	5th	25th	Median	75th	95th
Days:	4	12	26	54	116

Reproduced with permission from Reed. www.mdguidelines.com.

Chapter 14

Table 14-14 Ventricular Tachycardia

ICD-9-CM: 427.1

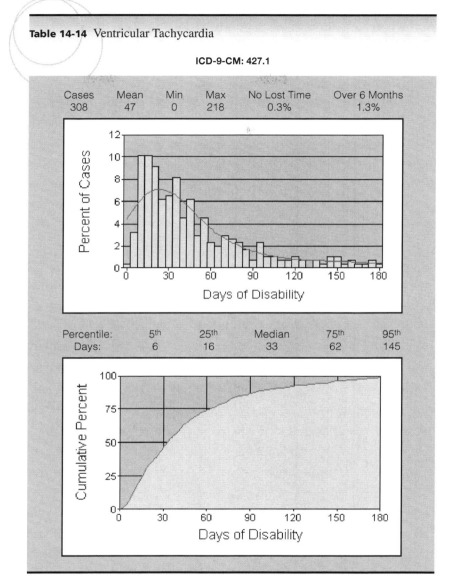

Cases	Mean	Min	Max	No Lost Time	Over 6 Months
308	47	0	218	0.3%	1.3%

Percentile:	5th	25th	Median	75th	95th
Days:	6	16	33	62	145

Reproduced with permission from Reed. www.mdguidelines.com.

Aneurysm of the Aorta and Peripheral Arterial Disease

Presumed Disability

The SSA listing for aneurysm of the aorta or major branches requires dissection demonstrated by appropriate medically acceptable imaging and not controlled by prescribed treatment. This may be due to any cause (eg, atherosclerosis, cystic medial necrosis, Marfan syndrome, trauma, etc).

The SSA listing for disability due to peripheral arterial disease requires intermittent claudication, Doppler study evidence of peripheral arterial disease (PAD), and one of the following: resting ankle/brachial systolic blood pressure ratio (ABI) of less than 0.50, *or* a decrease in systolic blood pressure at the ankle on exercise of 50% or more of pre-exercise level and requiring 10 minutes or more to return to pre-exercise level, *or* resting toe systolic pressure of less than 30 mm Hg, *or* resting toe/brachial systolic blood pressure ratio of less than 0.40.

Risk Assessment

Abdominal aortic aneurysm: The natural history of abdominal aortic aneurysm (AAA) is to enlarge over time.[124] Most AAAs never rupture, but when rupture does occur, the mortality rate is 80%. The US Preventive Services Task Force (USPSTF) now recommends one-time screening with ultrasonography to detect asymptomatic AAA in 65- to 75-year-old men who have ever smoked.[125] Elective repair for patients with an AAA 5.5 cm or larger has been associated with significantly lower death rates from complications of the AAA and reductions in total mortality of borderline significance.[126]

Peripheral artery disease of the lower extremities (PAD): PAD, when defined as a resting ABI less than 0.9, was found in 12% of women and 16% of men in a recent multicommunity cohort.[128] The most significant predictor of decreased functioning in individuals with PAD was the presence of CVD (angina pectoris, myocardial infarction, stroke, heart failure). Other studies have also found that the majority of risk from PAD of the lower extremities comes from its association with coronary heart disease.[129] Thus treatment of claudication is directed not only at improving walking distance, but elimination of smoking and exposure to environmental tobacco smoke and control of dyslipidemias, hypertension, diabetes, and weight.

Confirmation of PAD in patients with a consistent history can be accomplished with ABIs and Doppler studies. Imaging with CT angiography, MRI, or digital subtraction angiography should be reserved for patients being considered for revascularization therapy. D-dimer and biomarkers of inflammation have been observed to increase in patients in the 1 to 2 years before death,[130] but how this information is to be used to manage individual patients is not yet clear.

Aspirin and clopidogrel prescribed individually have been shown to reduce mortality by about 25%.[131] However, prescribing both drugs simultaneously has no advantage over prescription of one drug alone. Cilostazol, a drug with vasodilator and modest antiplatelet effect, has been shown to increase walking distance by about 50% in randomized clinical trials.[132] Revascularization therapy (endovascular or surgical) is reserved for patients whose job performance or lifestyle is compromised by claudication, patients who do not have a response to exercise and pharmacotherapy, and patients for whom the risk-benefit ratio with revascularization is favorable.[133] Because they are no longer limited in their physical activity by leg pain, patients may be able to exercise enough to develop angina pectoris after peripheral revascularization.

Capacity

Asymptomatic AAA by definition will not limit physical work capacity, provided blood pressure is adequately controlled during exercise. Capacity in patients with PAD is assessed with treadmill testing. Randomized trials of walking programs have demonstrated that they can increase maximum walking distance by 150%. Supervised programs produce results that are superior to unsupervised programs, and typically 1 to 2 months are required for patients to notice a benefit from the program.[134]

Tolerance

Because an unruptured AAA is asymptomatic, tolerance is not an issue. With PAD of the legs, however, tolerance is highly dependent on the job classification.[135] For individuals in a sedentary occupation, length of disability ranges from 7 to 28 days. If the individual is in a medium-activity occupation, the range is 7 to 42 days. Individuals whose occupational activities require heavy or very heavy physical activity may be indefinitely disabled by PAD. Among 936 reference cases, the median time lost from work was 53 days; less than 1% experienced no lost time on the job, and 6.5% lost more than 6 months (Table 14-15). New endovascular techniques can be expected to reduce the recovery time for successful revascularization procedures, but the disease is progressive and may lead to limb loss, particularly in individuals who continue to smoke.

Walking programs that increase a patient's ability to walk require that the patient repeatedly walk to pain and then rest.[136] Because of the pain associated with exercise programs, many patients do not like the programs, and drop-out rates are high.

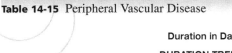

Table 14-15 Peripheral Vascular Disease

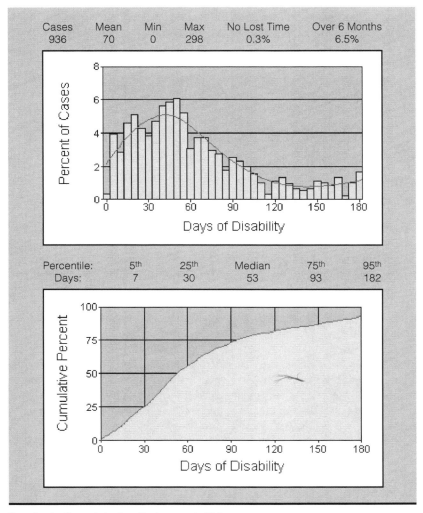

Duration in Days

DURATION TRENDS

ICD-9-CM: 443.9

Cases	Mean	Min	Max	No Lost Time	Over 6 Months
936	70	0	298	0.3%	6.5%

Percentile:	5th	25th	Median	75th	95th
Days:	7	30	53	93	182

Reproduced with permission from Reed. www.mdguidelines.com.

Summary

Cardiovascular conditions are common, and the key to evaluation is the selection of appropriate tests. The most definitive test of physical work capacity is the cardiopulmonary exercise test with measurement of gas exchange. While the SSA presumes disability for individuals who are unable to perform at 5 METs without signs of ischemia, have a left ventricular ejection fraction of less than 30%, or have severe atherosclerosis on coronary angiography, many of these patients can safely return to usually sedentary or light work after their ischemia and risk factors for disease progression have been addressed. The same is true for patients with arrhythmias and hypertension. Although less common than coronary artery disease, symptomatic PAD tends to be more debilitating. Assessment of disability is based on the disparity in systolic blood pressure between the arm and the lower extremity. Angiography is reserved for cases in which revascularization is being considered. Treatment of hypertension, dyslipidemia, and diabetes along with smoking cessation, a diet limited in saturated fat, avoidance of all tobacco smoke, adequate physical activity, and adherence to prescribed medication significantly increase both length and quality of life. As with other body system problems, patients with cardiovascular disease are rarely harmed by a return-to-work recommendation. The considerable benefits of returning to work usually significantly outweigh the risk.

References

1. American Heart Association. *Heart Disease and Stroke Statistics—2004 Update.* Dallas, TX: American Heart Association; 2003.

2. Cocchiarella L, Andersson GBJ, eds. *AMA Guides to the Evaluation of Permanent Impairment.* 5th ed. Chicago, IL: AMA Press; 2001:62–63, 112–114.

3. American College of Cardiology Guidelines, 2004. Available at: www.cardiosource.org. Accessed: February 2, 2011.

4. Fuster V, Alexander RW, O'Rourke RA, et al., eds. *Hurst's The Heart.* 10th ed. Columbus, OH: McGraw-Hill; 2001.

5. Beers MH, Berkow R, eds. *The Merck Manual of Diagnosis and Therapy.* Whitehouse Station, NJ: Merck & Co; 2004.

6. Barreiro TJ, Perillo I. An approach to interpreting spirometry. *Am Fam Physician.* 2004;69:1107–1114.

7. Sheffield LH. Exercise stress testing. In: *Braunwald's Heart Disease: A Textbook of Cardiovascular Medicine.* 3rd ed. Philadelphia, PA: WB Saunders Co, 1988:227.

8. Bruce RA, Kusumi F, Hosmer D. Maximal oxygen intake and nomographic assessment of functional aerobic impairment in cardiovascular disease. *Am Heart J.* 1973;85:546.

9. Fox SM III, Naughton JP, Haskell WL. Physical activity and the prevention of coronary artery disease. *Ann Clin Res.* 1971;3:404–432.

10. American College of Sports Medicine. *Guidelines for Graded Exercise Testing and Exercise Prescription.* Philadelphia, PA: Lea & Febiger; 1975:17.

11. Pollock ML, Wilmore JH, Fox SM. *Health and Fitness Through Physical Activity*. New York, NY: John Wiley & Sons; 1978.

12. Haskell WL. Design and implementation of cardiac conditioning programs. In: Wenger NK, Hellerstein H, eds. *Rehabilitation of the Coronary Patient*. New York, NY: John Wiley & Sons; 1978.

13. Astrand PO, Rodahl K. *Textbook of Work Physiology*. New York, NY: McGraw-Hill; 1977.

14. Wasserman K, Hansen JE, Sue DY, et al. *Principles of exercise testing and interpretation*. 4th ed. Philadelphia, PA: Lippincott Williams & Wilkins; 2005.

15. Cotes JE, Zejda J, King B. Lung function impairment as a guide to exercise limitation in work-related lung disorders. *Am Rev Respir Dis*. 1988;137: 1089–1093.

16. Haskell W, Brachfeld N, Bruce RA, et al. Task Force II: determination of occupational working capacity in patients with ischemic heart disease. *J Am Coll Cardiol*. 1989;14:4:1025–1034.

17. Ainsworth BE, Haskell WL, Leon AS, et al. Compendium of physical activities: classification of energy costs of human physical activities. *Med Sci Sports Exerc*. 1993;25:71–80.

18. Disability Evaluation Under Social Security (Blue Book, October 2008). *www.ssa.gov/disability/professionals/bluebook*. Accessed January 15, 2011.

19. Nishimura RA, Tajik AJ. Evaluation of diastolic filling of left ventricle in health and disease: Doppler echocardiography is the clinician's Rosetta Stone. *J Am Coll Cardiol*. 1997;30:8–18.

20. Jaffe WM, Roche AG, Coverdale HA, et al. Clinical evaluation versus Doppler echocardiography in quantitative assessment of valvular heart disease. *Circulation*. 1988;78:267–275.

21. Fleischmann KE, Hunink MG, Kuntz KM, et al. Exercise echocardiography or exercise SPECT imaging? A meta-analysis of diagnostic test performance. *JAMA*. 1998;280:913–920.

22. Cohn JN, Johnson GR, Shabetai R, et al. Ejection fraction, peak exercise oxygen consumption, cardiothoracic ratio, ventricular arrhythmias, and plasma norepinephrine as determinants of prognosis in heart failure. The V-HeFT VA Cooperative Studies Group. *Circulation*. 1993;87(6 Suppl):VI5–16.

23. Hall SL, Lorenc T. Secondary prevention of coronary artery disease. *Am Fam Physician*. 2010;81(3):289–296.

24. Melhorn JM, Ackerman B, eds. *Guides to Disease and Injury Causation*. Chicago, IL: AMA Press; 2008.

25. Social Security Administration. *Disability Evaluation Under Social Security*. SSA publication 64–039. Baltimore, MD: Social Security Administration; Jan 2003.

26. Criteria Committee of the New York Heart Association. *Diseases of the Heart and Blood Vessels: Nomenclature and Criteria for Disease*. 6th ed. Boston, MA: Little Brown; 1964.

27. Hammar N, Alfredsson L, Smedberg M, et al. Differences in the incidence of myocardial infarction among occupational groups. *Scand J Work Environ Health*. 1992;18:178–185.

28. Karasek RA, Brisson C, Kawakani N, et al. The job content questionnaire (JCQ): an instrument for internationally comparative assessments of psychosocial job characteristics. *J Occup Health Psychol*. 1998;3:322–355.

29. Karasek RA, Theorell T. *Healthy Work*. New York, NY: Basic Books; 1990.

30. Rosenstock L, Olsen J. Firefighting and death from cardiovascular causes. *N Engl J Med*. 2007;356(12):1261–1263.

31. Myers J, Prakash M, Froelicher V, et al. Exercise capacity and mortality among men referred for exercise testing. *N Engl J Med*. 2002;346:793–801.

32. Goroya T, Jacobsen S, Pellikka P, et al. Prognostic value of treadmill exercise testing in elderly persons. *Ann Intern Med*. 2000;132:11:862–870.

33. Giri S, Thompson P, Kiernan F, et al. Clinical and angiographic characteristics of exertion-related acute myocardial infarction. *JAMA*. 1999;282:18:1731–1736.

34. O'Connor C, Fiuzat M. Antidepressant use, depression, and poor cardiovascular outcomes. *Arch Intern Med*. 2009;169(22):2140–2141.

35. Whooley MA, de Jonge P, Vittinghoff E, et al. Depressive symptoms, health behaviors, and risk of cardiovascular events in patients with coronary heart disease. *JAMA*. 2008;300(20):2379–2388.

36. National Cholesterol Education Program. Risk Assessment Tool for Estimating 10-Year Risk of Developing Hard CHD (Myocardial Infarction and Coronary Death). Available at: http://hin.nhlbi.nih.gov/atpiii/calculator.asp?usertype=prof. Accessed January 15, 2011.

37. Mosca L. Novel cardiovascular risk factors: do they add value to your practice? *Am Fam Physician*. 2003;67:264.

38. Zhang R, Brennan ML, Fu X, et al. Association between myeloperoxidase levels and risk of coronary artery disease. *JAMA*. 2001;286:2136–2142.

39. Heeschen C, Dimmeler S, Fichtlscherer S, et al. Prognostic value of placental growth factor in patients with acute chest pain. *JAMA*. 2004;291:435–441.

40. Peters RJG, Boekholdt SM. Gene polymorphisms and the risk of myocardial infarction: an emerging relation. *N Engl J Med*. 2002;347:1963–1965.

41. Ridker PM. Evaluating novel cardiovascular risk factors: can we better predict heart attacks? *Ann Intern Med*. 1999;130:933–937.

42. Pischon T, Girman CJ, Hotamisligil GS, et al. Plasma adiponectin levels and risk of myocardial infarction in men. *JAMA*. 2004;291:1730–1737.

43. Ansell BJ, Navab M, Hama S, et al. Inflammatory/anti-inflammatory properties of high-density lipoprotein distinguish patients from control subjects better than high-density lipoprotein cholesterol levels and are favorably affected by simvastatin treatment. *Circulation*. 2003;108:2751–2756.

44. Grundy SM, Brewer HB, Cleeman JI, et al. NHLBI/AHA Conference Proceedings. Definition of metabolic syndrome: report of the National Heart, Lung, and Blood Institute/American Heart Association Conference on scientific issues related to definition. *Circulation*. 2004;109:433–438.

45. Bonow RO. Prognostic applications of exercise testing. *N Engl J Med*. 1991; 325:805.

46. Froom P, Cohen C, Rashcupkin J, et al. Referral to occupational medicine clinics and resumption of employment after myocardial infarction. *J Occup Environ Med*. 1999;41:943–947.

Chapter 14

47. Thompson PD, Klocke FJ, Levine BD, et al. 26th Bethesda Conference: recommendations for determining eligibility for competition in athletes with cardiovascular abnormalities. Task force 5: coronary artery disease. *J Am Coll Cardiol.* 1994;24:888–892.

48. Morantz CA. ACC statement on preparticipation cardiovascular screening for competitive athletes. *Am Fam Physician.* 2005;72(3):523–527.

49. Blumenthal R, Connolly H, Gersh BJ, et al. *Cardivascular Advisory Panel Guidelines for the Medical Examination of Commercial Motor Vehicle Drivers.* Washington, DC: US Department of Transportation; 2003. Available at: www.fmcsa.dot.gov/pdfs/cardio.pdf. Accessed February 8, 2011.

50. Fletcher G, Oken K, Safford R. Comprehensive rehabilitation of patients with coronary artery disease. In: *Braunwaldís Heart Disease: A Textbook of Cardiovascular Medicine.* 6th ed. Philadelphia, PA: WB Saunders; 2001:1406–1417.

51. Dorn J, Naughton J, Imamura D, et al. Results of a multicenter randomized clinical trial of exercise and long-term survival in myocardial infarction patients: The National Exercise and Heart Disease Project (NEHDP). *Circulation.* 1999;100:1764–1769.

52. Agency for Healthcare Research and Quality. *Cardiac Rehabilitation.* Publication 96-0672. Washington, DC: US Department of Health and Human Services; October 1995.

53. Pavy B, Iliou MC, Meurin P, et al. Safety of exercise training for cardiac patients. *Arch Intern Med.* 2006;166:2329–2334.

54. Gatti JC. Exercise-based rehabilitation for coronary heart disease. *Am Fam Phys.* 2004;70(3):485–486.

55. Hammill BG, Curtis LH, Schulman KA, Whellan DJ. Relationship between cardiac rehabilitation and long-term risks of death and myocardial infarction among elderly medicare beneficiaries. *Circulation.* 2010;121:63–70.

56. Milani RV, Lavie CJ. Impact of cardiac rehabilitation on depression and its associated mortality. *Am J Med.* 2007;120:799–806.

57. Taylor DO, Edwards LB, Boucek MM, et al. Registry of the international society for heart and lung transplantation: twenty-fourth official adult heart transplant report. *J Heart Lung Transpl.* 2007;26(8):769–781.

58. Hlatky MA, Boothroyd D, Horine S, et al. Employment after coronary angioplasty or coronary bypass surgery in patients employed at the time of revascularization. *Ann Intern Med.* 1998;129:543–547.

59. Schnall PL, Landsbergis PA, Baker D. Job strain and cardiovascular disease. *Ann Rev Public Health.* 1994;15:381–411.

60. Siegrist J. Adverse health effects of high effort–low reward conditions. *J Occup Health Psychol.* 1996;1:27–41.

61. Williams RB, Barefoot JC, Schneiderman N. Psychosocial risk factors for cardiovascular disease: more than one culprit at work. *JAMA.* 2003;290:2190–2192.

62. Bunker SJ, Colquhoun DM, Esler MD, et al. Stress and coronary heart disease: psychosocial risk factors. *Med J Aust.* 2003;178:272–276.

63. Bigos SJ, Battie MC, Spengler DM, et al. A prospective study of work perceptions and psychosocial factors affecting the report of back injury. *Spine.* 1991;16:1–6.

64. Cats-Baril WL, Frymoyer JW. Identifying patients at risk of becoming disabled because of low-back pain: the Vermont Rehabilitation Engineering Center predictive model. *Spine*. 1991;16:6:605–607.

65. Williams C, ed. Social factors, work, stress and cardiovascular disease prevention in the European Union. Brussels, Belgium: European Heart Network; 1998.

66. ENRICHD Investigators. Effects of treating depression and low perceived social support on clinical events after myocardial infarction: the Enhancing Recovery in Coronary Heart Disease Patients (ENRICHD) randomized trial. *JAMA*. 2003;289:3106–3116.

67. Thombs BD, deJonge P, Coyne JC, et al. Depression screening and patient outcomes in cardiovascular care. *JAMA*. 2008;300(18):2161–2171.

68. Glassman AH, Bigger JT. Antidepressants in coronary heart disease. *JAMA*. 2007;297(4):411–412.

69. 20th Bethesda Conference: insurability and employability of the patient with ischemic heart disease. *J Am Coll Cardiol*. 1989;14:1003–1044.

70. Reed P. The Medical Disability Advisor: Workplace Guidelines for Disability Duration. 5th ed. Westminster, CO: Reed Group Ltd; 2005.

71. Berg AO, chair; US Preventive Services Task Force. Screening for high blood pressure: recommendations and rationale. *Am J Prev Med*. 2003;25:159–164.

72. Sheridan S, Pignone M, Donahue K. Screening for high blood pressure. *Am J Prev Med*. 2003;25:151–158.

73. Chobanian AV, Bakris GL, Black HR, et al. The seventh report of the Joint National Committee on the Detection, Evaluation, and Treatment of High Blood Pressure: the JNC 7 report. *JAMA*. 2003;289:2560–2572.

74. Jones DW, Appel LJ, Sheps SG, et al. Measuring blood pressure accurately: new and persistent challenges. *JAMA*. 2003;289:1027–1030.

75. Clement DL, De Buyzere ML, De Bacquer DA, et al. Prognostic value of ambulatory blood-pressure recordings in patients with treated hypertension. *N Engl J Med*. 2003;348:2407–2415.

76. White WB. Ambulatory blood pressure monitoring in clinical practice. *N Engl J Med*. 2003;348:2377–2378.

77. Ernst ME, Bergus GR. Ambulatory blood pressure monitoring: technology with a purpose. *Am Fam Physician*. 2003;67:2262–2270.

78. Bobrie G, Chatellier G, Genes N, et al. Cardiovascular prognosis of masked hypertension detected by blood pressure self-measurement in elderly treated hypertensive patients. *JAMA*. 2004;291:1342–1349.

79. Palmieri V, de Simone G, Arnett DK, et al. Relation of various degrees of body mass index in patients with systemic hypertension to left ventricular mass, cardiac output, and peripheral resistance (the Hypertension Genetic Epidemiology Network Study). *Am J Cardiol*. 2001;88:1163–1168.

80. Devereux RB. Therapeutic options in minimizing left ventricular hypertrophy. Cardiac protection: the evolving role of ARBS. *Am Heart J*. 2000;139: S9–S14.

81. Carethon MR, Gidding SS, Nehgme R, et al. Cardiorespiratory fitness in young adulthood and the development of cardiovascular disease risk factors. *JAMA*. 2003;290:3092–3100.

Chapter 14

82. Stevens VJ, Obarzanek E, Cook NR, et al. Long-term weight loss and changes in blood pressure: results of the Trials of Hypertension revention phase II. *Ann Intern Med*. 2001;134:1–11.

83. Pickering TG. Lifestyle modification and blood pressure control: is the glass half full or half empty? *JAMA*. 2003;289:16:2131–2132.

84. Whelton PK, He J, Appel LJ, et al. Primary prevention of hypertension: clinical and public health advisory from the National High Blood Pressure Education Program. *JAMA*. 2002;288:1882–1888.

85. August P. Initial treatment of hypertension. *N Engl J Med*. 2003;348:610–616.

86. Aiyer AN, Kip KE, Mulukutia SR, et al. Predictors of significant short-term increases in blood pressure in a community-based population. *Am J Med*. 2007; 120:960–967.

87. Al'Absi M, Devereux R, et al. Blood pressure responses to acute stress and left ventricular mass (the Hypertension Genetic Epidemiology Network Study). *Am J Cardiol*. 2002;89:536–540.

88. Burke V, Beilin LJ, Cutt HE, et al. A lifestyle program for treated hypertensives improved health-related behaviors and cardiovascular risk factors, a randomized controlled trial. *J Clin Epidemiol*. 2007;60:133–141.

89. Markovitz JH, Matthews KA, Kannel WB, et al. Psychological predictors of hypertension in the Framingham study. *JAMA*. 1993;270:2439–2443.

90. Pickering TG, Devereux RB, James GD, et al. Environmental influences on blood pressure and the role of job strain. *J Hypertens*. 1996;14(suppl): S179–S185.

91. Yan LL, Liu K, Matthews KA, et al. Psychosocial factors and risk of hypertension: the Coronary Artery Risk Development in Young Adults (CARDIA) study. *JAMA*. 2003;290:2138–2148.

92. Devereux RB, Roman MJ, Paranicas M, et al. A population-based assessment of left ventricular systolic dysfunction in middle-aged and older adults: the strong heart study. *Am Heart J*. 2001;141:3:439–446.

93. Hall MJ, DeFrances CJ. 2001 National Hospital Discharge Survey: Advanced Data From Vital and Health Statistics. No. 332. Hyattsville, MD: National Center for Health Statistics; 2003.

94. Givertz MM, Colucci WS, Braunwald E. In *Braunwald's Heart Disease: A Textbook of Cardiovascular Medicine*. 6th ed. Philadelphia, PA: WB Saunders; 2001.

95. Lee DS, Austin PC, Stukel TA, et al. Dose-dependent impact of recurrent cardiac events on mortality in patients with heart failure. *Am J Med*. 2009;122:162–169.

96. Jessup M, Brozena S. Heart failure. N Engl J Med. 2003;348:20:2007–2018.

97. Gislason GH, Rasmussen JN, Abildstrom SZ, et al. Increased mortality and cardiovascular morbidity associated with use of nonsteroidal anti-inflammatory drugs in chronic heart failure. *Arch Intern Med*. 2009;169(2):141–149.

98. Flynn KE, Pina IL, Whellan DJ, et al. Effects of exercise training on health status in patients with chronic heart failure. *JAMA*. 2009;301(14):1451–1459.

99. O'Connor CM, Whellan DJ, Lee KL, et al. Efficacy and safety of exercise training in patients with chronic heart failure. *JAMA*. 2009;301(14):1439–1450.

100. Hlatky MA, Massie BM. Cardiac resynchronization for heart failure. *Ann Intern Med*. 2004;141(5):399–400.

101. Leichman JG, Wilson EB, Scarborough T, et al. Dramatic reversal of derangements in muscle metabolism and left ventricular function after bariatric surgery. *Am J Med*. 2008;121:966–973.

102. Hardy SE, Gill TM. Recovery from disability among community-dwelling older persons. JAMA. 2004;291:13:1596–1602.

103. Fonarow GC for the ADHERE Scientific Advisory Committee. The acute decompensated heart failure registry (ADHERE): opportunities to improve care of patients hospitalized with acute decompensated heart failure. *Rev Cardiovasc Med*. 2003;4(supl 7):S21–S30.

104. Klein L, O'Connor CM, Gattis WA, et al. Pharmacologic therapy for patients with chronic heart failure and reduced systolic function: review of trials and practical considerations. *Am J Cardiol*. 2003;91:18F–40F.

105. Rubart M, Zipes DP. Genesis of cardiac arrhythmias: electrophysiologic considerations. In *Braunwald's Heart Disease: A Textbook of Cardiovascular Medicine*. 6th ed. Philadelphia, PA: WB Saunders; 2001.

106. Adan V, Crown LA. Diagnosis and treatment of sick sinus syndrome. *Am Fam Physician*. 2003;67:8:1725–1732.

107. Epstein AE, DiMarco JP, Ellenbogen KA, et al. ACC/AHA/HRS 2008 Guidelines for Device-Based Therapy of Cardiac Rhythm Abnormalities: a report of the American College of Cardiology/American Heart Association Task Force on Practice Guidelines (Writing Committee to Revise the ACC/AHA/NASPE 2002 Guideline Update for Implantation of Cardiac Pacemakers and Antiarrhythmia Devices) developed in collaboration with the American Association for Thoracic Surgery and Society of Thoracic Surgeons. *J Am Coll Cardiol*. 2008;51(21):e1–62.

108. Braunwald's Heart Disease: A Textbook of Cardiovascular Medicine, 6th ed. Philadelphia, PA: WB Saunders; 2001.

109. Cain ME, Curtis AB. Rhythm control in atrial fibrillation-one setback after another. *N Engl J Med*. 2008;358(25):2725–2727.

110. McNamara RL, Tamariz LJ, Segal JB, Bass EB. Management of atrial fibrillation: review of the evidence for the role of pharmacologic therapy, electrical cardioversion, and echocardiography. *Annals of Internal Medicine*. 2003;139:1018–1033.

111. Rietbrock S, Heeley E, Plumb J, van Staa T. Chronic atrial fibrillation: incidence, prevalence, and prediction of stroke using the congestive heart failure, hypertension, age >75, diabetes mellitus, and prior stroke or transient ischemic attack (CHADS2) risk stratification scheme. *Am Heart J*. 2008; 156(1):57–64.

112. Wilber DJ, Pappone C, Neuzil P, et al. Comparision of antiarrhythmic drug therapy and radiofrequency catheter ablation in patients with paroxysmal atrial fibrillation. *JAMA*. 2010;303(4):333–340.

Chapter 14

113. Mokdad AH, Marks JS, Stroup DF, et al. Actual causes of death in the United States, 2000. *JAMA*. 2004;291:10:1238–1245.

114. McGinnis JM, Foege WH. The immediate vs the important. *JAMA*. 2004;291: 10:1263–1264.

115. Goldenberg I, Jonas M, Tenenbaum A, et al. Current smoking, smoking cessation, and the risk of sudden cardiac death in patients with coronary artery disease. *Arch Intern Med*. 2003;163:2301–2305.

116. Bardy GH, Lee KL, Mark DB, et al. Amiodarone or an implantable cardioverter-defibrillator for congestive heart failure. *N Engl J Med*. 2005; 352(3):225–237.

117. Epstein AE, DiMarco JP, Ellenbogen KA, et al. ACC/AHA/HRS 2008 Guidelines for device-based therapy of cardiac rhythm abnormalities: a report of the American College of Cardiology/American Heart Association Task Force on Practice Guidelines (Writing Committee to Revise the ACC/AHA/ NASPE 2002 Guideline Update for Implantation of Cardiac Pacemakers and Antiarrhythmia Devices) developed in collaboration with the American Association for Thoracic Surgery and Society of Thoracic Surgeons. *J Am Coll Cardiol*. 2008;51(21):e1–62.

118. Echt DS, Liebson PR, Mitchell LB, et al. Mortality and morbidity in patients receiving encainide, flecainide, or placebo. The cardiac arrhythmia suppression trial. *N Engl J Med*. 1991;324:781–788.

119. Waldo AL, Camm AJ, deRuyter H, et al. Effect of d-sotalol on mortality in patients with left ventricular dysfunction after recent and remote myocardial infarction. The SWORD investigators. Survival with oral d-sotalol. *Lancet*. 1996;348:9019:7–12.

120. Gregoratos G, Cheitlin MD, Conill A, et al. ACC/AHA guidelines for the implantation of cardiac pacemakers and antiarrythmic devices: executive summary-a report of the American College of Cardiology/American Heart Association task force on practice guidelines (committee on pacemaker implantation). *Circulation*. 1998;97:1325–1335.

121. Miller JM, Zipes DP. Management of the patient with cardiac arrhythmias. In *Braunwald's Heart Disease: A Textbook of Cardiovascular Medicine*. 6th ed. Philadelphia, PA: WB Saunders; 2001.

122. Zipes DP, Garson A. 26th Bethesda conference: recommendations for determining eligibility for competition in athletes with cardiovascular abnormalities. Task force 6: arrhythmias. *J Am Coll Cardiol*. 1994;24:4:892–899.

123. Barsky AJ. Palpitations, arrhythmias, and awareness of cardiac activity. *Ann Intern Med*. 2001;134:832–837.

124. Abdominal Aortic Aneurysm. *Annals of Internal Medicine*. 2009;150(9 %U http://www.annals.org/content/150/9/ITC5-1.abstract):ITC5-1.

125. Calonge N, Allan J, et al. Screening for abdominal aortic aneurysm: recommendation statement. *Ann Intern Med*. 2005;142(3):198–202.

126. Kim LG, RA PS, Ashton HA, Thompson SG. A sustained mortality benefit from screening for abdominal aortic aneurysm. *Ann Intern Med*. 2007;146(10): 699–706.

Working With Common Pulmonary Problems

Mark H. Hyman, MD and Philip Harber, MD, MPH

This chapter explores several common pulmonary problems encountered in clinical return-to-work evaluations. Table 15-1 summarizes the major categories. Lung difficulties are rising in prevalence. The estimated prevalence of asthma in the US population is 7.2%, and at least 11 million people have a chronic lung disease.[1,2] As the workforce ages, physicians will be increasingly confronted with disability determinations in patients with these pulmonary conditions that accompany aging. Lung conditions have a significant effect on the workforce.

One of the greatest effects on health in general, and pulmonary conditions in particular, is cigarette smoking.[1,2] In addition to the well-known effects of tobacco use, occupational exposures and air pollution are increasingly recognized as a cause of many pulmonary disorders, including Chronic Obstructive Pulmonary Disease (COPD).[3] Nevertheless, tobacco is still by far the greatest contributor to many pulmonary disorders. From a global perspective, biomass fuel burning is likely to be the second most important cause of lung disease.[4]

General Considerations

Assessment of work disability depends upon comparing the patient's functional ability with the job demands. Pulmonary function testing provides objective measurements of functional status. Table 15-2 summarizes the common tests and shows applicability to the various classes of respiratory disease. The most commonly used pulmonary function tests include spirometry and diffusing capacity of the lung for carbon monoxide (CO). Measurement of lung volumes is often useful in differentiating obstructive from restrictive disorders. Spirometry is generally available and can be conducted reproducibly. If the baseline test is abnormal, it is generally repeated after administration of an inhaled bronchodilator; significant increase following bronchodilators strongly suggests a component of asthma.

Table 15-1 Categories of Respiratory/Lung Diseases

Airway disorders
Asthma
Chronic obstructive pulmonary disease
Interstitial lung disease
Pneumoconiosis
Idiopathic pulmonary fibrosis
Immunologic (eg, hypersensitivity pneumonitis, chronic beryllium disease)
Pulmonary vascular disease
Primary
Secondary to collagen vascular disease or COPD
Venous thromboembolism related
Respiratory control disorders

Other pulmonary function tests are also frequently useful. Methacholine challenge testing can determine the degree of airway reactivity and is useful in patients with suspected asthma. Patients with asthma may occasionally have near-normal spirometry even though their airways are extremely reactive.

Cardiopulmonary exercise testing is useful if adequate information cannot be obtained from the basic lung function tests (spirometry, diffusing capacity for CO, and lung volumes). In addition to helping quantify the degree of limitation, exercise testing may help to diagnostically separate limitation from pulmonary disease, cardiac disease, simple physical deconditioning, and psychological factors. The testing may include measurement of the anaerobic threshold as well as assessment for exercise-related hemoglobin desaturation. COPD or prolonged inactivity may lead to skeletal muscle atrophy.

Standards for performing the pulmonary function tests have been established by the American Thoracic Society/European Respiratory Society[5–7] and by the American College of Occupational and Environmental Medicine.[8] To be accurate, spirometry must be properly performed with adequate patient motivation. Occasionally, accurate test data may not be available. In particular, reproducibility of the spirometry test is a good measure of the validity of the data. Examination of the actual tracings is also an important part of test interpretation. Pulmonary function tests must be interpreted in relationship to the expected normal results for an individual with the patient's age, height, gender, and race. In the United States,

Table 15-2 Major Pulmonary Function Tests

| | Disease Class | | | | |
---	Asthma	COPD	ILD	PVD	RCD
Spirometry					
Baseline	***	***	*		
Baseline plus postbronchodilator	****	****			
Diffusing capacity for CO		**	***	****	
Lung volumes (less-frequently necessary)		**	***		
Methacholine challenge testing	***				
6-minute walk		***	***	***	
Oxygen saturation		**	**		***
Arterial blood gas analysis (less-frequently necessary)		*	*	**	
Cardiopulmonary exercise test measures (Oxygen consumption, CO_2 production, End expiratory CO_2, Cardiac rhythm, Oxygen saturation)		*	**	***	
Exercise-induced bronchospasm test	**				
Epworth sleepiness score					**
Nocturnal polysomnography					****

The table summarizes applicability of the most common pulmonary function tests for the major disease categories. *ILD* = interstitial lung disease; *PVD* = pulmonary vascular disease; *RCD* = respiratory control disorders (eg, sleep apnea).

the prediction equations derived from the National Health and Nutrition Examination Survey are currently considered the most appropriate for spirometry interpretation.[9] Different protocols can be used in evaluating a patient's performance, the second most common probably being that of Morris et al.[10] Patient effort is the cornerstone for test interpretation. The American Thoracic Society and European Respiratory Society (ATS/ERS) have identified standards for assessing patient effort and interpreting results.[11] Every pulmonary function test must follow these standards to be fully interpretable. The test should indicate the data obtained as well as the best of three trials a patient performed. There should be a clear section on this report of reproducibility measures. Tables 15-1 and 15-2 outline available pulmonary function tests. Sample reports and their basic interpretation are shown in Tables 15-3, 15-4, 15-5, and 15-6.

Table 15-3 Sample Pulmonary Function Test Results for a Normal 37-Year-Old Patient

		Spirometry				
		Pre-Results 05/03/2004 14:35		Post-Results 05/03/2004 14:56		
Parameter	Predicted	Best: #2	% Predicted	Best: #3	% Predicted	% Difference
FVC	2.86	3.09	107.94	3.06	106.89	−0.97
FEV$_{.5}$	1.93	2.17	112.63	2.14	111.08	−1.38
FEV$_1$	2.45	2.67	109.00	2.66	108.60	−0.37
FEV$_3$	2.79	2.98	106.65	2.99	107.01	−0.34
PEFR	5.17	7.06	136.58	7.01	135.61	−0.71
FEF 25%–75%	2.90	3.28	113.03	3.09	106.48	−5.79
FEV$_1$/FVC	0.85	0.86	100.77	0.87	101.94	1.16
FEV$_3$/FVC	0.97	0.96	98.64	0.98	100.69	2.08
FET		5.29		5.58		5.48

MVV	87.46	87.00	99.48			
Reproducibility:	%	Volume	Criteria Met	%	Volume	Criteria Met
FVC (5%/200 mL)	1.29	0.04	Y	0.33	0.01	Y
FEV$_1$ (5%/200 mL)	1.12	0.03	Y			Y
PEFR (15%/300 mL)	10.06	0.71	Y	2.28	0.16	Y

Lung Volumes			05/03/2004 14:44
Parameter	Predicted	Test 1	% Predicted
TLC	4.12	4.03	97.82
FRC	2.23	1.75	78.48
RV	1.26	1.11	88.10
RV/TLC	0.30	0.28	93.33
SVC	2.86	2.92	102.10
IC	1.90	2.27	119.47
ERV	0.97	0.64	65.98
TV		0.91	
FRCT		2.47	

(Continued)

Table 15-3 *(Continued)*

Diffusion Capacity		05/03/2004	14:50
Notice: DLco results are based on the following values: Hb = 14.6 g/dL, COHb = 0 g/dL			
Parameter	**Predicted**	**Test 1**	**% Predicted**
DLco	23.68	24.81	104.77
VA	4.15	4.02	96.87
DLco/VA	5.90	6.17	104.58
IV		2.94	
BHt		9.64	
Sample Volume		0.94	

BHt indicates breath hold time; COHb, carboxyhemoglobin; DLco, carbon monoxide diffusion capacity; ERV, end residual volume; FEF, forced expiratory flow; FET, forced expiratory time; FEV_5, forced expiratory volume for .5 second; FEV_1, forced expiratory volume for 1 second; FEV_3, forced expiratory volume for 3 seconds; FRC, functional residual capacity; FRCT, functional residual capacity time (also called helium equilibration time); FVC, forced vital capacity; Hb, hemoglobin; IC, inspiratory capacity; IV, inspiratory volume; MVV, maximal voluntary ventilation; PEFR, peak expiratory flow rate; RV, residual volume; SVC, slow vital capacity; TLC, total lung capacity; TV, tidal volume; VA, alveolar ventilation.

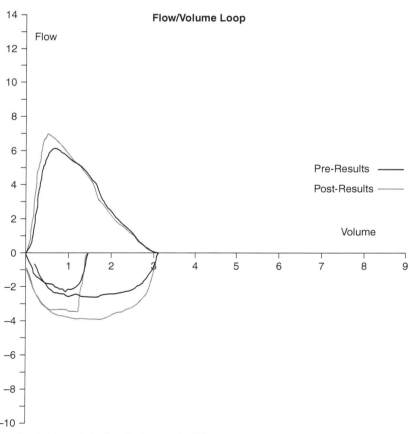

Reproduced with permission from Reed. www.mdguidelines.com.

Chapter 15

Table 15-4 Sample Pulmonary Function Test Results for a 44-Year-Old Patient With Chronic Obstructive Pulmonary Disease

		Spirometry				
		Pre-Results 02/05/2004 12:37		Post-Results 02/05/2004 12:54		
Parameter	Predicted	Best: #3	% Predicted	Best: #1	% Predicted	% Difference
FVC	5.23	5.72	109.39	5.73	109.59	0.17
FEV$_1$	4.20	3.45	82.09	3.68	87.57	6.67
FEV$_3$	4.94	4.86	98.31	4.91	99.32	1.03
PEFR	9.42	9.08	96.40	9.06	96.19	0.22
FEF 25%–75%	4.14	1.66	40.10	2.02	48.79	21.69
FEV$_1$/FVC	0.80	0.60	74.67	0.64	79.64	6.67
FEV$_3$/FVC	0.94	0.85	90.04	0.86	91.10	1.18
FET		10.29		8.99		12.63

MVV	141.33	148.88	104.72			
Reproducibility:	%	Volume	Criteria Met	%	Volume	Criteria Met
FVC (5%/200 mL)	2.62	0.15	Y	0.52	0.03	Y
FEV$_1$ (5%/200 mL)	0.29	0.01	Y	0.54	0.02	Y
PEFR (15%/300 mL)	3.41	0.31	Y	6.73	0.61	Y

Lung Volumes			02/05/2004 12:43
Parameter	Predicted	Test 1	% Predicted
TLC	7.23	8.84	122.27
FRC	3.58	4.94	137.99
RV	2.05	3.15	153.66
RV/TLC	0.28	0.36	128.57
SVC	5.23	5.68	108.60
IC	3.64	3.89	106.87
ERV	1.53	1.79	116.99
TV		2.05	
FRCT		2.80	

(Continued)

Table 15-4 *(Continued)*

Diffusion Capacity		02/05/2004	12:50
Notice: DLco results are based on the following values: Hb = 14.6 g/dL, COHb = 0 g/dL			
Parameter	**Predicted**	**Test 1**	**% Predicted**
DLco	38.39	28.28	73.67
VA	7.28	8.15	111.95
DLco/VA	5.48	3.47	63.32
IV		5.55	
BHt		10.30	
Sample Volume		1.02	

BHt indicates breath hold time; COHb, carboxyhemoglobin; DLco, carbon monoxide diffusion capacity; ERV, end residual volume; FEF, forced expiratory flow; FET, forced expiratory time; FEV_1, forced expiratory volume for 1 second; FEV_3, forced expiratory volume for 3 seconds; FRC, functional residual capacity; FRCT, functional residual capacity time (also called helium equilibration time); FVC, forced vital capacity; Hb, hemoglobin; IC, inspiratory capacity; IV, inspiratory volume; MVV, maximal voluntary ventilation; PEFR, peak expiratory flow rate; RV, residual volume; SVC, slow vital capacity; TLC, total lung capacity; TV, tidal volume; VA, alveolar ventilation.

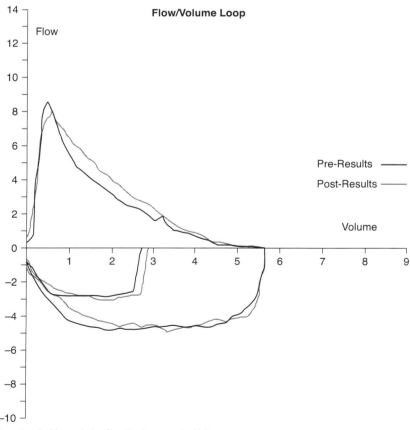

Table 15-5 Sample Pulmonary Function Test Results for a 61-Year-Old Patient With Restrictive Lung Disease

		Spirometry				
		Pre-Results 10/07/2002 16:34		Post-Results 10/07/2002 16:48		
Parameter	Predicted	Best: #2	% Predicted	Best: #3	% Predicted	% Difference
FVC	4.52	2.47	54.60	2.35	51.95	−4.86
FEV$_5$	2.81	1.25	44.49	1.22	43.43	−2.40
FEV$_1$	3.49	1.73	49.60	1.64	47.02	−5.20
FEV$_3$	4.16	2.26	54.36	2.01	48.35	−11.06
PEFR	8.11	3.94	48.59	3.91	48.22	−0.76
FEF 25%–75%	3.10	1.13	36.43	0.94	30.30	−16.81
FEV$_1$/FVC	0.77	0.70	91.17	0.70	91.17	
FEV$_3$/FVC	0.91	0.91	99.50	0.86	94.03	−5.49
FET		5.44		6.59		21.14

MVV	116.06	39.00	33.60				
Reproducibility:	%	Volume	Criteria Met	%	Volume	Criteria Met	
FVC (5%/200 mL)	6.07	0.15	N	16.17	0.38	N	
FEV$_1$ (5%/200 mL)	3.47	0.06	Y	17.07	0.28	N	
PEFR (15%/300 mL)	1.02	0.04	Y	2.30	0.09	Y	

Lung Volumes			10/07/2002 16:41
Parameter	Predicted	Test 1	% Predicted
TLC	6.70	4.68	69.85
FRC	3.48	2.69	77.30
RV	2.19	2.51	114.61
RV/TLC	0.33	0.54	163.64
SVC	4.52	2.17	48.01
IC	3.22	1.99	61.80
ERV	1.29	0.18	13.95
TV		0.67	
FRCT		1.55	

(Continued)

Table 15-5 *(Continued)*

| Diffusion Capacity | | 10/07/2002 | 16:45 |

Notice: DLco results are based on the following values: Hb = 14.6 g/dL, COHb = 0 g/dL

Parameter	Predicted	Test 1	% Predicted
DLco	32.25	22.32	69.21
VA	6.71	5.25	78.24
DLco/VA	4.92	4.25	86.38
IV		2.76	
BHt		10.01	
Sample Volume		0.43	

BHt indicates breath hold time; COHb, carboxyhemoglobin; DLco, carbon monoxide diffusion capacity; ERV, end residual volume; FEF, forced expiratory flow; FET, forced expiratory time; FEV$_5$, forced expiratory volume for .5 second; FEV$_1$, forced expiratory volume for 1 second; FEV$_3$, forced expiratory volume for 3 seconds; FRC, functional residual capacity; FRCT, functional residual capacity time (also called helium equilibration time); FVC, forced vital capacity; Hb, hemoglobin; IC, inspiratory capacity; IV, inspiratory volume; MVV, maximal voluntary ventilation; PEFR, peak expiratory flow rate; RV, residual volume; SVC, slow vital capacity; TLC, total lung capacity; TV, tidal volume; VA, alveolar ventilation.

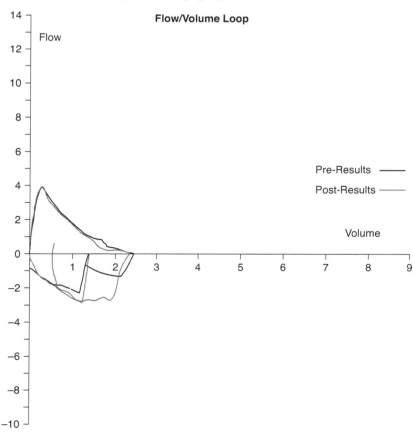

Reproduced with permission from Reed. www.mdguidelines.com.

Table 15-6 Sample Pulmonary Function Test Results for a 23-Year-Old Patient With Nonphysiologic Test*

| | | Spirometry | | | | |
| | | Pre-Results 05/05/2004 16:13 | | Post-Results 05/05/2004   16:24 | | |
Parameter	Predicted	Best: #3	% Predicted	Best: #2	% Predicted	% Difference
FVC	2.99	2.88	96.24	3.41	113.95	18.40
FEV$_{.5}$	2.09	1.62	77.69	2.69	129.01	66.05
FEV$_1$	2.66	2.49	93.46	3.15	118.23	26.51
FEV$_3$	2.99	2.23	74.70	3.37	112.88	51.12
PEFR	5.34	3.74	70.04	8.53	159.75	128.07
FEF 25%–75%	3.41	2.38	69.81	4.94	144.89	107.56
FEV$_1$/FVC	0.89	0.86	96.10	0.92	102.81	6.98
FEV$_3$/FVC	1.00	0.77	77.08	0.99	99.11	28.57
FET		1.70		4.56		168.24

| MVV | | | | | | | |
Reproducibility:	%	Volume	Criteria Met	%	Volume	Criteria Met
FVC (5%/200 mL)	2.08	0.06	Y	0.29	0.01	Y
FEV$_1$ (5%/200 mL)	18.07	0.45	N	0.32	0.01	Y
PEFR (15%/300 mL)	40.11	1.50	N	0.70	0.06	Y

| Lung Volumes | | | 05/05/2004   16:15 |
Parameter	Predicted	Test 1	% Predicted
TLC	3.96	3.86	97.47
FRC	2.10	1.64	78.10
RV	0.97	0.74	76.29
RV/TLC	0.24	0.19	79.17
SVC	2.99	3.12	104.35
IC	1.87	2.22	118.72
ERV	1.13	0.90	79.65
TV		0.52	
FRCT		2.36	

(Continued)

Table 15-6 *(Continued)*

Diffusion Capacity		05/05/2004	16:20
Notice: DLco results are based on the following values: Hb = 14.6 g/dL, COHb = 0 g/dL			
Parameter	**Predicted**	**Test 1**	**% Predicted**
DLco	24.81	20.82	83.92
VA	3.98	3.66	91.96
DLco/VA	6.30	5.69	90.32
IV		2.09	
BHt		9.64	
Sample Volume		0.41	

* Note the poor prebronchodilator effort resulting in irregular flow/volume loop, failed reproducibility, large apparent reversibility, and low MVV.

BHt indicates breath hold time; COHb, carboxyhemoglobin; DLco, carbon monoxide diffusion capacity; ERV, end residual volume; FEF, forced expiratory flow; FET, forced expiratory time; FEV_5, forced expiratory volume for .5 second; FEV_1, forced expiratory volume for 1 second; FEV_3, forced expiratory volume for 3 seconds; FRC, functional residual capacity; FRCT, functional residual capacity time (also called helium equilibration time); FVC, forced vital capacity; Hb, hemoglobin; IC, inspiratory capacity; IV, inspiratory volume; MVV, maximal voluntary ventilation; PEFR, peak expiratory flow rate; RV, residual volume; SVC, slow vital capacity; TLC, total lung capacity; TV, tidal volume; VA, alveolar ventilation.

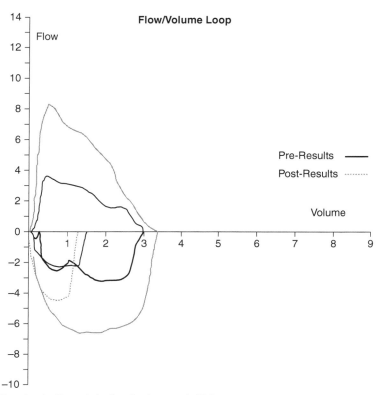

Reproduced with permission from Reed. www.mdguidelines.com.

Refinements to asthma/COPD diagnosis and screening have been promulgated.[6–8,12,13] In addition to pulmonary testing, cardiovascular evaluation is frequently necessary. This may include exercise stress testing, echocardiography, and other methods.

Reactive Airway Disease/Chronic Obstructive Pulmonary Disease

Presumed Disability
The presumed level of disability for asthma or COPD as outlined by the SSA is shown in Table 15-7. Note that this figure contains less detail than impairment tables normally used in disability evaluation.

Risk Assessment
The potential risk of continuing to work despite lung disease may be significant if the disease was either caused or aggravated by exposure to a chemical or biological agent encountered in the workplace.

Examples include work-related asthma and hypersensitivity pneumonitis. Work-related asthma includes: (a) work-exacerbated asthma, where work conditions produce temporary or permanent change in the asthmatic status even if the asthma was not caused by work; and (b) occupational asthma, in which the work exposures directly caused the asthma. Occupational asthma may be due to sensitization or to exposure to high levels of irritants (sometimes called *irritant induced asthma* or *reactive airways dysfunction syndrome,* RADS). Material safety data sheets may be helpful in identifying agents with which the patient works. Cigarette smoking, atopy, and other personal factors affect the risk of some, but not all, of these disorders.

Certain industries and occupations are associated with asthma or COPD; these include certain manufacturing operations and baking.[11] Pneumoconiosis may develop from exposures to silica, coal dust, asbestos, and many other agents.

The evaluating physician should carefully assess occupational exposures of the pulmonary disease patient. In many instances, identifying the work-related etiology can prevent subsequent exposures of the patient to inciting agents. This is particularly important in occupational asthma if the patient has become allergically sensitized to a workplace chemical or biological agent. The physician should consider recommending either work restrictions to eliminate

Table 15-7 Social Security Administration Presumed Disability in Pulmonary Conditions

3.01 Category of Impairments, Respiratory System

3.02 *Chronic Pulmonary Insufficiency*

A. Chronic obstructive pulmonary disease due to any cause, with the FEV_1 equal to or less than the values specified in Table I corresponding to the person's height without shoes. (In cases of marked spinal deformity, see 3.00E.)

Table I

Height Without Shoes (cm)	Height Without Shoes (in)	FEV_1 Equal to or Less Than (L, BTPS)
154 or less	60 or less	1.05
155–160	61–63	1.15
161–165	64–65	1.25
166–170	66–67	1.35
171–175	68–69	1.45
176–180	70–71	1.55
181 or more	72 or more	1.65

Or

B. Chronic restrictive ventilatory disease, due to any cause, with the FVC equal to or less than the values specified in Table II corresponding to the person's height without shoes. (In cases of marked spinal deformity, see 3.00E.)

Table II

Height Without Shoes (cm)	Height Without Shoes (in)	FVC Equal to or Less Than (L, BTPS)
154 or less	60 or less	1.25
155–160	61–63	1.35
161–165	64–65	1.45
166–170	66–67	1.55
171–175	68–69	1.65
176–180	70–71	1.75
181 or more	72 or more	1.85

Or

C. *Chronic impairment of gas exchange due to clinically documented pulmonary disease. With:*

1. Single breath DLCO (see 3.00F1) less than 10.5 mL/min/mm Hg or less than 40% of the predicted normal value. (Predicted values must either be based on data obtained at the test site or published values from a laboratory using the same technique as the test site. The source of the predicted values should be reported. If they are not published, they should be submitted in the form of a table or nomogram); or

(Continued)

Table 15-7 *(Continued)*

2. Arterial blood gas values of PO_2 and simultaneously determined PCO_2 measured while at rest (breathing room air, awake, and sitting or standing) in a clinically stable condition on at least two occasions, three or more weeks apart within a six-month period, equal to or less than the values specified in the applicable Table III-A or III-B:

Table III-A

(Applicable at test sites less than 3,000 feet above sea level)

Arterial PCO_2 (mm Hg)	Arterial PO_2 Equal To or Less Than (mm Hg)
30 or below	65
31	64
32	63
33	62
34	61
35	60
36	59
37	58
38	57
39	56
40 or above	55

Table III-B

(Applicable at test sites 3,000 through 6,000 feet above sea level)

Arterial PCO_2 (mm Hg)	Arterial PO_2 Equal To or Less Than (mm Hg)
30 or below	60
31	59
32	58
33	57
34	56
35	55
36	54
37	53
38	52
39	51

FEV_1 indicates forced expiratory volume for 1 second; FVC, forced vital capacity; PO_2, partial pressure of oxygen; PCO_2, partial pressure of carbon dioxide.

Adapted from Social Security Administration.[14]

future exposure or workplace exposure controls such as ventilation or respirator use. If a patient's lung disease is clearly recognized as work related, then the physician evaluating the individual's work ability has the responsibility to prevent further exposure to the involved substance through work restrictions or workplace exposure modification. (Restrictions are based on risk.)

There are many forms of lung disease that a physician may confront in disability assignments. The most common are asthma, COPD, and interstitial lung disease. The diagnosis of these conditions as occupational diseases is beyond the scope of this text. Links between the occupational environment and lung disease continue to be described.

Capacity

Work conditions may affect the disease course even if the disease itself was not caused by work exposures. The patient's capacity to continue working in a particular job should be determined by comparing his or her measured physiologic capacity to the demands of the job. Two distinct types of evaluation are appropriate to assess work capacity.

a. Does the patient have sufficient cardiopulmonary capacity to meet the physical demands of the job? This is particularly relevant in individuals with largely irreversible lung disorders such as interstitial lung disease and COPD.

b. Will the patient overreact to workplace irritants or allergic exposures? Such assessment is particularly relevant to asthma cases.

For asthma, a careful history of workplace and home-related triggers should generally be complemented by physiologic testing. Testing of airway hyper responsiveness may generally be conducted by measuring spirometry before and after administration of an aerosolized bronchodilator according to a standard protocol.

The American Thoracic Society recommends considering three criteria: (1) How severe is the residual FEV_1 reduction after bronchodilator administration? (2) How severe is the hyper responsiveness of the airways? (3) How much medication is necessary to control the asthma?

For asthma patients, spirometry should be conducted both before and after administration of an aerosolized bronchodilator. The degree of improvement after the bronchodilator indicates how severe the hyperresponsiveness is. Also, the postbronchodilator FEV_1 is considered a more accurate measure of functional ability than is the prebronchodilator FEV_1.

Direct measurement of airway hyper responsiveness is provided by metha-choline challenge testing. In this test, baseline spirometry is performed, and the patient is then given small doses of inhaled methacholine. The dose that produces a 20% decline in the FEV_1 is the provocative concentration-20 (PC^{20}). A low PC^{20} implies that the patient is very sensitive to irritants. Therefore, methacholine challenge is useful both for determining whether or not asthma is actually present as well as for determining how severe it is.

Less frequently, workplace testing is necessary. If the patient's symptoms have a suspected work-related asthma occupational component, then test-ing at the work site or at a nearby easily assessable facility may be neces-sary. This would allow documentation of a more severe impairment than is appreciated by testing in a physician's office.

In very unusual circumstances, specific agent bronchoprovocation testing is necessary. In this test, the patient is given very small doses of a chemical or biological agent to which he or she may be sensitized. The response of FEV_1 may show that the person is highly sensitive to very low concentra-tions of a provocative material. Under such circumstances, the individual should generally be removed from even low dose exposure to such material. Specific agent bronchoprovocation testing is complex and should be carried out only by physicians with particular expertise. It is very rarely necessary or feasible in disability assessments in the United States.

Tolerance

Dyspnea at low workloads, not accompanied by objective signs like tac-hypnea or reduced oxygen saturation, suggests that psychosocial factors and subjective responsive or tolerance, rather than risk or capacity, may be the underlying issues. As seen in cardiovascular discussions, psychosocial factors such as job satisfaction affect a patient's decision to work.[15] Patient and physician ability to base work recommendations on tolerance are poor, especially when seen in an emergency setting.[16,17] There are descriptions of psychological factors precipitating acute asthmatic attacks and psychological symptoms affecting COPD.[18] The evaluating physician should determine if the patient is receiving optimal treatment. Proper treatment of respiratory dis-orders, particularly asthma, may significantly reduce the level of disability. Treatment guidelines are available to guide clinicians in assessing whether a claimant has been adequately treated. Parallel to the discussion in the cardio-vascular chapter, rehabilitation protocols may also help with COPD.[19,20]

Disability Duration

The Medical Disability Advisor has disability duration tables for common lung conditions.

Table 15-8 Disability Duration Trends in Asthma

Medical treatment, acute asthma attack (mild to moderate)			
DURATION IN DAYS			
Job Classification	**Minimum**	**Optimum**	**Maximum**
Sedentary	0	3	7
Light	0	3	7
Medium	0	3	10
Heavy	0	3	14
Very Heavy	0	3	14

DURATION TRENDS

ICD-9-CM: 493, 493.0, 493.00, 493.1, 493.2, 493.9

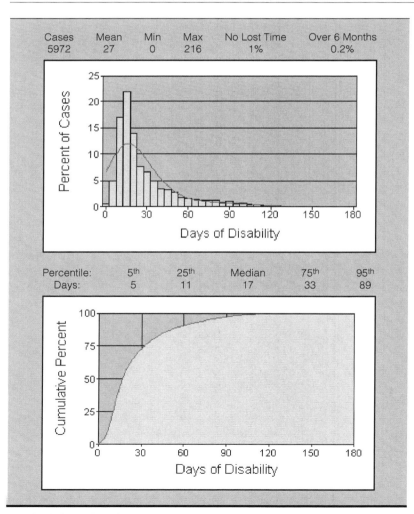

Cases	Mean	Min	Max	No Lost Time	Over 6 Months
5972	27	0	216	1%	0.2%

Percentile:	5th	25th	Median	75th	95th
Days:	5	11	17	33	89

Reproduced with permission from Reed. www.mdguidelines.com.

Table 15-9 Disability Duration Trends in COPD

Medical treatment, acute exacerbation			
DURATION IN DAYS			
Job Classification	Minimum	Optimum	Maximum
Sedentary	5	7	21
Light	5	7	21
Medium	5	10	21
Heavy	5	14	28
Very Heavy	5	14	28

DURATION TRENDS

ICD-9-CM: 496

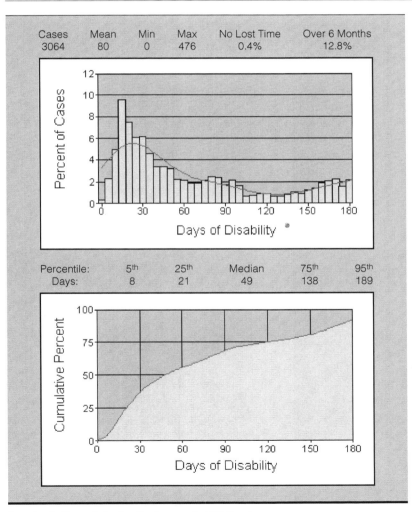

Cases	Mean	Min	Max	No Lost Time	Over 6 Months
3064	80	0	476	0.4%	12.8%

Percentile:	5th	25th	Median	75th	95th
Days:	8	21	49	138	189

Reproduced with permission from Reed. www.mdguidelines.com.

Interstital Lung Disease

Interstitial lung disease may be work related (eg, asbestosis, silicosis, coal workers pneumoconiosis, chronic beryllium disease) or may be naturally occurring (such as idiopathic pulmonary fibrosis or scleroderma lung disease).

Risk

The extent of the disease and its functional limitations should be determined as a guide to work ability. In advanced cases, the abnormality of the spirometry and diffusing capacity for CO may be so great that the additional testing is unnecessary. Frequently, however, the functional capacity is best determined using a pulmonary exercise test. Methodological criteria are available in recommendations of the ATS/ERS. Generally, a pulmonary exercise test should include direct measurement of the maximum oxygen consumption, ventilation, oxygen saturation, and continuously monitored exhaled carbon dioxide concentrations as well as cardiac monitoring. Many resources exist to aid in test interpretation.[21,22]

Capacity

Cardiopulmonary exercise testing may quantify the patient's capacity. In addition, it may greatly aid the differential diagnosis among airway disease, interstitial lung disease, pulmonary vascular disease, cardiac disease, and deconditioning as the cause of exercise functional limitation. In many patients, deconditioning and obesity are the major limiting factors for exercise limitation. Literature has now shown that a main reason for limitation in COPD patients is skeletal muscle atrophy that occurs with deconditioning from this prolonged respiratory condition.[23] Parallel to the discussion in the cardiovascular chapter, rehabilitation protocols may also help with COPD.[24,25]

Imaging studies are occasionally useful for identifying interstitial lung disease. High-resolution CAT scanning is also useful for providing insight into the particular type of disorder present. However, routine pulmonary function testing and exercise testing generally provide a greater amount of information concerning the actual workplace limitations.

If the patient's interstitial lung disease was caused by work, special work restrictions are necessary. Even if the patient is physically capable of meeting the job demands, exposure to the causative agent should be significantly reduced or eliminated. Even simple pneumoconiosis, which is generally not associated with significantly abnormal pulmonary function tests, places an individual at higher risk of developing advanced disease if exposure continues. Similar considerations apply to chronic beryllium disease, chronic hypersensitivity pneumonitis, and similar immunologic disorders.

Tolerance and Disability Duration

Patient limits in tolerance are often reflective of concerns that a work environment continues to expose the patient to offending pulmonary substances. Verification of a clean work environment or regular follow-up visits after a work shift may provide needed documentation and reassurance for work viability.

Pulmonary Vascular Disease

Pulmonary vascular disease is increasingly recognized. It may occur as a primary disorder or may be secondary to another disorder. Primary pulmonary hypertension, scleroderma associated pulmonary hypertension, and consequences of a single large or multiple small pulmonary emboli are common. Persons with significant pulmonary hypertension have functional limitations and dyspnea that appear disproportionate to the abnormalities on routine function testing.

Clinical examination may show signs of right heart strain, loud P2, or a suprasternal thrill. However, echocardiography and electrocardiography are much more accurate. Cardiopulmonary exercise testing is also useful in assessing limitation in patients with pulmonary vascular disorders.

Pulmonary thromboembolism is a common problem and is often undetected. Chronic pulmonary hypertension may develop from multiple pulmonary emboli. In addition, a single episode of a major pulmonary embolism may produce permanent pulmonary hypertension if it is not adequately recanalized. Generally, the echocardiogram, electrocardiogram, and perhaps a cardiopulmonary exercise test can quantify the extent of physiologic impairment and consequent work ability/disability. Right ventricular dysfunction as shown echocardiographically[13] is a serious indicator of long-term functional impairment.

Risk

From the occupational work ability standpoint, a history of prior pulmonary embolus requires careful consideration about whether the occupation constitutes a significant risk for recurrence. There has been considerable concern about air travel, particularly if prolonged, as a risk factor for pulmonary embolus. This is a particular concern when the employee's job requires air travel of greater than 6 hours duration.[15] Although the data are limited, some term this the "economy class syndrome," implying that the risk is greater in more cramped space.[18,19] Personal factors, in addition to the nature of the work, inform assessment of the risk of recurrence. For example, d-dimer test results after resolution of the acute episode significantly predict the likelihood of recurrence.[20]

Therefore, in assessing safe return to work or disability, the evaluating physician should consider three factors: (1) permanent physiologic impairment, particularly right ventricular dysfunction or pulmonary hypertension; (2) occupational factors that may increase the risk of recurrence; and (3) personal factors affecting likelihood of recurrence, including obesity, hypercoagulability, or evidence of ongoing clotting disorders, such as elevated d-dimer levels.

Capacity
Generally with pulmonary vascular disease conditions, the same principles of cardiopulmonary exercise evaluation would lead to a determination of a patient's work ability.

Tolerance and Disability Duration
Tolerance is generally not an issue with these conditions, as the objective testing would indicate what a patient can and cannot do.

Table 15-10 Disability Duration Trends in Pulmonary Embolism

	Medical treatment, pulmonary embolism		
	DURATION IN DAYS		
Job Classification	**Minimum**	**Optimum**	**Maximum**
Sedentary	7	14	28
Light	7	14	28
Medium	14	21	35
Heavy	28	42	49
Very Heavy	28	42	49

Surgical treatment, pulmonary embolectomy.

(Continued)

Table 15-10 *(Continued)*

Medical treatment, pulmonary embolism			
DURATION IN DAYS			
Job Classification	**Minimum**	**Optimum**	**Maximum**
Sedentary	42	56	112
Light	42	56	112
Medium	56	70	Indefinite
Heavy	56	84	Indefinite
Very Heavy	56	112	Indefinite

Surgical treatment, prophylaxis - vena cava interruption, intravascular, IVC umbrella.

DURATION IN DAYS			
Job Classification	**Minimum**	**Optimum**	**Maximum**
Sedentary	7	14	42
Light	7	14	56
Medium	14	21	84
Heavy	84	91	112
Very Heavy	84	98	112

Surgical treatment, prophylaxis - distal vein ligation.

DURATION IN DAYS			
Job Classification	**Minimum**	**Optimum**	**Maximum**
Sedentary	14	21	56
Light	14	21	91
Medium	28	35	140
Heavy	84	112	168
Very Heavy	84	112	182

Surgical treatment, prophylaxis - open vena cava interruption.

DURATION IN DAYS			
Job Classification	**Minimum**	**Optimum**	**Maximum**
Sedentary	28	35	56
Light	28	35	91
Medium	42	49	140
Heavy	84	112	168
Very Heavy	84	112	182

Reproduced with permission from Reed. www.mdguidelines.com.

Respiratory Control Disorders

Sleep Apnea

Sleep apnea is a common problem particularly in individuals with obesity, male gender, and in middle-aged or older individuals. In addition to causing pulmonary hypertension and increased cardiovascular risk, the major functional effect of sleep apnea is daytime hypersomnolence. Persons with sleep apnea constitute a significant public safety risk if they drive commercially. The Federal Motor Carrier Safety Administration of the Department of Transportation provides regulatory requirements for assessing individuals involved in interstate commerce. Such lack of alertness may also prevent individuals using dangerous machinery from working safely and effectively. Several recent consensus documents suggest work ability/disability assessment procedures for clinicians.[26]

In individuals at risk (eg, with significant obesity), the Epworth Sleepiness Score is a useful questionnaire screening instrument. However, definitive testing generally requires an overnight sleep study with polysomnography. Sleep apnea is often responsive to therapy, and therefore permanent impairment/disability should not be assessed until the patient has had an adequate trial of appropriate therapy (eg, nocturnal CPAP).

Summary

Pulmonary conditions are common, and return-to-work assessment in individuals with these conditions are challenging. Using information that is available will help physicians think through the issues of risk, capacity, and tolerance. As with other body system problems, patients with pulmonary disease are often capable of continuing to work. However, particular workplace risks must be considered when making a return-to-work recommendation. The considerable benefits of returning to work often outweigh any risks associated with working.

References

1. American Lung Association. Trends in Asthma Morbidity and Mortality; Trends in Chronic Bronchitis and Emphysema; Morbidity and Mortality – April 2004. New York, NY: American Heart Association; 2004.

2. Centers for Disease Control and Prevention. Behavioral Risk Factor Surveillance System (BRFSS); 2002 Asthma Data: Prevalence Tables and Maps. Available at: www.cdc.gov/asthma/brfss/02/brfssdata.htm. Accessed February 16, 2010.

Chapter 15

3. Balmes JR. Occupational contribution to the burden of chronic obstructive pulmonary disease. *J Occup Environ Med.* 2005;47(2):154-160.

4. Eisner MD, et al. An Official American Thoracic Society Public Policy Statement: Novel Risk Factors and the Global Burden of Chronic Obstructive Disease.

5. Macintyre N, et al. Standardisation of the single-breath determination of carbon monoxide uptake in the lung. *Eur Respir J.* 2005;26(4):720–735.

6. Wanger J, et al. Standardisation of the measurement of lung volumes. *Eur Respir J.* 2005;26(3):511–522.

7. Miller MR, et al. Standardisation of spirometry. *Eur Respir J.* 2005;26(2): 319–338.

8. Townsend MC. Evaluating pulmonary function change over time in the occupational setting. *J Occup Environ Med.* 2005;47(12):1307–1316.

9. Hankinson JL, Odencrantz JR, Fedan KB. Spirometric reference values from a sample of the general U.S. population. *Am J Respir Crit Care Med.* 1999;159:179–187.

10. Morris AH, Kanner RE, Crapo RO, et al. *Clinical Pulmonary Function Testing: A Manual of Uniform Laboratory Procedure.* 2nd ed. Denver, CO: Intermountain Thoracic Society; 1984.

11. American Thoracic Society. Standardization of spirometry: 1994 update. *Am J Respir Crit Care Med.* 1995;152:1107–1136.

12. Hnizdo E, et al. Association between chronic obstructive pulmonary disease and employment by industry and occupation in the US population: a study of data from the Third National Health and Nutrition Examination Survey. *Am J Epidemiol.* 2002;156(8):738–746.

13. Nici L, et al. American Thoracic Society/European Respiratory Society statement on pulmonary rehabilitation. *Am J Respir Crit Care Med.* 2006;173(12):1390–1413.

14. Social Security Administration. *Disability Evaluation Under Social Security.* Baltimore, MD: Social Security Administration: January 2003. SSA Publication 64–039.

15. Lavoie Kl, Bacon SL, Cartier A, et al. What's worse for asthma: mood disorders, anxiety disorders, or both? *Chest.* 2006;130:1039–1047

16. Nowak RM. National and international guidelines for the emergency management of adult asthma. In: Brenner BE, ed. *Emergency Asthma.* New York, NY: Marcel Dekker Inc; 1999.

17. Edmond SD, Camargo CA, Nowak RM. Advances, opportunities, and the new asthma guidelines. *Ann Emerg Med.* 1998;31:590–594.

18. Ng TP, Niti M, Tan WC, et al. Depressive symptoms and chronic obstructive pulmonary disease. *Arch Intern Med.* 2007;167:60–67

19. Goldhaber SZ. Pulmonary embolism. *Lancet,* 2004;363(9417):1295–1305.

20. Philbrick JT, et al. Air travel and venous thromboembolism: a systematic review. *J Gen Intern Med.* 2007;22(1):107–114.

21. Hansen JE, Wasserman K. Intergrated cardiopulmonary exercise testing. In: Demeter SL, Andersson GBJ, Smith GM, eds. *Disability Evaluation.* St Louis, MO: Mosby-Year Book: 1996.

22. Townsend MC. Technique and equipment pitfalls in spirometry testing: serious threats to your respiratory surveillance program. In: NORA Medical Surveillance Workshop. Available at: www.cdc.gov/niosh/sbw/osh prof/townsendhandout.html. Accessed May 18, 2004.

23. Lehmann R, et al. Incidence, clinical characteristics, and long-term prognosis of travel-associated pulmonary embolism. *Eur Heart J.* 2009;30(2):233–241.

24. Feltracco P, et al. Economy class syndrome: still a recurrent complication of long journeys. *Eur J Emerg Med.* 2007;14(2):100–103.

25. Verhovsek M, et al. Systematic review: D-dimer to predict recurrent disease after stopping anticoagulant therapy for unprovoked venous thromboembolism. *Ann Intern Med.* 2008;149(7):481-490, W94.

26. Talmage JB, et al. Consensus criteria for screening commercial drivers for obstructive sleep apnea: evidence of efficacy. *J Occup Environ Med.* 2008;50(3):324–329.

Working With Common Neurologic Problems

Edwin H. Klimek, MD

This chapter addresses return to work issues and risks to individuals and workplaces among persons of working age (arbitrarily designated 16 to 65 years) for conditions including primary and secondary headache syndromes, epilepsy (recurrent seizures vs first-time witnessed seizure), acquired brain injury, and progressive neurodegenerative conditions (eg, multiple sclerosis [MS] and hereditary neuropathies).

Physician-Certified Absenteeism for Neurologic Illness

Physician-certified absenteeism for neurologic illness may arise out of occupational health evaluations or within ongoing attending care without compromising the patient care relationship or casting doubt upon the advocacy role of the physician. This certification both arises from and is limited by the following circumstances:

- The patient stops work when he or she believes that illness or injury justifies absence.

- The physician certifies restricted work or modified work status.

- The patient returns to work when sufficiently recovered.

- Management attempts to provide accommodation and work autonomy.

- Insurers support this system by providing economic benefits for partial disability.

Patients confound this model by endorsing pain as a sign of a serious injury. Some are unprepared to attempt to return to work until all indicators of illness have resolved. They express a belief that the presence of pain or manifestations of neurologic illness is inconsistent with returning to work. An enabling philosophy of care among certifying physicians discounts the therapeutic affiliation of work-related activities compared to the hazards of daily life. Certifying physicians express concern of risk of injury during the attempt to return to work placing the onus on the certifying physician to disprove the risk. In all cases this is a misleading, if not an erroneous, assertion. The physician and individual should be reminded that the decision is not whether a return to work imposes a risk, but rather whether a return to work imposes a risk unacceptably greater than that of not returning to work.

For most musculoskeletal illnesses, guidelines for injury-specific recovery times are available from medical and scientific literature or are developed through consensus opinion of medical experience.[1] These guidelines frequently are based on return to work in job classifications of sedentary, light, medium, heavy, and very heavy activities. Unfortunately, the performance characteristics affected by neurologic illness related to motor coordination, sensation, and mental competence manifest in measurement of speed, accuracy, and reproducibility of the task are not as readily available.

This chapter assesses capacity to undertake gainful employment, which is regular attendance in a nonsheltered environment requiring competitive employment with or without accommodations that are feasible and realistic. Return to work may be possible through either modifications to the workplace or work autonomy.

The concept of work autonomy, or the ability of the worker to pace the work to suit the limitations of a continuing illness or injury, is slightly different from (although related to) workplace modifications. Return to modified work presumes residual work capacity and availability of adequate workplace alterations. The employer establishes the minimum performance reasonably necessary to accomplish a legitimate work-related purpose. In failing to accept an employee back to work, the employer demonstrates it is impossible to accommodate individual employees sharing the characteristics of the claimant without imposing undue hardship on the employer or a serious safety risk to the individual, coworkers, or the general public.

Patients are also assumed to be mentally competent despite neurologic illness and have primary responsibility to be informed enough about their condition to thoughtfully consider modified work opportunities available from the employer. The employer and patient should accept and understand the philosophies of partial disability and rapid return to work, as well as the role of modified work opportunities in achieving this goal.

Neurologic Illness: General

In general terms, neurologic illness may be episodic, static, or slowly deteriorating. In many situations, determination, motivation, and effort overcome persistent neurologic handicaps. This results in opportunities for reevaluation of evolving symptoms causally related with confidence to the original injury. If the presence of newly identifiable organic changes is entirely explained by the persisting neurologic illness, the trial of return to work is reassessed and encouraged. However, if a clear link to the workplace can be established for the worsening of the neurologic condition (risk), a continued return to work with or without suitable accommodation to reduce the risk of recurrence is a matter for informed discussion. Shift work and sleep cycle alteration, which may normally elicit fatigue, may be a cause of unavoidable deterioration. In the latter case, medical advice against a return to work may be given.

In musculoskeletal injury a combination of medical, sociodemographic, and psychological variables predict nonreturn. Presumably similar considerations apply to neurologic illness. Fear-avoidance variables, taken alone, provide a 70% correct prediction of continuing sick leave for patients with back pain at 12 months after treatment.[2] Intercurrent employment-related factors associated with poor outcome of a trial of return to work include a job in the public sector, a longer time in the occupation, and multiple job changes and periods of unemployment. Failure to return to work may also be associated with work factors, eg, job dissatisfaction.[3–5] Some patients do not return to work simply because it is more rewarding not to work, both financially and psychologically.[6–8] Self-determination and the will to be sick remain powerful predictors of an unsuccessful trial of return to work.

Headache

Persistent daily nondebilitating headaches are likely to be tension-type or mixed headaches, including migraine. Migraine is a common, chronic, incapacitating neurovascular disorder, characterized by attacks of severe headache, autonomic nervous system dysfunction, and, in some patients, an aura involving neurologic symptoms. This characteristic pattern of stereotypical recurrence is required to support the diagnosis.

Persistent debilitating daily headache is rare in clinical neurologic practice outside of infectious illness, abnormality of cerebrospinal fluid pressure, temporal arteritis, or head trauma. The hallmark of these conditions is abnormality of rheumatologic serology, cerebrospinal fluid contents, or opening pressure obtained by lumbar puncture after neuroimaging studies. The clinical characteristics of the headache are insufficient to rule out the possibility of intracranial disease.[9]

Undertaking neuroimaging studies as a risk management strategy for the examiner should be considered in all adult patients with headache of recent onset or in previously headache-free individuals in whom a trial of return to work is being considered. Detection of significant and treatable lesions is the goal of neuroimaging, but there are other important considerations that should be noted in the context of occupational health settings. Neuroimaging may relieve the patient's anxiety about having an underlying pathologic condition as well as improve the patient's overall satisfaction with his or her care, especially if the patient has an expectation of that type of test. This position is inherent in and consistent with practice guidelines of professional organizations, which suggest that there is insufficient evidence to make recommendations in patients for headaches other than migraine.[10,11]

Typically the neurologic examination is entirely normal in headache syndromes such as migraine. Studies suggest the incidence of clinically important findings on neuroimaging studies to be low (between 0.4% and 2.4%) in patients with acute headaches without head trauma.[10] However generalizing this data to the occupational health setting is problematic in light of false-positive findings on magnetic resonance (MR) imaging screening of self-declared normal volunteers.[12] This results in a large part from the white-matter hyperintensities present in asymptomatic individuals.[13] Accordingly, worrisome but predictable false positive studies should be discussed before the testing. The other considerations of an inadequate study missing intercurrent disease, risks of contrast media, radiation exposure with CT and over-sedation in claustrophobic patients having MRI scans are also part of informed consent.[14]

How the migraine pain is triggered and the cascade of events that follow are not well understood, and discussion of these issues is beyond the scope of this chapter. The initial diagnostic evaluation of all headache syndromes including posttraumatic headaches rests on a carefully obtained history including pain character, location, onset, precipitants, aura, other associated symptoms, duration, frequency, and time course followed by a focused neurologic examination to identify the red flags that warrant intensive or invasive investigations.[15]

Headache occurring in close temporal association to trauma may be considered posttraumatic headache (PTH), acute or chronic. Chronic PTHs, the headaches that persist for more than 3 months according to the International

Headache Society (IHS), occur infrequently. The preceding head injury may vary from minimal to severe and does not correlate with the duration or intensity of headache.[16] By the definition put forth by the IHS, headaches must start within 7 days of the injury itself.[17]

Chronic PTH has no special features but is symptomatically identical to other headaches such as chronic tension-type headache or migraine without aura.[18,19] This suggests that PTHs are generated by the same processes that cause the natural headaches, not by intracranial derangement from head blows or jolts.[20] The incidence of this entity is not clearly defined, with advocates indicating that it is found in most patients with postconcussional syndrome and skeptics suggesting it is nearly nonexistent in countries where possibilities for monetary compensation are minimal.[21]

Posttraumatic headache is often seen as part of the postconcussion syndrome.[22] Postconcussion syndrome refers to a large number of symptoms and signs usually following mild traumatic brain injury (MTBI).[23] The most common complaints are headaches, dizziness, fatigue, irritability, anxiety, insomnia, loss of consciousness and memory, and noise sensitivity.[24] While some proportion of difficult-to-manage cases may be malingerers or frauds or have compensation neurosis, most patients nevertheless have genuine complaints, in part resembling depression or dissociative phenomena, not all of which are cured by a verdict or any recommended treatment.[25–28]

Advocates of all sides seem to accept a bona fide presentation of an initial isolated migraine or an increased frequency of previously existing migraine headaches subsequent to an injury.[29] Essentially this accords with the belief that anyone may have a migraine attack occasionally without necessarily being a migraine patient. In the absence of trait markers specific to migraine or its subtypes, the classification of migraine headache is guided by diagnostic criteria.[30] That PTH is a diagnostic challenge may be inferred from the extreme frequency of headaches in the general population, affecting about eight of nine people at some time in their life, thereby diluting the presentation.[31]

Risk
In primary headache syndromes, risk is not an issue. Headaches secondary to structural disease are uncommon and are beyond the scope of this chapter.

Capacity
Capacity is rarely an issue in headache patients. They can perform activities, but they dislike doing so because of symptoms (pain, nausea, fatigue).

Tolerance

Tolerance for activity despite symptoms is the problem for patients with primary headache syndromes. In keeping with the philosophy outlined in Chapters 1 and 2, physicians should typically work with patients to minimize the frequency and severity of headaches and certify disability only for the specific days of severe headache. Many migraine patients work despite migraine. There is no objective way for a physician to determine, and thus certify, that a given headache is severe enough to justify missing work on a given day.

Sample Case: Headache

A middle-aged woman employed as a front desk receptionist for a large commercial enterprise feels unable to return to work as a result of debilitating headaches subsequent to a thyroid operation (tolerance). Headaches occur on a daily basis, with a severe headache that is described as a migraine about once a week. When a severe headache occurs, she is effectively housebound and chooses not "to do anything" because of severe pain. Before the surgery, a similar very bad headache occurred about once a year. For this problem she has been referred to a neurologist, who injected botulinum toxin on four occasions for headaches.

At the time of the encounter, the patient is having one of her daily headaches, for which she took two tablets of oxycodone before coming to the office. No other medication is taken regularly.

The history confirms that family members had headaches. The general medical and neurologic examinations are unremarkable. Neuroimaging studies are normal. Serologic evaluation, including thyroid function studies, is normal.

Indicators of superimposed depression or traits of avoidant personality are not found. Although the patient accepts a trial of interval therapy to reduce the frequency and severity of the migraine, she does not wish to reduce daily analgesic use. A trial of increased activity and progressive return to work is obstructed by family commitments to child care.

In this case the diagnosis of daily headaches and common migraine was supported. Daily analgesic use raised the possibility of medication-induced rebound headaches. Maximal medical therapy was not established. While continuing to advocate for a trial of return to work and compliance with treatment, her attending physician was not able to certify her as disabled for her usual occupation.

To prepare for a return to work for patients who report chronic disabling headache, a challenge of graded activity and exercise while keeping a headache diary or using a headache scale is advisable.[32] The failure to adhere to a graded increase in exercise allows social and personal barriers to emerge and be addressed without being complicated by workplace stressors. Identification of the benefits of increased activity on most headaches is underscored.

Debilitating chronic headache rarely occurs without amplification of other normal body sensations. Patients who experience chronic headache also seem to confuse responsible therapeutic drug use with drug misuse for symptoms common to everyday life, which they misunderstand as warning signs of serious disease. Some thereby express emotional distress constrained only by cultural and familial rules.

There are more reviews of treatment options in the literature than original clinical research outlining the incidence, characteristics, and effectiveness of therapy for PTH. This may be in part because the clinical distinction between PTH and other headache subtypes is obscured by the substantial degree of overlap in the symptoms, by the ways in which these headache subtypes evolve over time, and by the use of retrospective symptom histories to assign clinical diagnosis.[33,34] This is further blurred when diagnostic suspicion and acumen are focused on existing criteria for diagnosis of headache that may in themselves not be adequate in either primary or posttraumatic headaches.[35]

Responses to therapeutic intervention are diagnostically unreliable, because there may be an undue lag in response that may be contaminated by external events and by the natural course of headaches and underlying medical illness.[36,37] The risk to the workplace of a trial of return to work in headache is typically limited to lack of productivity attributable to unreliable or unpredictable attendance rather than damage of product or hazard to coworkers.

Epilepsy

Epilepsy is distinct among diseases for fleeting yet severe effect on employment, social life, and the sense of well-being. It is complicated by the balance between a person's right to manage his or her seizures and guard his or her confidentiality against the employer's knowledge. In the United Kingdom, 53% of employed people with epilepsy chose to conceal their illness.[38] The employer is often reluctant to allow these individuals to continue at the workplace, fearing workplace disruption or repercussion of potential workplace injury. A difficulty commonly encountered in epilepsy is that employers are hesitant to recognize that employees, despite having epilepsy, are able to return to work if reasonable accommodations can be made. The reasonableness of the accommodation is not a medical issue.

Sample Case: Seizure

A factory worker has a witnessed first-time seizure without focal onset or prolonged postictal period. It is unaccompanied by indication of substance misuse or previous childhood or family history of seizure. Physical examination limited to the neurologic system reveals no abnormality. Magnetic resonance imaging (MRI) and electroencephalography (EEG) are unremarkable. After discussion of the options, anticonvulsant therapy is not initiated. The employer is keen to temporarily provide employment alternatives ensuring no use of machinery and no work activities that could result in injury if a seizure occurred during work.

Although in many such presentations confirmation of the diagnosis may be medically and ethically challenging,[39,40] the crux of this problem is prognostication of recurrence so that work tasks can be addressed. Prognosis and treatment of the first seizure depend on diagnostic accuracy in identification of a specific epilepsy syndrome, yet patients with first seizures are generally falsely regarded as a homogeneous group.[41] Studies of seizure recurrence after a first tonic-clonic seizure give conflicting predictions of recurrence, with a meta-analysis suggesting a 2-year risk of recurrence as high as 40%.[42]

Assessment of adults should comprise rigorous clinical evaluation with explicit questions about previous minor epileptic symptoms, early EEG (ideally within 24 hours of the seizure), sleep-deprived EEG if the first EEG is nondiagnostic, and MR imaging for all patients except those for whom idiopathic generalized epilepsy is confirmed on their EEG or those with benign rolandic epilepsy.[43]

In part this extensive emphasis on investigations reflects the uncertainty and unreliability of the investigation in prognostication. Electroencephalography is most useful in the management of patients with suspected epilepsy. In patients without a diagnosis, the EEG presence of "epileptiform" activity does not establish the diagnosis beyond doubt because similar activity may be found in about 2% of individuals who have never had a seizure.[44] Similarly, in patients with undoubted epilepsy, multiple recordings may fail to demonstrate epileptiform activity in 8%.

A problematic issue sometimes confused with the capacity to work is the privilege to drive. Patients who should not be driving or who should be driving only under certain circumstances should be so advised. This does not preclude them from gainful employment, except employment as the operator of a motor vehicle. Most physicians have a standard warning letter about driving (or a form providing advice for multiple risks, including driving) and many provide the patient with a copy.

While the confidential nature of the physician-patient relationship is of the utmost importance, under certain circumstances physicians are required by law to report particular events or patient conditions to the appropriate government or regulatory agency. These requirements generally state that any physician who diagnoses or treats a person with epilepsy must report that person's name, age, and address and may grant physicians immunity in compliance with the law.

In planning a return to work for patients with seizures, one should consider the predictability of the disorder and aura that may precede the loss of consciousness. Spudis et al.[45] suggested that idiopathic isolated attacks should be treated more favorably than recurrent attacks with abnormal investigations. These might include a breakthrough seizure due to physician-directed medication change, an isolated seizure when the medical examination indicates that another episode appears unlikely, a seizure related to a temporary illness, a seizure due to an isolated incident of not taking medication, an established pattern of nocturnal seizures, an established pattern of seizures that do not impair driving ability, or an established pattern of an extended warning aura.

The major risk to the workplace of a trial of return to work in seizures is probably productivity reduction attributable to unreliable or unpredictable attendance. The risk to the patient from a seizure is similar to the risk were it to occur in a non-workplace setting. It is rare for damage of product or hazard to coworkers to be found during the ictus.

A common error in evaluating patients with a seizure disorder is misattribution of persistent concurrent cognitive impairment to seizures, rather than drug-induced side effects. Drowsiness in the workplace may be cause for work restriction. Shift work not only makes seizures more likely as a result of sleep deprivation but has the potential to intensify the drowsiness induced by therapy.

Risk
Typical work restrictions for patients with seizures include no driving, no climbing to heights, and no working with machinery or under conditions in which significant injury to self or others is predictable if a seizure occurred. Drowsiness from medications may be an additional issue of risk.

Capacity
Capacity in patients with seizure disorders is not affected. As long as risk is adequately addressed, these patients work without limitations.

Tolerance
Patients with seizure disorders may dislike working, fearing that seizures in the workplace will be embarrassing, but this is an issue of patient choice (to work or not to work) and not a reason for physician-certified work absence or disability.

Brain Injury

Brain injuries vary in severity. Severe traumatic brain injury is obvious to the layperson and is seldom misdiagnosed by health professionals.[46] Severe head injury may result in partial or complete paralysis, speech problems, impaired cognitive functioning, disability from employment, long periods of coma, and long-term care requirements. The injury will be apparent in changes on computed tomography, MR imaging, and other brain imaging. Disability after closed head injury varies depending on the injury mechanism, neuropathology, and other factors, such as medical complications.[46]

Patients with mild traumatic brain injury (MTBI) describe a similar constellation of postinjury complaints. Symptoms may include headaches,[47] dizziness, lethargy, memory loss, irritability, personality changes, cognitive deficits, and/or perceptual changes. These symptoms have been characterized under various names, including minor head injury,[48] mild head injury,[49] closed head injury,[50] postconcussive syndrome,[51] postconcussional syndrome,[52] postconcussional disorder,[53] minor traumatic brain injury,[54] traumatic cephalgia, post–brain injury syndrome, and posttraumatic syndrome. The variability in neurobehavioral outcome after MTBI may be, in part, attributed to ascertainment bias, giving a wide variance to severity and dysfunction in individuals after MTBI.

Research studies show a wide variability in the degree and duration of disability after MTBI. For example, some clinical observations show that patients with MTBI (Glasgow Coma Scale score, 13–15), who are able to follow commands less than 1 hour after injury, demonstrate no long-term persistent neuropsychological impairments.[55] Other research indicates that only 49% had a "good recovery."[56]

Individuals who were productive before injury may become unproductive after a MTBI. Patients with fractures of the skull, severe cerebral contusions, or large intracranial hematomas that are successfully treated can make uneventful and complete recoveries,[57] but patients with stable pre-accident psychological and work histories with no prior complaints may apparently develop functional impairments after MTBI. This is the "MTBI paradox": a so-called mild injury can result in apparently serious problems. Evidence indicates that 1 year after injury most patients (73%) return to work, even thought 84% report having complaints.[58]

Although patients with MTBI report similar clusters of symptoms and complaints, the precise etiology of symptoms is elusive, and many health professionals take an aggressive treatment approach and treat all reported symptoms. Others advise that the majority of symptoms will resolve within 90 days of the injury. In some cases, expectation may be the cause of these early symptoms.[59–61]

Risk
Patients with head injury, mild or severe, are not at risk of harm with work activities for which they have appropriate intellect and motor skills. The brain does not become injured or get worse with activity. There is no basis for work restrictions, unless posttraumatic seizures are present.

Capacity
Individuals with severe brain injury may lack the intellectual or motor skills to perform essential work functions. Their work limitations may preclude a return to employment. Functional testing or a trial of supervised work activity may be helpful in determining work ability.

Tolerance

Tolerance for symptoms like headache, malaise, and fatigue may be reasons cited by patients with brain injury for choosing not to work. These symptoms are not measurable or verifiable and are infrequently a basis for physician certification of work absence. Commonly, such symptoms can be satisfactorily addressed by work autonomy, in which the pace and rate of work are modified. Personality changes found in severe TBI may become significant obstacles to return to work because of changes in motivation and effort.

Multiple Sclerosis

In 1983, the Kurtzke Expanded Disability Status Scale (EDSS), shown in Table 16-1, considered eight functional systems intended to be independent of one another and that in combination reflect all the manifestations of neurologic impairment in multiple sclerosis (MS).[62] These functional groups or functional systems were pyramidal (P), cerebellar (Cll), brain stem (BS), sensory (S), bowel and bladder (BB), visual (V), cerebral or mental (Cb), and other or miscellaneous (O).

Table 16-1 Kurtzke Extended Disability Status Scale[62]

0.0	Normal neurologic examination (all grade 0 in all functional system [FS] scores)
1.0	No disability, minimal signs in one FS (ie, grade 1)
1.5	No disability, minimal signs in more than one FS (more than one grade 1)
2.0	Minimal disability in one FS (one FS grade 2, others 0 or 1)
2.5	Minimal disability in two FSs (two FSs grade 2, others 0 or 1)
3.0	Moderate disability in one FS (one FS grade 3, others 0 or 1); or mild disability in three or four FSs (three or four FSs grade 2, others 0 or 1) though fully ambulatory
3.5	Fully ambulatory but with moderate disability in one FS (one grade 3) and one or two FSs grade 2; or two grade 3 (others 0 or 1); or five grade 2 (others 0 or 1)
4.0	Fully ambulatory without aid, self-sufficient, up and about some 12 hours a day despite relatively severe disability consisting of one FS grade 4 (others 0 or 1); or combination of lesser grades exceeding limits of previous steps; patient should be able to walk >500 m without assist or rest
4.5	Fully ambulatory without aid, up and about much of the day, may otherwise require minimal assistance; characterized by relatively severe disability usually consisting of one FS grade 4 (others 0 or 1); or combinations of lesser grades exceeding limits of previous steps; walks >300 m without assist or rest
5.0	Ambulatory without aid for at least 200 m; disability severe enough to impair full daily activities (eg, working a full day without special provision) (usual FS equivalents are one grade 5 alone, others 0 or 1; or combinations of lesser grades); patient walks >200 m without aid or rest

(Continued)

Table 16-1 *(Continued)*

5.5	Ambulatory without aid for at least 100 m; disability severe enough to preclude full daily activities (usual FS equivalents are one grade 5 alone, others 0 or 1; or combinations of lesser grades). Enough to preclude full daily activities. (Usual FS equivalents are one grade 5 alone, others 0 or 1; or combinations of lesser grades).
6.0	Intermittent or unilateral constant assistance (cane, crutch, brace) required to walk at least 100 m (usual FS equivalents are combinations with more than one FS grade 3)
6.5	Constant bilateral assistance (canes, crutches, braces) required to walk at least 20 m (usual FS equivalents are combinations with more than one FS grade 3)
7.0	Unable to walk at least 5 m even with aid, essentially restricted to wheelchair; wheels self and transfers alone; up and about in wheelchair some 12 hours a day (usual FS equivalents are combinations with more than one FS grade 4+; very rarely pyramidal grade 5 alone)
7.5	Unable to take more than a few steps; restricted to wheelchair; may need aid in transfer; wheels self but cannot carry on in wheelchair a full day (usual FS equivalents are combinations with more than one FS grade 4+; very rarely pyramidal grade 5 alone)
8.0	Essentially restricted to chair or perambulated in wheelchair, but out of bed most of day; retains many self-care functions; generally has effective use of arms (usual FS equivalents are combinations, generally grade 4+ in several systems)
8.5	Essentially restricted to bed most of day; has some effective use of arm(s); retains some self-care functions (usual FS equivalents are combinations, generally 4 in several systems)
9.0	Helpless, bed-ridden patient; can communicate and eat (usual FS equivalents are combinations, mostly grade 4+)
9.5	Totally helpless, bed-ridden patient; unable to communicate effectively or eat or swallow (usual FS equivalents are combinations, almost all grade 4+)
10.0	Death due to MS

Within the EDSS, the principle of objective abnormality with no impairment of function is accepted, with step 3.0 being mild impairment without impeding normal functions except in rare individuals (steeplejacks or concert pianists). The lowest grades (up to step 4.0) presume the ability to ambulate fully for 500 m and carry out full daily activities. The EDSS correlates with the MR imaging–defined volume of plaque burden most closely for the pyramidal subscores. This probably reflects that factors other than volumetrically determined lesion load are important determinants for disability.[63]

Sample Case: Multiple Sclerosis

A 30-year-old female laboratory technician with known clinically definite MS presents with a flare of optic neuritis in the left eye and ataxia. She has an EDSS score of 4.0 at the time of relapse. She has worked for 10 years with the disorder. She and her husband have made a conscious decision not to inform her employer and her family of the disorder so that she will not be treated "differently." She has been on immunomodulating therapy for much of the time.

In this case a temporary medical absence for suppression of the relapse is undertaken. A remission is expected and occurs, with resumption of full-time work in 3 weeks.

In planning a return to work for patients with established MS, the temporal profile of the disorder can predict future recurrence and loss of ability. Early in the course of the disorder the presentation is less reliable; however, patients with prominent cerebellospinal signs have a less favorable prognosis. The benefits of established disease predicting future response to therapy are fortunately present in the previous case example. Chronic progressive MS with an EDSS score of 4.0 is often inconsistent with regular competitive employment.

Significant temporary relapses treated with intravenous corticosteroid infusions are likely inconsistent with workplace attendance during the relapse. Corticosteroids are also a psychoactive stimulant, and a withdrawal depression may be noted that may prolong the work absence.

The risk to the workplace of a trial of return to work in MS is dependent on the extent of the incoordination and corticospinal involvement. Unilateral visual dysfunction is rarely relevant except when strict binocular vision is a rigid task prerequisite. Damage to product or hazard to coworkers may ensue from incoordination. Therapeutic intervention including self-injection of immunomodulating therapy is unlikely to produce disabling side effects. Transient influenza-like reactions and local soreness may occur.

Disability From Multiple Sclerosis

The US Social Security Administration's (SSA) criteria for total disability from MS are as follows:

A. Disorganization of motor function, meaning significant and persistent disorganization of motor function in two extremities, resulting in sustained disturbance of gross and dexterous movements, or gait and station

B. Significant visual impairment (as described in the vision criteria) or significant mental impairment (as described in the mental illness criteria)

C. Significant, reproducible fatigue of motor function with substantial weakness on repetitive activity, demonstrated on physical examination (not just by patient history), resulting from neurologic dysfunction in areas of the central nervous system known to be pathologically involved by the MS process

Risk

Patients with MS are not at risk of harm with work activities for which they have appropriate intellect and motor skills. The brain does not become injured or get worse with activity. There is no basis for work restrictions.

Capacity

Patients with MS may be deconditioned from inactivity, but their current exercise ability, although measurable by treadmill testing, may be capable of increasing with progressive exercise or with progressively more difficult work. Fatigue or muscle weakness that can be documented on physical examination (and not merely reported by the patient) is an issue of work limitation based on capacity. If patients lack the necessary visual, auditory, sensory, motor, or intellectual function for the job in question, they usually have appropriate lesions on MR images. This loss of neurologic function, corroborated by the presence of appropriate lesions on MR images, may be the basis for physician certification of disability based or work limitations (due to capacity).

Magnetic resonance images do not predict disability. The plaque burden affecting the corticospinal tract approximates the EDSS score. Ataxia or incoordination may result in work limitations. Typically this is seen in older males presenting with spasticity who have a predominance of spinal and cerebellar involvement. They tend to have a gradually progressive downhill course.

The EDSS is intended to reflect all manifestations of MS in a hierarchical fashion; however, the arithmetic appearance may be misleading, because an EDSS score of 4 is not "twice as bad" as an EDSS score of 2. Chronic progressive MS with an EDSS score of 4.0 is often inconsistent with regular competitive employment (based on capacity).

Tolerance

Tolerance for symptoms like headache, malaise, weakness, and fatigue may be reasons cited by patients with MS for choosing not to work. These symptoms are not measurable or verifiable and are infrequently a basis for physician certification of work absence. The common complaint of fatigue in MS is of practical significance with impaired motor function, because there is typically no mental fatigue in the early stages of MS. Fatigue or weakness that cannot be documented on physical examination but is reported by the patient is an issue of tolerance and not capacity. As such, it is not generally a reason for physician-imposed work limitations. The choice to work or not to work despite subjective fatigue is the patient's choice.

Commonly, such symptoms can be satisfactorily addressed by work autonomy, in which the pace and rate of work are modified. Personality changes found in MS may become significant obstacles to return to work through changes in motivation and effort. Without a limitation of walking (manifest with an EDSS score of 4.0), this is rarely an obstacle to function.

Polyneuropathy

Diabetes is the most common disorder presenting with prominent signs and symptoms of neuropathy. The police officer at the practice range who discharges his weapon accidentally because he is unable to sense the trigger of the revolver poses a great hazard to himself and others. Driving skills are unlikely to be affected by diabetic neuropathy, although the concomitant hypoglycemia of overmedication and visual disturbance of retinal disease must be considered.

Sample Case: Polyneuropathy

A 35-year-old carpenter presents for evaluation with Charcot-Marie-Tooth disease, a familial polyneuropathy. He notes that he is unable to ascend or descend ladders because his plantar flexion at the ankle is weak (capacity) and the perception of the rungs through his steel-toe and steel-shank work boots is unreliable (risk). He has inexplicably dropped windows carried in the grip of the hand (capacity). Although he enjoys his job, he is concerned that he may not be able to drive because of foot pedal miscue (risk).

In the case given, the worker has a mismatch of occupational and personal expectations with the medical illness. He should be considered for retraining as the requirements of his job are inconsistent with personal safety (risk).

In planning a return to work for patients with established polyneuropathy, the temporal profile of the disorder can predict the loss of ability. Early in the course of the disorder, the neuropathic symptoms may be distracting but of limited functional importance. As the disease progresses, difficulty manipulating objects, such as starting threaded connections, is a common complaint of those working in trades.

Therapeutic interventions in familial polyneuropathies are generally of limited benefit. If the cause is diabetes, the systemic medical illness must be considered.

The risk to the workplace of a trial of return to work in polyneuropathy is dependent on the extent of the incoordination and motor weakness that develops late in the disease. The damage to product or hazard to coworkers ensues from the incoordination.

Risk

The risk to patients with peripheral neuropathy relates to the sensory deficit and to the motor deficit. If gait and coordinated activity are impaired, the individual may be at risk climbing to heights, walking on narrow surfaces, and working with hazardous equipment. These factors would be a basis for physician-imposed activity restrictions. Prolonged standing or walking on feet that lack sensation may lead to skin ulceration and is a basis for work restrictions on standing, walking, and carrying.

Capacity

Individuals with peripheral neuropathy may no longer be capable of the walking or coordinated activity required to meet the essential functions of the job in question. This would be the basis for a work limitation. Functional testing or a trial of supervised work activity may be helpful in determining work ability.

Tolerance

There are usually no issues of work tolerance in individuals with peripheral neuropathy. If they have the capacity to work at acceptable risk, they may work. If the neuropathy is painful, the decision to work or not to work despite pain is the patient's choice. Pain is not measurable and thus is not a basis for a physician to impose work restrictions or work limitations.

Summary

Persistent neurologic illness may be remitting-relapsing (episodic), static, or slowly deteriorating. These patterns result in opportunities for reevaluation of evolving concerns causally related with confidence to the original injury or illness. In most situations, determination, motivation, and effort overcome established neurologic handicaps. Temporary work absence to permit treatment or convalescence may be required. Permanent work restriction may allow the worker to continue productive activity. Long-term avoidance of return to accommodated work can be detrimental.[1] A trial of supervised work activity may be helpful in determining work ability.

References

1. Reed P. Workplace guidelines for disability duration. In: *The Medical Disability Advisor*. 3rd ed. Boulder, CO: Reed Group Ltd; 2001.

2. Klenerman L, Slade PD, Stanley M, et al. The prediction of chronicity in patients with an acute attack of low back pain in a general practice setting. *Spine*. 1995;20:478–484.

3. Deyo RA. Practice variations, treatment fads, rising disability: do we need a new clinical research paradigm? *Spine*. 1993;18:2153–2162.

4. Deyo RA, Andersson G, Bombardier C, et al. Outcome measures for studying patients with low back pain. *Spine*. 1994;19(suppl):S2032-S2036.

5. Nachemson A. Newest knowledge of low back pain: a critical look. *Clin Orthop*. 1992;279:8–20.

6. Eaton MW. Obstacles to the vocational rehabilitation of individuals receiving workers' compensation. *J Rehabil*. 1979;45:59–63.

7. Lamb HR, Rogawski AA. Supplemental security income and the sick role. *Am J Psychiatry*. 1978;35:1221–1224.

8. McIntosh G, Melles T, Hall H. Guidelines for the identification of barriers to rehabilitation of back injuries. *J Occup Rehabil*. 1995;5:195–201.

9. Duarte J, Sempere AP, Delgado JA, Naranjo G, Sevillano MD, Claveria LE. Headache of recent onset in adults: a prospective population-based study. *Acta Neurol Scand*. 1996;94:67–70.

10. Quality Standards Subcommittee of the American Academy of Neurology. Practice parameter: the utility of neuroimaging in the evaluation of headache in patients with normal neurologic examinations [summary statement]. *Neurology*. 1994;44:1353–1354.

11. Solomom GD, Cady RG, Klapper JA, Ryan RE. National Headache Foundation: standards of care for treating headache in primary care practice. *Cleve Clin J Med*. 1997:64;373–383.

12. Katzman GL, Dagher AP, Patronas NJ. Incidental findings on brain magnetic resonance imaging from 1000 asymptomatic volunteers. *JAMA*. 1999; 282: 36–39.

13. Lindgren A, Roijer A, Rudling O, et al. Cerebral lesions on magnetic resonance imaging, heart disease, and vascular risk factors in subjects without stroke: a population-based study. *Stroke*. 1994;25:929–934.

14. Vernooil MW, Ikran MA, Tanghe HL, et al. Incidental findings on brain MRI in the general population. *N Engl J Med.* 2007;357:1821–1828.

15. Kaniecki R. Headache assessment and management: contempo update. *JAMA.* 2003;289:1430–1433.

16. Warner JS. Posttraumatic headache: a myth? *Arch Neurol.* 2000;57:1778–1780.

17. Olesen J, Bousser MG, Diener HC., et al. International Classification of Headache Disorders, 2nd ed. Blackwell Publishing. http://www.ihs-classification. org/en/02_klassifikation/03_teil2/05.02.00_necktrauma.html. Accessed February 5, 2011.

18. Couch JR, Bearss C. Chronic daily headache in the posttrauma syndrome: relation to extent of head injury. *Headache.* 2001;41:559–564.

19. Radanov BP, Di Stefano G, Augustiny KF. Symptomatic approach to posttraumatic headache and its possible implications for treatment. *Eur Spine J.* 2001;10:403–407.

20. Haas DC. Chronic post-traumatic headaches classified and compared with natural headaches. *Cephalalgia.* 1996;16:486–493.

21. Mickeviciene D, Schrader H, Surkiene D, Kunicka R, Stovner LJ, Sand T. A historical cohort study on posttraumatic headache outside the medicolegal context. *Cephalgia.* 2001;21:524.

22. Packard RC. Epidemiology and pathogenesis of posttraumatic headache. *J Head Trauma Rehabil.* 1999;14:9–21.

23. Evans RW. The postconcussion syndrome and the sequelae of mild head injury. *Neurol Clin.* 1992;10:815–847.

24. NIH Consensus Development Panel on Rehabilitation of Persons with Traumatic Brain Injury. Consensus conference from the National Institutes of Health: rehabilitation of persons with traumatic brain injury. *JAMA.* 1999;282:974–983.

25. Binder LM, Rohling ML. Money matters: a meta-analytic review of the effects of financial incentives on recovery after closed-head injury. *Am J Psychiatry.* 1996;153:7–10.

26. Rosenthal M, Christensen BK, Ross TP. Depression following traumatic brain injury. *Arch Phys Med Rehabil.* 1998;79:90–103.

27. Mittenberg W, DiGiulio DV, Perrin S, Bass AE. Symptoms following mild head injury: expectation as aetiology. *J Neurol Neurosurg Psychiatry.* 1992;55:200–204.

28. Mooney G, Peed JS. The association between mild traumatic brain injury and psychiatric conditions. *Brain Inj.* 2001;15:865–877.

29. Rasmussen BK, Jensen R, Schrod M, Olesen J. Epidemiology of headache in a general population: a prevalence study. *J Clin Epidemiol.* 1991;44:1147–1157.

30. Pryse-Phillips WE, Dodick DW, Edmeads JG, et al. Guidelines for the diagnosis and management of migraine in clinical practice. *CMAJ.* 1997;156:1273–1287.

31. Stewart WF. Epidemiology of migraine. *Am J Manage Care.* 1999;5(suppl):S63–S72.

Chapter 16

32. Goadsby PJ, Lipton RB, Ferrrari MD. Migraine: current understanding and therapy. *N Engl J Med.* 2002;346:257–270.

33. Ferrari MD. Migraine. *Lancet.* 1998;351:1043–1051.

34. Merikangas KR, Dartigues JF, Whitaker A, Angst J. Diagnostic criteria for migraine: a validity study. *Neurology.* 1994;44(suppl 4):Sll.

35. Smetana GW. The diagnostic value of historical features in primary headache syndromes: a comprehensive review. *Arch Intern Med.* 2000;160:2729–2737.

36. Warner JS. Time required for improvement of an analgesic rebound headache. *Headache.* 1998;38:229–230.

37. Hansson L, Smith DHG, Reeves R, Lapuerta P. Headache in mild-to-moderate hypertension and its reduction by irbesartan therapy. *Arch Intern Med.* 2000; 160:1654–1658.

38. Dalrymple J, Appleby J. Cross sectional study of reporting of epileptic seizures to general practitioners. *BMJ.* 2000;320:94–97.

39. Zaidi A, Clough P, Scheepers B, Fitzpatrick A. Treatment resistant epilepsy or convulsive syncope? *BMJ.* 1998;317:869–870.

40. Whitaker JN. The confluence of quality of care, cost-effectiveness, pragmatism, and medical ethics in the diagnosis of nonepileptic seizures: a provocative situation for neurology. *Arch Neurol.* 2001:58;2066–2067.

41. Van Ness PC. Therapy for the epilepsies. *Arch Neurol.* 2002;59:732–735.

42. Berg AT, Shinnar S. The risk of seizure recurrence following a first unprovoked seizure: a quantitative review. *Neurology.* 1991;41:965–972.

43. King MA, Newton MR, Jackson GD, et al. Epileptology of the first-seizure presentation: a clinical, electroencephalographic, and magnetic resonance imaging study of 300 consecutive patients. *Lancet.* 1998;352:1007–1011.

44. Aminoff MJ. *Electrodiagnosis in Clinical Neurology.* 2nd ed. New York, NY: Churchill Livingstone; 1986, p. 42.

45. Spudis EV, Penry JK, Gibson P. Driving impairment caused by episodic brain dysfunction. *Arch Neurol.* 1986;43:558–564.

46. Macciocchi SN, Reid DB, Barth JT. Disability following head injury. *Curr Opin Neurol.* 1993;6:773–777.

47. Martelli MF, Grayson RL, Zasler ND. Posttraumatic headache: neuropsychological and psychological effects and treatment implications. *J Head Trauma Rehabil.* 1999;14:49–69.

48. King N. Mild head injury: neuropathology, sequelae, measurement and recovery. *Br J Clin Psychol.* 1997;36:161–184.

49. Beers SR. Cognitive effects of mild head injury in children and adolescents. *Neuropsychol Rev.* 1992;3:281–320.

50. Capruso DX, Levin HS. Cognitive impairment following closed head injury. *Neurol Clin.* 1992;10:879–893.

51. Bohnen N, Jolles J. Neurobehavioral aspects of postconcussive symptoms after mild head injury. *J Nerv Ment Dis.* 1992;180:683–692.

52. Jacobson RR. The post-concussional syndrome: physiogenesis, psychogenesis and malingering: an integrative model. *J Psychosom Res.* 1995;39:675–693.

53. Anderson SD. Postconcussional disorder and loss of consciousness. *Bull Am Acad Psychiatry Law.* 1996;24:493–504.

54. Katz RT, DeLuca J. Sequelae of minor traumatic brain injury. *Am Fam Physician.* 1992;46:1491–1498.

55. Dikmen SS, Machamer JE, Winn HR, et al. Neuropsychological outcome at 1-year post head injury. *Neuropsychology.* 1995;9:80–90.

56. Thornhill S, Teasdale GM, Murray GD, et al. Disability in young people and adults one year after head injury: prospective cohort study. *BMJ.* 2000;320: 1631–1635.

57. Graham DI, Adams JH, Nicoll JA, et al. The nature, distribution and causes of traumatic brain injury. *Brain Pathol.* 1995;5:397–406.

58. van der Naalt J, van Zomeren AH, Sluiter WJ, Minderhoud JM. One year outcome in mild to moderate head injury: the predictive value of acute injury characteristics related to complaints and return to work. *J Neurol Neurosurg Psychiatry.* 1999;66:207–213.

59. Mittenberg W, DiGiulio DV, Perrin S, et al. Symptoms following mild head injury: expectation as aetiology. *J Neurol Neurosurg Psychiatry.* 1992;55(3): 200–204.

60. Gasquoine PG. Postconcussion symptoms. *Neuropsychol Rev.* 1997;7:77–85.

61. Satz PS, Alfano MS, Light RF, et al. Persistent post-concussive syndrome: a proposed methodology and literature review to determine the effects, if any, of mild head and other bodily injury. *J Clin Exp Neuropsychol.* 1999;21:620–628.

62. Kurztke JF. Rating neurologic impairment in multiple sclerosis: an Expanded Disability Status Scale (EDSS). *Neurology.* 1983;33:144–152.

63. Riahi F, Zijdenbos A, Narayanan S, et al. Improved correlation between scores on the Expanded Disability Status Scale and the cerebral lesion load in relapsing-remitting multiple sclerosis: results of the application of new imaging methods. *Brain.* 1998;121:1305–1312.

Chapter 16

Working With Common Rheumatologic Problems

David Silver, MD and Stuart Silverman, MD

Rheumatic diseases are the leading cause of work-related disability in the United States.[1-3] These illnesses represent more than 100 different types of arthritis, autoimmune diseases, and pain syndromes, which can be regional or systemic. The degree of disability relates to disease severity, systemic features of the disease, and psychosocial factors. Overlap among autoimmune diseases is seen in up to 25% of patients.[4] In addition, between 15% and 25% of individuals with rheumatoid arthritis and systemic lupus erythematosus have fibromyalgia, with potential for decreasing tolerance as a result (see Chapter 23).[5-8] Well-done studies examining the issue of disability and rheumatic disease are somewhat limited, but data suggest that patients who return to paid work have better disease outcomes.[9]

Rheumatoid Arthritis

Rheumatoid arthritis (RA) is the most common systemic rheumatic condition, affecting between 0.5% and 1% of the US population. Women are more commonly affected than men, with peak incidence occurring between the ages of twenty and forty.[4,10] For reasons that are unclear, both the incidence and severity of rheumatoid arthritis have been diminishing over the past 30 years. In addition, improvements in treatment have further reduced disability as a result of rheumatoid arthritis.[11,12] Unfortunately, individuals whose diagnosis was made more than 15 years ago may have already suffered severe joint damage prior to the advent of these newer therapies and have significant impairments as a result. Disability can occur early in disease and, without appropriate treatment, progresses with duration and severity of disease. Although previous studies document the effect of RA on work loss and work reduction, the reasons are not clearly elucidated.[13,14]

Disease severity, which correlates directly with work disability, can be quantified in numerous ways. The simplest is a tender and swollen joint count, an effective measure of disease activity (but not necessarily disease severity), yet it does not account for all joint deformities and ankylosis that is responsible for limitations. A modified Sharp score, which utilizes x-ray criteria to look at joint narrowing and erosions, may overestimate the degree of symptoms if active inflammation is not present. The DAS score directly correlates with level of function but is extremely difficult to administer in the office setting. The HAQ and SF-36 are self-assessment questionnaires that can be used not only in RA but also other diseases as well and are often useful in determining individuals' level of physical function.[15,16] Symptoms can be worsened by anemia as measured in standard blood count studies or restricted lung capacity, which can be measured by formal pulmonary function testing. In some people, pulmonary exercise stress tests can provide greater insight into the degree of impairment.

Risk

Work restriction would depend on the severity of disease as it relates to joint deformities and their subsequent loss of motion, strength, and stability. Individuals with active synovitis should avoid highly repetitive activities, as they may damage an already inflamed joint or cause a tendon rupture. For example, if an individual has significant swelling of their PIP, MCP, and wrist joints and has ulnar deviation, a job involving frequent typing and fine motor manipulation of the hands would not be appropriate as it may lead to further injury.[13,14,17] Individuals with significant joint instability may also benefit from restrictions based on risk. For example, those with significant knee instability from rheumatoid arthritis may be given restrictions to preclude heavy lifting and carrying. Operation of heavy machinery should be avoided, and individuals with diminished range of motion due to joint deformities should avoid being around hazardous materials. Many of the antirheumatic medications can have significant immunosuppressive effects, and individuals should avoid exposure to infectious agents. People with advanced rheumatoid arthritis may have significant subluxations at C1-2. Forceful flexion and extension of the neck can lead to transection of the spinal cord, so avoidance of occupations that involve sudden extreme head movements must be pursued.

Capacity

Improvement in treatment has greatly limited the number of individuals with marked joint deformities and allows individuals with RA to have improved work capacity. Individuals with joint deformities will have decreased strength and loss of range of motion, which can greatly reduce capacity to do certain job-related tasks. With active disease and deformities, individuals can have significant limitation in activities such as typing, pinching, grasping, and writing, as well as climbing ladders or stairs if the lower extremity disease is extensive. Individuals with extensive anemia or lung involvement often have diminished exercise capacity.[18] Often these limitations can be

Table 17-1 Disability Duration, Medical Treatment, Rheumatoid Arthritis[16]

Job Classification	Minimum	Optimum	Maximum
Sedentary	1	14	84
Light	3	28	84
Medium	7	56	112
Heavy	42	140	Indefinite
Very Heavy	64	180	Indefinite

Reproduced with permission from Reed. www.mdguidelines.com.

accommodated, and individuals with RA can remain gainfully employed with appropriate work restrictions in place. See Table 17-1.

Tolerance

Individuals with RA, as well as individuals with other rheumatic diseases, will complain of fatigue and pain, and these symptoms often are more debilitating than the joint swelling and deformities. These symptoms can be compounded by anemia or restricted lung capacity. New treatments may give a more immediate effect on the fatigue symptoms, even prior to seeing a reduction in synovitis or pain.

Workplace modifications and use of adaptive devices can often allow individuals with RA to remain in the workplace. Ergonomic assessment is especially important for individuals with arthritis, and work with vocational rehabilitation counselors can provide support in maintaining employment, even with seeming high levels of deformities.

Systemic Lupus Erythematosus

Systemic lupus erythematosus (SLE) affects about 0.3% of all Americans and is significantly more common in women than men (9:1 ratio).[4] African-Americans are three times more likely than Caucasians to suffer with lupus, and their disease severity is greater. About two-thirds of individuals with SLE will have mild disease, affecting the skin, joints, and serosa. Common manifestations of disease include pain, fatigue, cognitive impairment, and mood disturbances. One-third of individuals will have more significant disease including renal, bone marrow, or central nervous system (CNS) involvement in addition to the other manifestations. Individuals may also have isolated cutaneous disease without internal manifestations.[19] Tools for measuring disease activity are not typically utilized in clinical practice, but looking for evidence of major organ system involvement is essential as treatment is radically different for those individuals. Often cognitive issues (eg, lupus cerebritis) are significant in individuals with SLE and can lead to greater difficulty than joint symptoms, which are painful, but not usually deforming.[20,21] Depression and other mood changes are commonly observed as well, likely as a result of low-grade inflammation, and must be considered regardless of disease severity. Neuropsychiatric testing may play an important role in determining level of capacity/disability.

Risk

Severity of disease is usually observed soon after onset, and individuals with early severe disease clearly are at greater risk for work-related disability. In addition, individuals with lower socioeconomic status or education level and individuals with increased physical strength requirements for the job have greater disability.[22] Up to 50% of individuals with SLE will become disabled at some point, frequently soon after diagnosis.[23]

Sun exposure has been well documented to cause rashes but can also increase SLE activity, often within 15 minutes. Jobs with significant sun exposure should be avoided, unless there is opportunity to apply sunscreen frequently and sun protective clothing can be worn. High emotional stress has been linked to lupus flares and should be avoided.[24] Individuals with SLE should also be restricted from work with agents that are known to trigger lupus or cause flares (aromatic amines, hydrazines, Tartrazine, and hair dyes), as well as certain heavy metals (mercury, cadmium, and gold).[25]

Individuals with SLE who have cognitive impairment and reduced executive function can be limited from occupations that involve high-level brain function, especially those that involve safety issues.

Capacity

Endurance can not only be limited by deconditioning, but if individuals have serositis, lung, or cardiac involvement, they may experience decreased work capacity. In addition, anemia is a common finding in lupus and may limit work abilities. Individuals with impaired renal function may experience peripheral edema and cognitive slowing.[26] Complications of medication, many of which are immunosuppressive, can lead to infections, bone marrow suppression, and other complications. Thus patients taking these drugs should avoid high–infection risk environments.

Tolerance

Work tolerance can be a significant issue for patients with SLE. Fatigue is experienced by the vast majority of individuals, even if therapy has been

Table 17-2 Disability Duration, Medical or Supportive Treatment, Systemic Lupus Erythematosus[16]

Job Classification	Minimum	Optimum	Maximum
Sedentary	1	14	42
Light	1	21	64
Medium	7	42	91
Heavy	42	63	140
Very Heavy	42	70	182

Reproduced with permission from Reed. www.mdguidelines.com.

effective in controlling other symptoms. Medications may further worsen the fatigue or anemia. Most people with SLE do not develop joint deformities, but synovitis can lead to pain, stiffness, and decrease work tolerance. Educating individuals that joint damage is unlikely may help to overcome this obstacle. Myalgias and arthralgias are common and may become a factor as well. Patients may experience life threatening complications of disease during flare ups, which can result in short-term disability, but does not prevent them from ultimately returning to the workplace.[20] Appropriate workplace accommodations, such as being able to change positions at will and frequent rest breaks to account for these factors, can allow patients with SLE to remain gainfully employed. See Table 17-2.

Ankylosing Spondylitis

Ankylosing spondylitis (AS) is a chronic progressive rheumatic disorder that involves inflammation of the spine, sacroiliac joints, and peripheral joints.[27] AS is part of the spondyloarthropathies, which also include Reiter's syndrome, the arthritis associated with inflammatory bowel disease (Crohn's, ulcerative colitis), psoriatic arthritis, and reactive arthritis. Individuals with AS typically have pain, stiffness, and motion loss in the spine and peripheral joints. They may also have eye inflammation (iritis), fatigue, or anemia of chronic disease. AS affects about 1.4% of the US population. Prevalence is linked to the genetic marker, HLA-B27, seen in about 8% of the US population.[27]

Work disability occurs in about 18.5% of patients with spondyloarthropathy.[28] In those patients given anti-TNF therapy, disability is higher at 41%,[29] probably because they have more severe disease. Of those who continue to work, productivity decreases 8.3%.[28]

The burden of active disease in AS may be assessed with a Bath Ankylosing Spondylitis Disease Activity Index (or BASDAI), which can be used to assess the need for additional therapy such as biologic therapy. Functional impairment due to disease may also be assessed with the BASFI, which assesses the functional impairment due to disease as well as improvements following therapy. BASG is the Bath Ankylosing Spondylitis Global assessment.

Disability may be permanent. Disability depends on age of onset, time since diagnosis, delay in diagnosis, duration of disease, disease activity, hip involvement, spinal deformity, and spinal mobility.[30] In other studies, disability was related to chest expansion, BASFI, and Bath AS radiologic index.[31] Disability is associated with poorer global health status and greater comorbidities.[28] Work disability is also associated with type of work, with greater disability for manual workers.[29] Prognosis for AS is variable. However, prognosis has improved over time with the availability of newer biological agents that may limit peripheral joint involvement and possibly axial skeletal involvement. In one study by Barkham et al.,[32] Etanercept decreased risk of job loss in a double blind placebo controlled trial. In another study of 121 male patients, 38 (41%) were able to continue work, 54 patients (45%) changed to a lighter work, and 29 (24%) were retired.[30]

Losses in productivity are correlated with HAQ, BASFI, BASDAI, and BAS-G.[28] See Table 17-3.

Risk

At the onset of disease, few restrictions are needed for individuals who are doing sedentary or light work. Individuals may need to take breaks from sitting or standing or to do stretching or breathing exercises. Workers with decreased lung capacity should avoid environmental exposure to smoke and fumes.

Table 17-3 Disability Duration, Ankylosing Spondylitis[16]

DISABILITY DURATION IN DAYS (MDG 2010)			
Job Classification	Minimum	Optimum	Maximum
Sedentary	0	7	28
Light	0	14	42
Medium	0	112	Indefinite
Heavy	0	168	Indefinite
Very Heavy	0	168	Indefinite

Reproduced with permission from Reed. www.mdguidelines.com.

Capacity

Individuals with AS have decreased capacity based on limited motion of the cervical, thoracic, and lumbar spine and SI joints. They may have limited chest expansion resulting in decreased lung capacity.[27] Pulmonary capacity can be measured as outlined in the chapter on pulmonary conditions. Individuals who have more severe disease may not be able to do medium work, and are usually incapable of heavy work. Peripheral joint involvement may result in separate limitations based on the joints involved.[16]

Tolerance

Tolerance factors in ankylosing spondylitis include fatigue and stiffness with prolonged sitting or standing.[27] To assist them in tolerating their environment, patients with decreased lung capacity due to spinal involvement should be encouraged to stop smoking.

Osteoarthritis

Osteoarthritis is the most common disease affecting Americans, with 70 million people, almost one out of four, suffering with the disease.[4,19,33] Osteoarthritis risk increases with age, therefore a significant percentage of individuals with OA may have already left the workplace due to their age rather than disease severity. However, individuals who have had previous joint injuries may develop OA at an earlier stage, leading to significant work limitations.

OA can occur in a single joint or multiple joints and is not necessarily symmetric.[4,19] Highly physical jobs with heavy mechanical loads may be related to developing OA, especially in the hips or knees.[34,35] A hereditary form of OA can lead to accelerated joint deformities as early as age 40. Workplace disability may be greater in patients with lower extremity involvement. See Tables 17-4 through 17-7.

Table 17-4 Disability Duration, Medical Treatment, Hip[16]

Job Classification	Minimum	Optimum	Maximum
Sedentary	0	0	7
Light	0	0	14
Medium	0	0	14
Heavy	0	7	Indefinite
Very Heavy	0	14	Indefinite

Reproduced with permission from Reed. www.mdguidelines.com.

Table 17-5 Disability Duration, Medical Treatment, Knee[16]

Job Classification	Minimum	Optimum	Maximum
Sedentary	0	0	7
Light	0	0	14
Medium	0	0	14
Heavy	0	14	Indefinite
Very Heavy	0	21	Indefinite

Reproduced with permission from Reed. www.mdguidelines.com.

Table 17-6 Disability Duration, Medical Treatment, Wrist[16]

Job Classification	Minimum	Optimum	Maximum
Sedentary	0	1	7
Light	0	3	10
Medium	0	7	14
Heavy	0	14	21
Very Heavy	0	21	28

Reproduced with permission from Reed. www.mdguidelines.com.

Table 17-7 Disability Duration, Medical Treatment, Shoulder[16]

Job Classification	Minimum	Optimum	Maximum
Sedentary	0	0	3
Light	0	0	7
Medium	0	3	10
Heavy	0	7	14
Very Heavy	0	7	21

Reproduced with permission from Reed. www.mdguidelines.com.

Risk

Much of the disability related to OA depends on the joints involved. Further complicating matters is that specific types of exercise, such as quadriceps strengthening for the knees, actually decreases symptoms of osteoarthritis, but incorrect or excessive activity may increase symptoms.[36] Symptoms are tolerance issues, while disease progression is a risk issue. Individuals with joint replacement of the hip or knee should be restricted from doing heavy work, as this might lead to implant loosening. Individuals who have advanced OA of the hips or knees should be limited to sedentary or light work to avoid further damage.[16] Upper extremity OA, depending on the joint or joints affected, can lead to different issues. In patients with OA of the spine, prophylaxic lifting restrictions may need to be in place if there is significant neurological compromise (spinal stenosis).

Capacity

Decreased muscle mass due to deconditioning can lead to diminished work capacity, but a graduated exercise program may help to reverse this.[37]

Work capacity may be diminished by decreased strength and range of motion. Often adaptive devices, such as a tract ball computer mouse or splinting, can help to alleviate some of these issues.

Individuals with extensive OA of the spine frequently have decreased range of motion in the cervical and lumbar regions. If there is significant shoulder involvement, work limitations based on range of motion may limit occupations that involve substantial reaching above shoulder level. Also, if there is involvement of the hands or wrist, depending on the degree of joint motion and stability, there may be limitations on fine motor activities.

Tolerance

Most of the decrease in work ability is related to pain and stiffness.

Pain, which can lead to deconditioning and decrease motion beyond what would be expected, can decrease work tolerance. Stiffness can make patients fearful of moving joints beyond a certain range of motion, even though there is little if any risk of damage.[37] Appropriate treatment with exercise to improve endurance, strength, and flexibility and simple analgesics can help to restore function and improve work capacity.[38]

Osteoporosis

Osteoporosis is common and expensive and results in significant loss of quality of life.[39] About one-half of all women over age 50 will experience an osteoporotic fracture in their lifetimes.[40] The incidence of osteoporotic fractures in women exceeds the combined risk of breast cancer, stroke, and heart attack. About one in four men over age 50 will experience an osteoporotic fracture.[40] The incidence of osteoporotic fractures is similar to the incidence of prostate cancer or myocardial infarction.

Osteoporosis is diagnosed two ways: by the presence of a fragility fracture or by use of central bone density measurement referred to as Dual energy X-ray Absorptiometry (DXA). Fracture risk depends on bone mineral density (BMD) and clinical risk factors.

Risk

Disability in individuals with osteoporosis is a consequence of the development of fragility fractures. The length of disability depends on the location and type of fracture, underlying diseases, the treatment or surgical intervention, the ability to ambulate, and the job requirement.[16] Spinal fractures result in loss of height and tolerance issues like pain with prolonged sitting, prolonged standing, or heavier work. Patients with prior spinal fractures have greater disability and loss of quality of life with further fracture.[41] Hip fractures may impair mobility and may limit (capacity) manual work.[16] For patients with significant osteoporosis (DXA T scores >2 standard deviations below the mean), even with no history of fragility fracture (yet), physicians may impose restrictions on very heavy activity like jumping and heavy lifting, due to the risk of vertebral fracture. See Tables 17-8 and 17-9.

Table 17-8 Disability Duration, Femoral Neck Fracture[16]

Job Classification	Minimum	Optimum	Maximum
Sedentary	21	42	56
Light	42	56	84
Medium	56	84	112
Heavy	91	112	154
Very Heavy	112	154	182

Reproduced with permission from Reed. www.mdguidelines.com.

Table 17-9 Disability Duration, Vertebral Fracture[16]

Job Classification	Minimum	Optimum	Maximum
Sedentary	21	28	42
Light	42	49	56
Medium	70	77	84
Heavy	Indefinite	Indefinite	Indefinite
Very Heavy	Indefinite	Indefinite	Indefinite

Reproduced with permission from Reed. www.mdguidelines.com.

Individuals with osteoporosis are at risk of fracture if they fall and may not be able to work heights or balance.[16]

Capacity

Work capacity may be impaired by reduced lung capacity from thoracic compression fractures.

Tolerance

Individuals with vertebral compression fractures will describe fatigue with prolonged sitting or standing.[39] They often have decreased self esteem due to inability to do the physical function requirements of their daily roles.[39]

Summary

Rheumatic diseases are a common cause of work-related disability. Studies have demonstrated that with appropriate accommodations, most patients with rheumatic disease are capable of remaining gainfully employed. With data emerging regarding improved disease outcomes in patients doing paid work, appropriate measures should be implemented to allow patients with rheumatic disease to remain in the workplace.

References

1. Yelin E, Meenan R, Nevitt M, et al. Work disability and rheumatoid arthritis: Effects of disease, social and work factors. *Ann Int Med*. 1980;93:551–6.

2. Straaton KV, Maisiak R, Wrigley JM, et al. Variants to return to work among persons unemployed due to arthritis and musculoskeletal disorders. *Arth Rheum*. 199;39:101–9.

3. Prevalence of disabilities and associated health conditions among adults-United States, 1999. *MMWR*. 2001;50:120–5.

4. Kelley's Textbook of Rheumatology, Seventh Edition. Elsevier Saunders. 2005:1258.

5. Dhir V, Lawrence A, Aggarwal A, et al. Fibromyalgia is common and adversely affects pain and fatigue perception in North Indian patients with rheumatoid arthritis. *J Rheum*. 2009;36:2443–8.

6. Ranzolin A, Brenol JC, Bredemeier M, et al. Association of concomitant fibromyalgia with worse disease activity score in 28 joints, health assessment questionnaire, and short form 36 scores in patients with rheumatoid arthritis. *Arth Rheum*. 2009;61:794–800.

7. Coury F, Rossat A, Tebib A, et al. Rheumatoid arthritis and fibromyalgia: a frequent unrelated association complicating disease management. *J Rheum*. 2009;38: 58–62.

8. Wolfe F, Petri M, Alarcón GS, et al. Fibromyalgia, systemic lupus erythematosis (SLE), and evaluation of SLE activity. *J Rheum*. 2009;36:82–8.

9. Grenning K, Redevand E, Steinsbekk A. Paid work is associated with improved health-related quality of life in patients with rheumatoid arthritis. *Clin Rheum*. 2010; in print.

10. Olofsson T, Engulnd M, Saxne T, et al. Decrease in sick leave among patients with rheumatoid arthritis in the first 12 months after start of treatment with tumor necrosis factor antagonists: a population-based controlled cohort study. *Ann Rheum Dis*. 2010 Dec;69(12):2131–6.

11. Hazes JM, Taylor P, Strand V, et al. Physical function improvements and relief from fatigue and pain are associated with increased productivity at work and at home in rheumatoid arthritis patients treated with certolizumab pegol. *Rheumatology* (Oxford). 2010 Oct;49(10):1900–10.

12. Scheneeberger EE, Citera G, et al. Factors associated with disability in patients with rheumatoid arthritis. *J Clin Rheum*. 2010;16:215–8.

13. Macedo A, Oakley S, Gullick N, et al. An examination of work instability, functional impairment, and disease activity in employed patients with rheumatoid arthritis. *J Rheum*. 2009;36:225–30.

14. Strand V. Longer term benefits of treating rheumatoid arthritis: assessment of radiographic damage and physical function in clinical trials. *Clin Exp Rheum*. 2004;22:S57–64.

15. Sokka T. How should rheumatoid arthritis disease activity be measured today and in the future in clinical care? *Rheum Dis Clin N Am*. 2010;243–57.

16. Adapted from Medical Disability Guidelines, 2010. www.mdguidelines.com.

17. Ascherman DP. Interstitial lung disease in rheumatoid arthritis. *Curr Rheum Rep*. 2010;12:363–9.

18. Kelley's Textbook of Rheumatology, Seventh Edition. Elsevier Saunders. 2005

19. Klippel J, ed. *Primer on the Rheumatic Diseases*, 13th ed. Springer; 2009.

20. Sweet JJ, Doninger NA, Zee PC, et al. Factors influencing cognitive function, sleep, and quality of life in individuals with systemic lupus erythematosus: a review of the literature. *Clin Neuropsych*. 2004;18:132–147.

21. Baker K, Pope J. Employment and work disability in systemic lupus erythematosus: A systematic review. *Rheum*. 2009;48:281–284.

22. Baker K, Pope J, Fortin P, Silverman E, et al. Work disability in systemic lupus erythematosus is prevalent and associated with socio-demographic and disease related factors. *Lupus*. 2009;18:1281–1288.

23. Partridge A, Karlson E, Daltroy, L, et al. Risk factors for early work disability in systemic lupus erythematosus: results from a multicenter study. *Arth Rheum*. 1997;40:2199–2206.

24. Wallace DJ. The role of stress and trauma in rheumatoid arthritis and systemic lupus erythematosus. *Semin Arth Rheum*. 1987;16:153–157.

25. Cooper GS, Wither J, Bernatsky S, et al. Occupational and environmental exposures and risk of systemic lupus erythematosus: silica, sunlight, solvents. *Rheumatology* (Oxford). 2010 Nov;49(11):2172–80.

Chapter 17

26. Petri M. Clinical features of systemic lupus erythematosus. *Curr Opin Rheum.* 1985;7:395–401.

27. Van der Heijde D. Ankylosing spondylitis. Clinical Features. In *Primer on the Rheumatic Diseases* 2008, Springer, New York City. Klippel JH, Stone JH, Crofford LJ, White PH, editors. pp 193–199.

28. Rohekar S, Pope J. Assessment of work disability in seronegative spondyloarthritis. *Clin Exp Rheumatol.* 2010;28(1):35–40.

29. Verstappen SM, Watson KD, Lunt M, et al. Working status in patients with rheumatoid arthritis, ankylosing spondylitis and psoriatic arthritis: results from the British Society for Rheumatology Biologics Register. *Rheumatology (Oxford).* 2010;49(8):1570–1577. Epub 2010 May 5.

30. Cakar E, Taskaynatan MA, Dincer U, et al. Work disability in ankylosing spondylitis: differences among working and work-disabled patients. *Clin Rheumatol.* 2009;28(11):1309–1314. Epub 2009 Aug 16.

31. Ariza-Ariza R, Hernandez-Cruz B, Collantes E, et al. Work disability in patients with ankylosing spondylitis. *J Rheumatol.* 2009;36(11):2512–2516. Epub 2009 Oct 15.

32. Barkham N, Coates LC, Keen H, et al. Double blind placebo-controlled trial of etanercept in the prevention of work disability in ankylosing spondylitis. *Ann Rheum Dis* 2010;69(11):1926–1928.

33. Zhang Y, Jordan JM. Epidemiology of osteoarthritis. *Rheum Dis Clin N Am.* 2008;34:515–529

34. Cooper C, Snow S, McAlindon TE, et al. Risk factors for the incidence and progression of radiographic knee osteoarthritis. *Arthritis Rheum.* 2000 May;43(5):995–1000.

35. Pope DP, Hunt IM, Birrell FN, et al. Hip pain onset in relation to cumulative workplace and leisure time mechanical load: a population based case-control study. *Ann Rheum Dis.* 2003 Apr;62(4):322–6.

36. Sharma L, Dunlop D, Cahue S, et al. Quadriceps strength and osteoarthritis progression in malaligned and lax knees. *Ann Int Med.* 2003;138:613–619.

37. Silver DS. *Playing Through Arthritis: How to Conquer Pain and Enjoy Your Favorite Sports and Activities.* Contemporary Press. 2003.

38. Hunter DJ, Eckstein F. Exercise and osteoarthritis. *J Anat.* 2009;214:197–207.

39. Silverman SL, Minshall ME, Shen W, et al. Health Related Quality of Life Subgroup of the Multiple Outcomes of Raloxifene Evaluation Study. The relationship of health-related quality of life to prevalent and incident vertebral fractures in post-menopausal women with osteoporosis: results from the Multiple Outcomes of Raloxifene Evaluation (MORE) Study. *Arthritis Rheum.* 2001;44(11):2611–2619.

40. Harvey N, Dennison E, Cooper C. Epidemiology of osteoporotic fractures in primer on the metabolic bone diseases and disorders of bone metabolism. 7th Edition. American Society for Bone and Mineral Research 2008; pp 198–202.

41. Suzuki N, Ogikubo O, Hansson T. Previous vertebral compression fractures add to the deterioration of the disability and quality of life after an acute compression fracture. *Eur Spine J.* 2010;19(4):567–574. Epub 2009 Sep 18.

Chapter 17

Chapter 18

Working With Common Gastrointestinal Problems

Cynthia Ko, MD

Gastrointestinal diseases are extremely common in the United States, and a frequent cause of short-term absenteeism. Patients with gastrointestinal diseases have reduced productivity, increased use of sick leave, and increased indirect medical costs for employers and insurers.[1,2] However, there are limited studies or data on long-term disability related to gastrointestinal diseases. Assessment of disability related to gastrointestinal diseases is limited by a relative lack of objective measures of disability, the subjective nature of many symptoms, and the waxing and waning course of many of these disorders. In addition, there is often poor correlation between objective measures of disease and symptom severity.[3–8]

There is little evidence that most common gastrointestinal diseases are associated with increased risk from work or a decreased capacity for work. For example, although patients may report that stress causes exacerbations of the symptoms of irritable bowel syndrome, stress is not believed to be causative or lead to increased harm for patients with this disorder.[9] Work capacity may decrease in patients with anemia, malnutrition, or weight loss related to digestive disorders, although these complications are again rare with most common gastrointestinal illnesses such as gastroesophageal reflux disease (GERD) or irritable bowel syndrome. For most patients with digestive diseases, the issues surrounding disability are related to tolerance for work. Patients commonly report pain and fatigue related to gastrointestinal illnesses as the primary symptoms leading to considerations for disability. However, pain or fatigue are difficult to measure objectively and often do not correlate well with objective measures of disease activity or severity.[3,4] In addition, patients with chronic gastrointestinal diseases frequently have coexisting anxiety or depression,[9–12] which add to the complexity of assessing disability. Disability may arise more from these co-existing psychiatric issues than from the concomitant gastrointestinal illnesses, and such issues may need to be considered separately for disability. Finally, patients may need work accommodations, such as ready availability of bathroom facilities, rather than true work restrictions or limitations to continue to be productive employees.

The Social Security Administration (SSA) has defined disability criteria for the following gastrointestinal disorders: inflammatory bowel disease, liver disease, gastrointestinal hemorrhage, short bowel syndrome, and malnutrition.[13] Disability may be considered for other gastrointestinal conditions depending on the duration, severity, and response to treatment. The need for supplemental enteral or parenteral nutrition does not, by itself, indicate inability to do any gainful activity unless patients have short bowel syndrome. Likewise, surgical diversion, such as ileostomy or colostomy, does not preclude gainful employment except for those with co-existing malnutrition.[13]

This chapter will discuss the issues around working with common gastrointestinal diseases, such as gastroesophageal reflux disease, inflammatory bowel disease, and functional bowel diseases including irritable bowel syndrome. It will also discuss working with chronic liver disease and briefly cover other conditions qualified for disability under SSA guidelines.

Gastroesophageal Reflux Disease

Heartburn, the cardinal symptom of gastroesophageal reflux disease (GERD), is common, with up to 20% of the general population reporting heartburn or acid regurgitation at least weekly.[14] In addition, GERD is one of the most costly gastrointestinal disorders in terms of direct costs, with most expenses related to prescription medications needed for symptom control.[1,2] Lifestyle factors including obesity, alcohol use, diet, and smoking are commonly associated with GERD. Although the presence of poorly controlled GERD has significant effects on health-related quality of life and daily functioning,[15–17] there are not defined SSA criteria for disability for this condition. Nocturnal symptoms are frequent[16] and may have particular effect upon quality of life and work productivity[17] because of sleep disturbance.

Patients with GERD report decreased work productivity[17–19] with increased direct and indirect medical costs to employers. For example, Dean et al., found that 33% workers with GERD believed that these symptoms reduced their work productivity, with an overall 6% reduction in productivity.[17] Studies vary in regards to absenteeism in patients with GERD, with some studies reporting no significant increases in absenteeism,[17] but others reporting up to 3 hours per week of lost work time.[15,18] GERD has not generally been found to be a significant cause of short-term or long-term disability.[17,20] The effect of GERD upon work ability and productivity appears to increase with disease severity.[15–17,21] Using the Work Productivity and Activity Impairment questionnaire, Wahlqvist et al. found that 6% of patients with moderate GERD reported lost work time, with 25% reporting reduced productivity.[15] Eighteen percent of patients with severe GERD reported lost work time, with 32% reporting reduced work productivity. Adequate treatment of GERD symptoms may reduce, but not eliminate, absenteeism and "presenteeism" (that is, reduced productivity while at work).[19,22] Despite these data, patients with GERD rarely require long-term disability, and there is little objective basis for work restrictions or limitations due to this condition.

Risk

Risk is not an issue for patients with GERD, as there are no known work-related activities that may increase harm from this disorder. Therefore, GERD should not be a cause for work restrictions.

Capacity

Capacity in GERD is usually not an issue. GERD should not affect exercise capacity or functional abilities. Work capacity may be affected by other comorbid conditions, such as obesity, which frequently coexist with reflux disease. There is not an objective physical basis for work limitations directly related to GERD.

Tolerance

Patients may report increasing reflux symptoms with stressful environments. Tolerance for these subjective symptoms is required by the patient and is usually not sufficient to justify a certification of disability or inability to work. They may also choose to pursue a different work environment in order to decrease stress and avoid symptom exacerbations. The Reed Group has published guidelines for disability duration for medical or surgical treatment of GERD (Table 18-1).

Table 18-1 Length of Disability for Gastroesophageal Reflux Disease (GERD)[23]

	Minimum (days)	Optimum (days)	Maximum (days)
Medical Treatment of GERD			
Any work	0	1	3
Surgical Treatment – Laparoscopic Esophageal Fundoplication			
Any work	7	9	14

Reproduced with permission from Reed. www.mdguidelines.com.

Functional Bowel Diseases, including Irritable Bowel Syndrome and Functional Dyspepsia

Irritable bowel syndrome (IBS) is one of the most common reasons for physician visits.[1] It is a common condition, with estimates of prevalence between 5% and 20%, a range similar to the prevalence of asthma or hypertension. However, only a minority of patients with symptoms consistent with IBS actually seek medical care for this condition. The hallmark of IBS is abdominal pain associated with changes in bowel habits (either constipation or diarrhea) or associated with bowel movements in the absence of an organic etiology for symptoms.[24] Patients may have frequent diarrhea and fecal urgency. Functional dyspepsia is similar to IBS, with symptoms of upper abdominal pain, also in the absence of an organic etiology.[24] There is likely a considerable overlap between IBS and functional dyspepsia, and over time many patients will have symptoms consistent with both diagnoses. Although there are reliable and validated questionnaires to ascertain the presence of functional gastrointestinal disorders such as IBS,[24] there are few objective measures of pain or fatigue in these syndromes. It is common to use validated questionnaires such as the Short Form-36 to assess quality of life in these patients in research settings, but it is unclear how to assess daily function and ability to work with these syndromes in daily clinical practice. These disorders do not have a SSA listing for presumed disability.

The economic costs of the functional bowel disorders are considerable, but indirect costs, including reduced workplace productivity, have been estimated to represent up to 75% of the costs of this disorder.[1,25] Both IBS and functional dyspepsia are commonly seen in younger populations and as such potentially have a profound effect on work ability and productivity. Many studies have documented higher rates of absenteeism, increased medical and indirect costs, and reduced productivity in patients with IBS.[10,26–29] For example, one survey of random US households found that persons with IBS missed an average of 13.4 days from work or school per year, compared to 4.9 days for persons without gastrointestinal illnesses.[27,30] IBS may be the second leading cause of workplace absenteeism, behind the common cold.[27] However, this condition does not appear to be associated with higher rates of long-term work disability, as most patients with IBS tend to miss work sporadically.[20] Studies using the Work Productivity and Activity Impairment instrument have shown that 10% of patients with severe IBS report work time missed, with 39% reporting work impairment.[28,31] Patients with IBS report reduced productivity, with one study showing a reduced productivity rate of 21.1%, equivalent to working only 4 days of a 5-day workweek.[27] Direct medical costs to employers are up to 1.5 times higher for patients with IBS.[20] Functional dyspepsia is also associated with higher rates of sick leave and decreased productivity.[32,33] However, it is not associated with increases in short-term or long-term disability.[32] Among patients with IBS, women tend to report a greater disease burden, with more problems in workplace functioning and higher rates of long-term sick leave and disability than men.[10,34]

Anxiety, depression, and a history of prior physical, emotional, or sexual abuse are common with both IBS and functional dyspepsia, especially as severity of illness increases.[9,10,34] Severity of functional bowel diseases is often related to the degree of psychological distress. Therefore, appropriate assessment and treatment of coexisting psychiatric disorders is important for patients with functional bowel diseases and may improve health status and workplace functioning. The workplace environment may also play a role in disability assessments in these disorders. Patients will frequently report increases in symptoms with stressful environments. One study reported an association between low decision-making authority about working hours and planning work, as well as fewer learning opportunities at work, with IBS.[10] Modification of the work environment, or possibly a choice of a different work environment, may improve working ability and function for these patients.

Risk
Risk is not an issue with functional bowel diseases. There is little to no evidence that work causes these diseases or poses a potential for harm and objective worsening of symptoms in these syndromes in the absence of psychological distress.

Capacity
Capacity is not an issue with IBS or functional dyspepsia. Underlying fatigue is often related to coexisting depression or anxiety, which should be evaluated and managed separately. Patients can perform work-related activities but may not like to because of subjective increases in symptoms.

Tolerance
The issue for work-related disability in patients with functional bowel diseases is typically tolerance. Patients are capable of performing work-related duties but may have increases in pain related to such activities. Patients frequently report that the stressful environment related to work worsens these subjective symptoms. IBS may cause patients to make

Table 18-2 Length of disability for irritable bowel syndrome[23]

	Minimum (days)	Optimum (days)	Maximum (days)
Irritable Bowel Syndrome			
Any work	0	1	3
Medical Treatment of Dyspepsia			
Any work	0	1	5

Reproduced with permission from Reed. www.mdguidelines.com.

accommodations in work schedules, such as working fewer days or hours, or working from home.[26,35,36] However, patients can choose whether or not to work despite such symptoms. The patient's situation is similar to that of patients with other functional syndromes, such as fibromyalgia, with which significant symptoms exist but cannot be confirmed objectively. Physicians may choose to evaluate patients for disability based upon coexisting anxiety or depression. Guidelines for disability duration for irritable bowel syndrome are shown in Table 18-2. Although there are not similar guidelines for functional dyspepsia, it is reasonable to believe that disability duration should be similar.

Inflammatory Bowel Disease

SSA criteria for awarding disability for Crohn's disease include persistent or recurrent intestinal obstruction, persistent or recurrent systemic manifestations such as anemia or hypoalbuminemia, persistent perianal disease, weight loss, or need for supplemental daily enteral or parenteral nutrition.[13] There are not well-defined criteria for ulcerative colitis, but it is reasonable to believe that considerations would be similar. There may also be justifiable reasons for considering disability based on extraintestinal manifestations of inflammatory bowel disease, such as arthritis; hepatobiliary disease, including primary sclerosing cholangitis; or ocular involvement with uveitis or iritis.

The inflammatory bowel diseases—Crohn's disease or ulcerative colitis— are chronic autoimmune diseases typically characterized by periods of symptom flares and remission. Typical symptoms include abdominal pain, diarrhea, rectal bleeding, fatigue, and fevers. Diagnosis requires pathological confirmation. Patients with inflammatory bowel disease may also have extraintestinal manifestations such as ocular disease, hepatobiliary disease, inflammatory arthritis, or skin involvement including pyoderma gangrenosum or erythema nodosum. Patients with Crohn's disease may develop recurrent bowel obstructions related to intestinal strictures. Crohn's disease is not considered curable and recurrence can occur throughout life. In contrast, ulcerative colitis is considered curable by total colectomy. Patients may be hospitalized for management of symptom flares or for surgery. Treatment is generally with anti-inflammatory medications, such as 5-aminosalicylic acid derivates, or with immunosuppressive medications such as corticosteroids, azathioprine, or antibodies targeted against the inflammatory response.

Patients with Crohn's disease are at risk for reduced work productivity and short- or long-term disability.[37-39] Anathakrishnan et al., found that 5.7% of patients with Crohn's disease in a tertiary referral center had received Social Security disability, while a Canadian study found 25% of patients with Crohn's disease received disability payments.[39,40] Data for patients with ulcerative colitis are more limited, but generally these patients report less disability than those with Crohn's disease.[38] The number of hospitalizations, prior surgeries, and poor quality of life are associated with likelihood of Crohn's-related disability.[40] Demographic characteristics do not reliably predict disability, although some studies have shown that younger age is associated with disability.[39,40] A review of approved disability claims in Spain showed that perianal disease, presence of an ostomy, persistently active disease, fecal incontinence, and the number of associated diseases were associated with court-awarded disability.[41] Disease remission is associated with improved quality of life and employment status.[42]

For patients with inflammatory bowel disease, overall disease severity and course must be considered when assessing ability to work. Patients may have frequent symptom flares that make it difficult to attend work on a regular basis. Conversely, patients with a history of severe ulcerative colitis may have been cured with surgery and be able to return to work. Those with prior severe disease who enter remission with appropriate medications may also be able to return to work. Patients with ongoing moderate to severe disease may develop anemia and malnutrition that hinder the ability to work.

Depression and anxiety occur frequently in patients with inflammatory bowel disease and may impair their ability to work.[11,43] Such psychiatric issues may need to be addressed separately from the underlying gastrointestinal disease in regards to disability. Finally, patients may need workplace accommodations, such as ready access to bathroom facilities, in order to remain productive. They may also need short periods off work to recover from symptom flares, hospitalization, or surgery.

Chapter 18

Risk

Risk is not generally considered an issue for patients with inflammatory bowel disease. The pathogenesis of inflammatory bowel disease is poorly understood, as are the mechanisms and predisposing factors for disease flares. There is not clear evidence that work-related activities either cause inflammatory bowel diseases or lead to symptom exacerbations. There is modest data suggesting that psychological stress and adverse life events may worsen the course of inflammatory bowel diseases, but few studies have looked at the effect of stress reduction interventions on these diseases.[44-46] Therefore, work restrictions are typically not needed for patients with inflammatory bowel diseases, with the possible exception of restrictions to reduce work-related psychological stress. A clear pattern of worsened disease activity during periods of work and decreased disease activity during periods with accommodation designed to decrease workplace stress would justify such a restriction.

Capacity

Patients with inflammatory bowel disease may have reduced capacity for work-related activities due to fatigue, malnutrition, or anemia associated with the underlying condition. In addition, they may have decreased capacity for work-related activities while recovering from symptom flares, hospitalizations, or surgery. Guidelines for disability duration for medical or surgical treatment of inflammatory bowel disease are shown in Table 18-3. Work limitations may be appropriate in these situations.

Table 18-3 Length of Disability—Inflammatory Bowel Disease[23]

Job Classification	Minimum (days)	Optimum (days)	Maximum (days)
Medical Treatment, Crohn's Disease or Ulcerative Colitis			
Sedentary	7	14	21
Light	7	14	28
Medium	7	14	42
Heavy	7	14	63
Very Heavy	7	14	84
Surgical Treatment of Crohn's Disease, Ileostomy with Bowel Resection			
Sedentary	14	21	28
Light	21	28	35
Medium	28	42	56
Heavy	42	49	84
Very Heavy	42	56	91

(Continued)

Table 18-3 *(Continued)*

Surgical Treatment, Laparoscopic Partial Colon Resection		
Sedentary	10	14	21
Light	10	14	21
Medium	14	21	28
Heavy	14	35	42
Very Heavy	14	42	56
Surgical Treatment, Open Partial Colon Resection		
Sedentary	21	28	35
Light	21	28	42
Medium	28	35	56
Heavy	35	42	84
Very Heavy	42	42	91

Reproduced with permission from Reed. www.mdguidelines.com.

Tolerance

Patients may have reduced tolerance for work because of underlying symptoms such as abdominal pain. In addition, concerns over bowel symptoms such as diarrhea and fecal urgency may limit productivity in certain work environments. Workplace accommodations, such as ready access to restroom facilities, may be needed for patients with inflammatory bowel disease to maintain ability to work and productivity.

Chronic Liver Disease

Manifestations of end-stage liver disease that allow patients to qualify for disability under Social Security guidelines include recurrent gastrointestinal hemorrhage, ascites, spontaneous bacterial peritonitis, hepatorenal syndrome, or hepatopulmonary syndrome.[13] *Hepatorenal syndrome* is defined as functional renal failure with chronic liver disease in the absence of underlying intrinsic renal pathology. Criteria for disability include serum creatinine elevation of at least 2 mg/dL, oliguria with 24-hour urine output less than 500 mL, or sodium retention with urine sodium <10 mEq/liter. *Hepatopulmonary syndrome* is defined as arterial hypoxemia due to intrapulmonary arteriovenous shunting and vasodilation in patients with chronic liver disease in the absence of other causes of arterial deoxygenation. Patients may present with dyspnea, cyanosis, and clubbing. Criteria for disability include arterial oxygen desaturation or documentation of intrapulmonary arteriovenous shunting by contrast-enhanced echocardiography or lung perfusion scanning. Gastrointestinal hemorrhage from varices or portal hypertensive

Chapter 18

gastropathy, requiring hospitalization and transfusion of at least 2 units of blood, may allow patients to be eligible for disability for 1 year following the last documented transfusion. The presence of ascites, hydrothorax, or spontaneous bacterial peritonitis may also qualify patients for disability. Hepatic encephalopathy is an additional criterion for disability, requiring documentation of abnormal behavior, cognitive dysfunction, or altered levels of consciousness along with medical documentation of asterixis, an abnormal electroencephalogram, hypoalbuminemia, or coagulopathy. However, it is unclear whether the increasingly recognized entity of minimal hepatic encephalopathy meets these Social Security criteria for disability.[13]

Finally, the SSA will consider patients to be disabled for 1 year after liver transplantation. Further disability after that time point depends on adequacy of liver function, comorbid complications, and other adverse treatment effects.

It may be difficult to judge ability to work in patients with less advanced liver disease. Patients with mild liver disease are frequently asymptomatic or have vague, nonspecific symptoms. However, patients with mild to moderate liver disease may complain of fatigue that is out of proportion to documented objective findings.[3,4,47] In these cases, it may be difficult for physicians to certify disability based on either risk or capacity, and judgments may have to be made about patient's tolerance for work activities.

Treatment for hepatitis virus–related liver disease, either hepatitis B or hepatitis C, may cause significant adverse events. In particular, interferon treatment may cause fatigue, flu-like symptoms, fatigue, nausea, neutropenia, thrombocytopenia, and psychiatric disturbances. Treatment of hepatitis C with ribavirin can also cause anemia. These adverse events may have significant effects on ability to work while undergoing treatment. It may be appropriate to consider short-term disability related to these adverse effects while treatment is ongoing. However, these adverse effects usually wane within a few days to weeks after discontinuing treatment and are not a basis for long-term disability.

End-stage liver disease or cirrhosis from any etiology leads to similar symptoms and complications. Disability considerations become more important with advancing liver disease, as patients experience common complications such as hepatic encephalopathy, gastrointestinal bleeding, renal dysfunction, or ascites. However, there is little data about the prevalence and risk factors for disability amongst patients with mild to moderate liver disease or cirrhosis. Up to 70% of patients with end-stage liver disease may be disabled, but the prevalence of disability in patients with less severe liver disease is not well studied.[48,49]

The complication of advanced liver disease with potentially the greatest impact on work ability is hepatic encephalopathy. Encephalopathy is characterized by varying degrees of cognitive dysfunction and behavioral changes, with more severe encephalopathy manifesting as altered levels of consciousness and potentially coma. Recently, minimal hepatic encephalopathy has been increasingly recognized.[50] Its manifestations are believed to represent subcortical impairment, with particular deficits in attention and visuospatial domains.[50] Patients with minimal hepatic encephalopathy have subtle cognitive deficits, behavior changes such as irritability, and impaired judgment that may not be recognized clinically. However, minimal hepatic encephalopathy has significant effect on quality of life and ability to carry out activities of daily living.[51,52] For example, minimal hepatic encephalopathy results in increased risk of traffic accidents and impaired driving ability.[53,54] Minimal hepatic encephalopathy may be diagnosed with neuropsychological testing, including number connection tests and the critical flicker frequency.[55,56] However, there is no clear consensus on diagnostic criteria for this disorder. In assessing work ability, physicians may wish to consider screening for minimal hepatic encephalopathy and treating appropriately if it is present. Overt hepatic encephalopathy, which is generally not seen until there is advanced liver disease and cirrhosis, has clear effect on cognitive function and work ability[52] and is a clear criterion for disability. Nevertheless, treatment of hepatic encephalopathy leads to improvement in health-related quality of life.[57]

Risk

In general, work-related activities should not pose a risk to patients with chronic liver disease. The exception would be for patients with hepatic encephalopathy, for whom certain tasks such as driving or operating heavy machinery may be risky due to impaired judgment and cognitive defects. Work restrictions may be appropriate for these patients. Work restrictions to avoid exposure to potentially hepatotoxic chemicals, such as carbon tetrachloride, vinyl chloride, and polychlorinated biphenyls, may also be appropriate.

Capacity

Patients with advanced liver disease may have decreased exercise capacity from anemia, ascites, renal failure, or hepatopulmonary syndrome. Physician-prescribed work limitations may be appropriate for patients with these complications.

Tolerance

Patients with mild to moderate liver disease of many etiologies, including hepatitis C, nonalcoholic fatty liver disease, and primary biliary cirrhosis,

Table 18-4 Length of Disability - Chronic Liver Disease[23]

Job Classification	Minimum (days)	Optimum (days)	Maximum (days)
Medical Treatment, Cirrhosis of the Liver			
Sedentary	1	14	42
Light	1	14	56
Medium	1	14	Indefinite
Heavy	1	14	Indefinite
Very Heavy	1	14	Indefinite
Medical Treatment, Hepatitis B or C			
Any work	0	14	42
Sclerotherapy or Ligation, Esophageal Varices			
Sedentary	14	28	56
Light	28	42	70
Medium	42	63	84
Heavy	56	70	112
Very Heavy	56	70	112

Reproduced with permission from Reed. www.mdguidelines.com.

may complain of fatigue. Disease-related fatigue without other objective findings may impair a patient's tolerance for work activities but is not necessarily a cause for physician-certified disability according to the current biomedical model. Guidelines from the Reed Group for disability duration for treatment of chronic liver disease are shown in Table 18-4.

Gastrointestinal Hemorrhage

Social Security criteria for disability related to gastrointestinal hemorrhage include the requirement for blood transfusions of at least 2 units of packed red blood cells at least 3 times within a consecutive 6-month period.[13] The transfusions must be at least 30 days apart during this period. Patients meeting these criteria may qualify for disability for 1 year following the last documented transfusion, at which time re-evaluation is required. These criteria apply to patients with acute recurrent or chronic gastrointestinal hemorrhage, and not necessarily to those with an isolated episode of acute bleeding.

The most common causes of acute upper gastrointestinal bleeding include peptic ulcer disease, Mallory-Weiss tears, and erosive esophagitis due to GERD. The most common causes of acute lower gastrointestinal bleeding

Table 18-5 Length of Disability for Gastrointestinal Hemorrhage or Anemia[23]

Job Classification	Minimum (days)	Optimum (days)	Maximum (days)
Acute Upper Gastrointestinal Bleeding			
Sedentary	1	3	7
Light	1	3	7
Medium	3	7	14
Heavy	3	7	14
Very Heavy	3	7	14
Anemia – Supportive Treatment			
Any work	0	7	14

Reproduced with permission from Reed. www.mdguidelines.com.

include diverticulosis and angioectasias. In most patients, acute hemorrhage from these common causes is readily diagnosed and treated with low risk of recurrence after the initial event. Patients may have residual anemia after the initial episode, which may limit their work capacity temporarily. Work accommodations or short-term sick leave may be needed for these patients during the recovery period. However, long-term disability is not needed if the event is self-limited.

Some patients, however, develop chronic gastrointestinal hemorrhage, for example due to gastric, small intestinal, or colonic vascular ectasias, which cannot be completely controlled with medical or endoscopic therapy. These patients may have recurrent or persistent anemia and require periodic blood transfusions. Work capacity may decrease secondary to anemia, with fatigue, shortness of breath, and deconditioning. Typically, those with only mild anemia do not need work accommodations or limitations. If the anemia is moderate or severe leading to reduced work capacity, work limitations to reduce physical demands may be needed either temporarily or on a permanent basis. Guidelines for disability duration related to acute gastrointestinal hemorrhage or symptomatic treatment of anemia are shown in Table 18-5.

Summary

Gastrointestinal diseases are common in the general population and incur large direct and indirect medical costs. Despite this, there are few objective criteria or guidelines to assess risk, capacity, or tolerance for work in patients with these disorders. Disability may be certified in patients with chronic inflammatory bowel disease or with end-stage liver disease once

complications have occurred. In contrast, with the most common gastrointestinal conditions such as GERD and functional bowel diseases, there is no
basis for physician-imposed physical work restrictions or limitations based
on risk or capacity. Tolerance for working is the greater issue in these conditions, in which case patients may decide whether or not to work with their
symptoms, and physician-certified disability may not be required.

References

1. Sandler RS, Everhart JE, Donowitz M, et al. The burden of selected digestive
   diseases in the United States. *Gastroenterology*. 2002;122:1500–1511.

2. Shaheen NJ, Hansen RA, Morgan DR, et al. The burden of gastrointestinal and
   liver diseases, 2006. *Am J Gastroenterol*. 2006;101:2128–2138.

3. Goldblatt J, Taylor PJ, Lipman T, et al. The true impact of fatigue in primary
   biliary cirrhosis: a population study. *Gastroenterology*. 2002;122:1235–1241.

4. Newton JL. Systemic symptoms in non-alcoholic fatty liver disease. *Dig Dis Sci*.
   2010;28:214–219.

5. Papi C, Ciaco A, Bianchi M, Montanti S, Koch M, Capurso L. Correlation of
   various Crohn's disease activity indexes in subgroups of patients with primarily inflammatory or fibrostenosing clinical characteristics. *J Clin Gastroenterol*.
   1996;23:40–43.

6. Minderhoud IM, Samsom M, Oldenburg B. What predicts mucosal inflammation
   in Crohn's disease patients? *Inflamm Bowel Dis*. 2007;13:1567–1572.

7. Johnson DA, Fennerty MB. Heartburn severity underestimates erosive
   esophagitis severity in elderly patients with gastroesophageal reflux disease.
   Gastroenterology. 2004;126:660–664.

8. Locke GR, Zinsmeister AR, Talley NJ. Can symptoms predict endoscopic
   findings in GERD? *Gastrointest Endosc*. 2003;58:661–670.

9. Levy RL, Olden KW, Naliboff BD, et al. Psychosocial aspects of the functional
   gastrointestinal disorders. *Gastroenterology*. 2006;130:1447–1458.

10. Faresjo A, Grodzinsky E, Johansson S, Wallander MA, Timpka T, Akerlind I.
    A population-based case-control study of work and psychosocial problems in
    patients with irritable bowel syndrome—women are more seriously affected than
    men. *Am J Gastroenterol*. 2007;102:371–379.

11. Fuller-Thomson E, Sulman J. Depression and inflammatory bowel disease:
    findings from two nationally representative Canadian surveys. *Inflamm Bowel
    Dis*. 2006;12:697–707.

12. Bjornsson E, Simren M, Olsson R, Chapman RW. Fatigue in patients with
    primary sclerosing cholangitis. *Scand J Gastroenterol*. 2004;39:961–968.

13. Social Security Administration. *Disability Evaluation under Social Security*.
    SSA Pub. No. 64-039 (ICN 468600). Baltimore, MD: Social Security
    Administration; 2008.

14. Locke GR, 3rd, Talley NJ, Fett SL, Zinsmeister AR, Melton LJ, 3rd. Prevalence and clinical spectrum of gastroesophageal reflux: a population-based study in Olmsted County, Minnesota. *Gastroenterology*. 1997;112:1448–1456.

15. Wahlqvist P, Karlsson M, Johnson D, Carlsson J, Bolge SC, Wallander MA. Relationship between symptom load of gastro-esophageal reflux disease and health-related quality of life, work productivity, resource utilization and concomitant diseases: survey of a US cohort. *Aliment Pharmacol Ther*. 2008;27: 960–970.

16. Dean BB, Aguilar D, Johnson LF, et al. Night-time and daytime atypical manifestations of gastro-esophageal reflux disease: frequency, severity and impact on health-related quality of life. *Aliment Pharmacol Ther*. 2008;27:327–337.

17. Dean BB, Crawley JA, Schmitt CM, Wong J, Ofman JJ. The burden of illness of gastro-esophageal reflux disease: impact on work productivity. *Aliment Pharmacol Ther*. 2003;17:1309–1317.

18. Gisbert JP, Cooper A, Karagiannis D, et al. Impact of gastroesophageal reflux disease on work absenteeism, presenteeism and productivity in daily life: a European observational study. *Health Qual Life Outcomes*. 2009;7:90.

19. Gross M, Beckenbauer U, Burkowitz J, Walther H, Brueggenjuergen B. Impact of gastro-oesophageal reflux disease on work productivity despite therapy with proton pump inhibitors in Germany. *Eur J Med Res*. 2010;15:124–130.

20. Leong SA, Barghout V, Birnbaum HG, et al. The economic consequences of irritable bowel syndrome: a US employer perspective. *Arch Intern Med*. 2003;163:929–935.

21. Toghanian S, Wahlqvist P, Johnson DA, Bolge SC, Liljas B. The burden of disrupting gastro-oesophageal reflux disease: a database study in US and European cohorts. *Clin Drug Investig*. 2010;30:167–178.

22. Johnson DA, Orr WC, Crawley JA, et al. Effect of esomeprazole on nighttime heartburn and sleep quality in patients with GERD: a randomized, placebo-controlled trial. *Am J Gastroenterol*. 2005;100:1914–1922.

23. Medical Disability Advisor. Available at www.MDguidelines.com. Accessed August 9, 2010.

24. Drossman DA. The functional gastrointestinal disorders and the Rome III process. *Gastroenterology*. 2006;130:1377–1390.

25. Camilleri M, Williams DE. Economic burden of irritable bowel syndrome. Proposed strategies to control expenditures. *Pharmacoeconomics*. 2000;17: 331–338.

26. Cash B. Economic impact of irritable bowel syndrome: what does the future hold? *Am J Manag Care*. 2005;11:S4–6.

27. Cash B, Sullivan S, Barghout V. Total costs of IBS: employer and managed care perspective. *Am J Manag Care*. 2005;11:S7–16.

28. Pare P, Gray J, Lam S, et al. Health-related quality of life, work productivity, and health care resource utilization of subjects with irritable bowel syndrome: baseline results from LOGIC (Longitudinal Outcomes Study of Gastrointestinal Symptoms in Canada), a naturalistic study. *Clin Ther*. 2006;28:1726–1735; discussion 1710–1721.

Chapter 18

29. Schultz AB, Chen CY, Edington DW. The cost and impact of health conditions on presenteeism to employers: a review of the literature. *Pharmacoeconomics*. 2009;27:365–378.

30. Drossman DA, Li Z, Andruzzi E, et al. U.S. householder survey of functional gastrointestinal disorders. Prevalence, sociodemography, and health impact. *Dig Dis Sci*. 1993;38:1569–1580.

31. Reilly MC, Bracco A, Ricci JF, Santoro J, Stevens T. The validity and accuracy of the Work Productivity and Activity Impairment questionnaire—irritable bowel syndrome version (WPAI:IBS). *Aliment Pharmacol Ther*. 2004;20:459–467.

32. Brook RA, Kleinman NL, Choung RS, Melkonian AK, Smeeding JE, Talley NJ. Functional dyspepsia impacts absenteeism and direct and indirect costs. *Clin Gastroenterol Hepatol*. 2010;8:498–503.

33. Camilleri M, Dubois D, Coulie B, et al. Prevalence and socioeconomic impact of upper gastrointestinal disorders in the United States: results of the US Upper Gastrointestinal Study. *Clin Gastroenterol Hepatol*. 2005;3:543–552.

34. Chang L, Toner BB, Fukudo S, et al. Gender, age, society, culture, and the patient's perspective in the functional gastrointestinal disorders. *Gastroenterology*. 2006;130:1435–1446.

35. Silk DB. Impact of irritable bowel syndrome on personal relationships and working practices. *Eur J Gastroenterol Hepatol*. 2001;13:1327–1332.

36. Dancey CP, Backhouse S. Towards a better understanding of patients with irritable bowel syndrome. *J Adv Nurs*. 1993;18:1443–1450.

37. Bernklev T, Jahnsen J, Henriksen M, et al. Relationship between sick leave, unemployment, disability, and health-related quality of life in patients with inflammatory bowel disease. *Inflamm Bowel Dis*. 2006;12:402–412.

38. Boonen A, Dagnelie PC, Feleus A, et al. The impact of inflammatory bowel disease on labor force participation: results of a population sampled case-control study. *Inflamm Bowel Dis*. 2002;8:382–389.

39. Feagan BG, Bala M, Yan S, Olson A, Hanauer S. Unemployment and disability in patients with moderately to severely active Crohn's disease. *J Clin Gastroenterol*. 2005;39:390–395.

40. Ananthakrishnan AN, Weber LR, Knox JF, et al. Permanent work disability in Crohn's disease. *Am J Gastroenterol*. 2008;103:154–161.

41. Calvet X, Motos J, Montserrat A, Gallardo O, Vergara M. Analysis of court criteria for awarding disability benefits to patients with Crohn's disease. *Clin Gastroenterol Hepatol*. 2009;7:1322–1327.

42. Lichtenstein GR, Yan S, Bala M, Hanauer S. Remission in patients with Crohn's disease is associated with improvement in employment and quality of life and a decrease in hospitalizations and surgeries. *Am J Gastroenterol*. 2004;99:91–96.

43. Deter HC, Keller W, von Wietersheim J, Jantschek G, Duchmann R, Zeitz M. Psychological treatment may reduce the need for healthcare in patients with Crohn's disease. *Inflamm Bowel Dis*. 2007;13:745–752.

44. Lix LM, Graff LA, Walker JR, et al. Longitudinal study of quality of life and psychological functioning for active, fluctuating, and inactive disease patterns in inflammatory bowel disease. *Inflamm Bowel Dis*. 2008;14:1575–1584.

45. Rampton D. Does stress influence inflammatory bowel disease? The clinical data. *Dig Dis Sci*. 2009;27 Suppl 1:76–79.

46. Rogala L, Miller N, Graff LA, et al. Population-based controlled study of social support, self-perceived stress, activity and work issues, and access to health care in inflammatory bowel disease. *Inflamm Bowel Dis*. 2008;14:526–535.

47. Teuber G, Schafer A, Rimpel J, et al. Deterioration of health-related quality of life and fatigue in patients with chronic hepatitis C: Association with demographic factors, inflammatory activity, and degree of fibrosis. *J Hepatol*. 2008;49:923–929.

48. Kanwal F, Hays RD, Kilbourne AM, Dulai GS, Gralnek IM. Are physician-derived disease severity indices associated with health-related quality of life in patients with end-stage liver disease? *Am J Gastroenterol*. 2004;99:1726–1732.

49. Su J, Brook RA, Kleinman NL, Corey-Lisle P. The impact of hepatitis C virus infection on work absence, productivity, and healthcare benefit costs. *Hepatology*. 2010;52:436–442.

50. Stewart CA, Smith GE. Minimal hepatic encephalopathy. *Nat Clin Pract Gastroenterol Hepatol*. 2007;4:677–685.

51. Schomerus H, Hamster W. Quality of life in cirrhotics with minimal hepatic encephalopathy. *Metab Brain Dis*. 2001;16:37–41.

52. Arguedas MR, DeLawrence TG, McGuire BM. Influence of hepatic encephalopathy on health-related quality of life in patients with cirrhosis. *Dig Dis Sci*. 2003;48:1622–1626.

53. Wein C, Koch H, Popp B, Oehler G, Schauder P. Minimal hepatic encephalopathy impairs fitness to drive. *Hepatology*. 2004;39:739–745.

54. Bajaj JS, Saeian K, Hafeezullah M, Hoffmann RG, Hammeke TA. Patients with minimal hepatic encephalopathy have poor insight into their driving skills. *Clin Gastroenterol Hepatol*. 2008;6:1135–1139; quiz 1065.

55. Ferenci P, Lockwood A, Mullen K, Tarter R, Weissenborn K, Blei AT. Hepatic encephalopathy—definition, nomenclature, diagnosis, and quantification: final report of the working party at the 11th World Congresses of Gastroenterology, Vienna, 1998. *Hepatology*. 2002;35:716–721.

56. Sharma P, Sharma BC, Puri V, Sarin SK. Critical flicker frequency: diagnostic tool for minimal hepatic encephalopathy. *J Hepatol*. 2007;47:67–73.

57. Les I, Doval E, Flavia M, et al. Quality of life in cirrhosis is related to potentially treatable factors. *Eur J Gastroenterol Hepatol*. 2010;22:221–227.

Chapter 18

.

Chapter 19

Urologic Disease

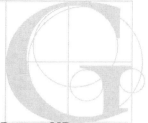

Christopher J. Welty, MD and Michael P. Porter, MD

Introduction

The overall burden of urologic disease in the United States population is large. Among adults in 2000, there were an estimated 19.4 million total physician visits, 2.5 million ER visits, and 617,904 hospital admissions for a primary urologic diagnosis.[1] The treatment of most urologic conditions falls along the entire spectrum of medical to surgical. How a disease state or treatment affects an individual's ability to work often depends on the chosen method of treatment. Accordingly, in this chapter we will address recovery, rehabilitation, and time off work on the basis of treatment modality; major surgery, minor surgery and endoscopy, or medical therapy.

There is little data regarding risk and capacity for work for most urologic conditions. There is some data on work tolerance following specific surgeries, such as prostatectomy, and this will be provided where appropriate. This chapter also provides guidelines for likely recovery times in the form of tables from the Medical Disability Advisor, when available.[2] These tables are based on medical disability claims data and expert opinion. In instances when no appropriate MDA table was available, tables were created from the author's opinion and are referenced as such. These recommendations represent reasonable recovery times, not strict guidelines. The minimal times represent the ideal recovery of an otherwise fit patient, while the maximum represents a time beyond which an explanation for further disability should be sought.

Major Surgery

Recovery from major surgery can be divided into three phases: acute, intermediate, and long-term. The duration and challenges of each phase vary by the specific surgery. The acute phase immediately follows surgery, involves control of incisional pain and return of bowel function, and is usually spent in the hospital. The intermediate phase usually involves improving strength and mobility to near pre-operative levels and occurs outside of the hospital, either at home or in a rehabilitation facility. This can take several weeks to several months, depending on the surgery. There may be a short-term decrease in work capacity during this time, due to surgeon imposed activity or lifting restrictions. The long-term phase involves further recovery of strength and adjusting to other surgery specific features.

Radical Prostatectomy

Background

Prostate cancer is the most common cancer to affect men in the United States, with an estimated 1 in 6 men diagnosed with prostate cancer over their lifespan.[3] Roughly one-third of all cases occur in men <65 years of age.[4] Due to a variety of factors, including long term cancer control, long term functional outcomes, and fitness to tolerate surgery, younger men (age 40–60) are more likely to receive radical prostatectomy than older men.[5] Surgery can be performed as open or with robotic assistance.

Recovery

The acute recovery from prostatectomy usually involves 1–3 days in the hospital for pain control, return of intestinal function, and assistance with ambulation. There is a slightly shorter hospitalization time for robotic surgery than for open surgery.[6–9] Discharge occurs when the patient is ambulating independently, has good pain control with oral narcotics, and is tolerating a diet. Patients are discharged with the urinary catheter in place and, less often, the surgical drain.

In the intermediate phase, the major barriers to returning to work after discharge are pain control, lifting restrictions, and the urinary catheter. Several studies have found that pain following open and robotic-assisted prostatectomy is generally low; as many as 25% of patients do not require narcotic pain medications after discharge.[10] Due to the risk of post-operative hernia, men are usually instructed to refrain from lifting more than 10 pounds for up to 6 weeks. This may lead to a temporary work restriction for men with jobs that require lifting. Sultan and colleagues analyzed a case series of 542 men undergoing open RRP with no specific restrictions and found a mean return to unrestricted activity of 34 days, with 25% of men returning to full activity before 3 weeks. The urinary catheter may decrease work tolerance due to catheter discomfort and leakage around

Chapter 19

the catheter.[11] In addition, men with active jobs may be instructed not to work until the catheter is removed due to the concern that the catheter could cause trauma to the operative site. While highly motivated men with sedentary jobs may return to work before the catheter is removed, most men will need at least 2 weeks off work as pain control and strength improve. The catheter is commonly removed 1–2 weeks after surgery. The ability to return to work after catheter removal will vary by the lifting and activity requirements of the job. Tables 19-1 and 19-2 show the expected recovery times available from the Medical Disability Advisor for open and robot assisted prostatectomy, respectively.[2] Currently, studies comparing the two surgical approaches do not support as large of a difference in recovery as is stated in these tables.

A patient's long-term recovery is affected by the recovery of urinary continence. Following both RRP and RALRP, most men are incontinent when

Table 19-1 Recommended recovery times following Radical Prostectomy[2]

Job Classification	DURATION IN DAYS		
	Minimum	Optimum	Maximum
Sedentary	7	21	35
Light	14	42	42
Medium	28	49	54
Heavy	42	56	70
Very Heavy	42	63	84

Table 19-2 Recommended recovery times following robot-assisted laparoscopic prostatectomy[2]

Job Classification	DURATION IN DAYS		
	Minimum	Optimum	Maximum
Sedentary	3	7	21
Light	7	14	28
Medium	10	21	35
Heavy	14	28	42
Very Heavy	21	35	42

Chapter 19

the catheter is initially removed. The rate at which continence returns is variable; some men experience return of urinary control within the first several days, while others may require several weeks to months and incontinence can continue to improve over the course of a year.[12,13] Long-term continence ranges from 85%–98%, although some continent men will have leakage with significant strain.[14] While leakage does not pose significant risk to the patient, if large it can affect the individual's tolerance of lifting. Because of this, a significant number of men with medium and heavy-duty work may need permanent work accommodations to decrease lifting and convenient access to a restroom.

Cystectomy and Urinary Diversion

Background

Cystectomy is most commonly performed for clinically invasive bladder cancer, although it can be performed for some benign diseases, such as intersitial cystitis, radiation cystitis, and neurogenic bladder. Bladder cancer incidence increases with age and affects males three times more commonly than females. Removal of the bladder requires construction of an alternate means for drainage of the urine, known as urinary diversion. The most common techniques for urinary diversion are conduit diversion and continent diversion. Conduit diversion involves creating an abdominal wall stoma from an isolated segment of bowel, similar to colostomy. The ureters are implanted into the bowel segment, and urine is continuously excreted in an appliance and collection device worn over the stoma. In continent diversion, an isolated bowel segment is used to construct a reservoir. The reservoir is either connected to the native urethra or to a continent stoma on the abdominal wall. Patients empty the reservoir through valsalva voiding or through intermittent catheterization. The choice of diversion has an impact on post-operative recovery. Ileal conduits account for about 85% of urinary diversions performed in the Medicare population, and this proportion has been relatively stable over the past decade. Continent diversion is more common in younger patients.[15]

Recovery

The recovery from cystectomy is the longest of the urologic procedures and is dependent on the early post-operative course. A recent review of the SEER cancer database revealed a rate of minor complication of 51% and rate of major complication of 13%.[16] Minor complications include delayed return of bowel function, wound infection/breakdown, and dehydration. Major complications include bowel obstruction requiring reoperation, organ failure, and chronic disability.

In the absence of complication, the acute, in-hospital recovery after cystectomy is 5–8 days. After discharge, patients may have a prolonged intermediate recovery time at home, with outpatient physical therapy, or with a brief inpatient rehabilitation stay. Patients who have undergone cystectomy have the additional challenge of learning to care for the urinary diversion and may benefit from further outpatient consultation with an enterostomal therapist.[17] Those with a continent diversion need to adjust to a new voiding pattern and may need to intermittently catheterize through the urethra to empty adequately. In addition, both groups of patients will likely need several follow-up visits in the first few months following surgery.

More than any other surgery discussed in this chapter, patients will likely have temporarily decreased work capacity and tolerance due to temporary work restrictions and deconditioning. Following the acute recovery, patients that follow specific physical activity and dietary guidelines have been shown to have a faster recovery and improved quality of life outcomes.[18] Return to work can be facilitated with several small accommodations. These include convenient access to restroom facilities, either for urostomy care or self-catheterization if needed, and reduction in required physical activity for several weeks.

Nephrectomy

Background
Nephrectomy is most commonly performed for renal cancer, although it is also less commonly performed for chronic infection or kidney stones with a non-functional kidney. The use of nephrectomy has increased over the past

Chapter 19

Table 19-3 Recommended recovery times following cystectomy[2]

Job Classification	DURATION IN DAYS		
	Minimum	Optimum	Maximum
Sedentary	42	49	56
Light	42	49	56
Medium	42	49	70
Heavy	56	63	84
Very Heavy	56	63	112

20 years due to increased kidney cancer detection through modern imaging technologies. Renal cancer is currently the seventh most common malignancy diagnosed in the United States.[4,19]

Nephrectomy can be performed either through an open or laparoscopic approach. With either approach, either the entire kidney (total nephrectomy, radical nephrectomy) or only the diseased portion of the kidney (partial nephrectomy) can be excised. As the recovery from these two approaches differs greatly, they will be discussed separately.

Open Nephrectomy

The acute recovery from open nephrectomy usually involves 3–7 days in hospital for pain control and mobilization. Because the abdominal wall musculature is divided, recovery time to full activity is longer than with prostatectomy. There is usually a temporary lifting restriction for 4–6 weeks following surgery. The average return to full activity following nephrectomy is around 60 days.[20,21] It is possible that with work accommodations, such as decreased demands for lifting and restarting part-time, a patient can return to work earlier than this.

Laparoscopic Nephrectomy

The principal advantage for laparoscopic nephrectomy is decreased recovery time and post-operative pain compared to open nephrectomy.[20,21,22,23] Acutely, patients usually spend 2–3 days in the hospital. The average return to full activity is 35–45 days, although patients can return to work sooner. Lifting restriction are usually imposed for 2 weeks following surgery, as opposed the 4–6 weeks following open surgery. Table 19-5 is adapted from the Medical Disability Advisor recommendations for laparoscopic

Table 19-4 Recommended recovery times following open nephrectomy[2]

Job Classification	DURATION IN DAYS		
	Minimum	Optimum	Maximum
Sedentary	14	28	42
Light	14	28	56
Medium	21	35	56
Heavy	28	42	70
Very Heavy	28	42	70

Chapter 19

Table 19-5 Recommended recovery times following laparoscopic nephrectomy[2]

Job Classification	DURATION IN DAYS		
	Minimum	Optimum	Maximum
Sedentary	3	7	14
Light	5	10	21
Medium	10	14	28
Heavy	14	28	35
Very Heavy	14	35	42

cholecystectomy.[2] Recovery from laparoscopic nephrectomy is likely to be slightly longer as the surgery usually takes longer, involves more dissection of the intra-abdominal organs, and requires an additional incision to remove the kidney.

Minor Surgery, Endoscopy, and Medical Therapy

Most urologic disease is not treated with major surgery. Treatments for one disease can often involve both long-term medical therapy and minor open or endoscopic procedures. The most common of these diagnoses and procedures are reviewed in this section.

Scrotal Surgery

The most common scrotal surgeries are hydrocelectomy, varicocelectomy, and, less commonly, radical orchiectomy. The recovery time from all three of these scrotal surgeries depends on the surgical approach. Table 19-6 is adapted from the Medical Disability Advisor and gives recovery guidelines for procedures performed through an inguinal incision.[2] For procedures performed through scrotal incisions, work tolerance may be temporarily limited by scrotal pain and swelling. Most patients will benefit from at least several days of limited activity with scrotal elevation. After that, men can usually resume activity as tolerated, although return to full activity usually takes 2–3 weeks as the scrotal swelling resolves. Following varicocelectomy and inguinal orchiectomy, some surgeons will impose lifting restrictions for up to 4 weeks to limit the risk of varicocele recurrence or hernia.

Chapter 19

Table 19-6 Recommended recovery times following inguinal approach scrotal surgery[2]

Job Classification	DURATION IN DAYS		
	Minimum	Optimum	Maximum
Sedentary	3	7	14
Light	3	7	21
Medium	7	14	21
Heavy	7	14	21
Very Heavy	7	14	21

Vasectomy

Vasectomy is the most common urologic procedure performed in the United States.[25] The procedure is commonly performed in the office setting under local anesthesia and is performed by both urologists and family practitioners. It is performed through one or two small scrotal incisions and involves division and ligation of the free ends of the vas deferens. Recovery is quick with low complication rates. Men can often return to work the following day. Those with more active jobs will benefit from light duty if possible and 3–4 days out of work.

Urinary Incontinence

Urinary incontinence is a common problem among women and represents a large disease burden in the United States.[26] Urinary incontinence is classified as either stress or urge incontinence based on the symptoms and inciting factors that accompany episodes of leakage. These categories are thought to relate to the underlying cause of incontinence and can be helpful in directing therapy, although many women present with mixed symptoms. Incontinence episodes do not present a medical risk to the patient. The degree to which incontinence affects work tolerance depends on frequency and volume of the episodes.

Stress Urinary Incontinence

Stress urinary incontinence (SUI) is characterized by leakage with movements that increase intrabdominal pressure, such as sneezing or lifting. These episodes range for leakage of a few drops of urine with significant straining to leaking large volumes with standing. For those with mild SUI, workplace accommodations such as decreasing heavy lifting and convenient access to bathroom factilities can greatly improve work tolerance.

Of the two type of incontinence, SUI is more amenable to surgical therapy as there is usually an identifiable anatomic abnormality that contributes to the disease process.[27] The lifetime risk of a woman having at least one surgery for urinary incontinence has been estimated to be 11%.[26] Many different approaches have been developed to treat urinary incontinence in an effort to minimize recovery time and maximize the result. The past 10 years have seen the development of minimally invasive sling procedures using synthetic mesh.

The sling procedure has rapidly become the most commonly performed procedure for incontinence due to a decrease in hospitalization, recovery time, and lower complication rates.[28] A urinary catheter is placed intraoperatively and removed before the patient leaves the hospital, usually the same day or after an overnight stay. A small percentage of women will be temporarily unable to void when the catheter is removed and will require a catheter on discharge. In general, pain control is good following this surgery and light activity can be resumed in the first week post-operatively. Some surgeons restrict heavy lifting for several weeks following surgery. It is also important to note that the ultimate goal of surgery is to decrease the frequency of stress urinary incontinence episodes, but not eliminate them completely. As such, these patients may still benefit from the work accommodations described above.

Urge Incontinence
Patients with urge incontinence, or overactive bladder (OAB), describe a sudden, uncontrollable urge to void and the need to void frequently. These

Chapter 19

Table 19-7 Recommended recovery times following tension-free vaginal tape (TVT). (Guidelines suggested by the authors.)

Job Classification	DURATION IN DAYS		
	Minimum	Optimum	Maximum
Sedentary	3	7	14
Light	3	7	14
Medium	14	21	28
Heavy	21	24	28
Very Heavy	21	24	28

episodes are often brought on by certain cues, such as running water or putting the key in the door at home. OAB is related to uncontrolled bladder contraction or poor bladder compliance and generally responds better to medical therapy than surgery. Though some surgical therapies are available for refractory OAB, they are not commonly used.[29] Non-surgical therapies for OAB may include behavior modification of fluid intake, pelvic floor physical therapy, and a wide variety of pharmacologic therapies aimed at decreasing the frequency of bladder contraction. Tolerance of pharmacologic therapies can be limited by common side effects such as dry mouth and constipation. The overall goal of therapy is to balance the improvement in quality of life from decreased urinary symptoms with the downside of side effects. OAB can greatly affect tolerance as the urge to void can be quite severe. The work place can be made more accommodating by decreasing triggers that lead to urinary urge (such as running water) and easy access to bathroom facilities.

Kidney Stones

Background
Kidney stones are relatively common in the United States. The diagnosis is about twice as common among men as women, and about 10% of men will have a kidney stone by age 60. The economic impact is significant. The average expenditure by private insurance for employees with kidney stones is about twice as for those without.[30]

Urinary stones usually form in the kidney from components naturally found in the urine. Patients become symptomatic when the stone migrates from the kidney into the ureter and blocks the flow of urine. Common symptoms are severe colicky pain, nausea, and vomiting. Most stones will pass spontaneously, and passage rates can be increased with medical expulsive therapy (MET).[31] Medical expulsive therapy involves aggressive oral hydration to increase urine output and administration of an oral alpha-blocker. Stones larger than 8mm are unlikely to pass.

Surgery
Two procedures, extracorporeal shockwave lithotripsy (ESWL) and ureteroscopy with stone manipulation and/or fragmentation, account for the vast majority of stone procedures in the United States. ESWL is the more common of the two procedures. Both are usually performed as outpatient procedures and have a short recovery time.

Recovery

Patients undergoing MET are unlikely to be able to work while passing a kidney stone secondary to pain and narcotic medication requirements. For this reason, trials of MET should be limited. Following surgery, most people will be able to return to work in 2–3 days. A minority of patients will experience significant discomfort from placement of a ureteral stent that will require time away from work. If this does occur, the individual's recovery may be prolonged depending on how long the stent needs to remain in place to safely manage and treat the stone.

Finally, up to 50% of patients will recur within 7.5 years of the initial diagnosis. Recurrences can be decreased, but not entirely eliminated, with

Table 19-8 Recommended recovery times for medical expulsive therapy[2]

	DURATION IN DAYS		
Job Classification	Minimum	Optimum	Maximum
Any Work	1	3	7

Table 19-9 Recommended recovery times for extracorporeal shockwave lithotripsy[2]

	DURATION IN DAYS		
Job Classification	Minimum	Optimum	Maximum
Any Work	1	2	7

Table 19-10 Recommended recovery times for ureteroscopy. (Guidelines suggested by the authors.)

	DURATION IN DAYS		
Job Classification	Minimum	Optimum	Maximum
Any Work	3	7	14

aggressive fluid intake and some medical therapies. Some occupations, such as airline pilot, have specific work restrictions for patients with kidney stones due to safety concerns from sudden attacks of severe pain. These restrictions are imposed by the employer and are not due to medical safety concerns. For occupations where this is a concern, specific guidelines from the employer should be used.[2]

Benign Prostatic Hyperplasia

Background

Nearly one quarter of Caucasian men in the United States aged 50–79 will experience symptoms resulting from BPH.[32] Symptoms of BPH are referred to as lower urinary tract symptoms (LUTS) and include urinary frequency, incomplete emptying of the bladder, frequent nighttime urination, strong sudden urges to urinate, urge urinary incontinence, weak stream, urinary hesitancy, and post void dribbling. Historically, BPH was often treated with surgery; transurethral prostatectomy (TURP) was the second most common procedure performed in the United States prior to 1990.[32] However, with the advent of effective medical therapy for BPH with alpha-blockers and 5-alpha-reductase inhibitors, the utilization of TURP decreased by 50% in the 1990s.[33] Medical management of LUTS is not always successful. If significant urinary obstruction persists, men can go on to develop worsening urge, urinary frequency, and chronic bladder dysfunction. Thus, TURP remains an important option for men who fail medical therapy for BPH.

Recovery

Patients usually spend one night in the hospital following TURP. The catheter placed in the operating room is usually removed the following day. Patients are usually discharged without a catheter, although a small percentage of men will be unable to void on post-operative day one and are discharged with a catheter in place that is removed 1 week later. Hospitalization and recovery time can be prolonged by persistent hematuria following surgery or significant blood loss requiring transfusion. Transfusion is necessary in 1–3% of cases.[34] Due to concerns for delayed bleeding, most surgeons will recommend limited activity for 1 to 2 weeks following surgery. In addition, most men will experience an exacerbation of lower urinary tract symptoms after TURP that resolves over 4–6 weeks post surgery. In the initial 7–14 days, these symptoms can be severe and result in frequent need to urinate and associated urge incontinence. Some men may require additional time off of work until these symptoms resolve.

Table 19-11 Recommended recovery times for transurethral resection of prostate[2]

	DURATION IN DAYS		
Job Classification	Minimum	Optimum	Maximum
Sedentary	7	9	14
Light	7	9	14
Medium	14	16	21
Heavy	21	24	28
Very Heavy	21	24	28

Endoscopic Management of Bladder Cancer

Background

Previously in this chapter, we reviewed cystectomy, which is used to treat muscle invasive bladder cancer. Prior to cystectomy, patients undergo trans-urethral resection of the bladder tumor (TURBT) at time of initial diagnosis. In addition, three-quarters of patients will have non-muscle invasive disease and never progress to cystectomy.[4]

TURBT

TURBT is an endoscopic procedure usually preformed as an outpatient or, less commonly, with an overnight stay. Recovery time from TURBT is generally less than that of TURP as the risk of delayed post-operative

Table 19-12 Recommended recovery times for transurethral resection of bladder tumor. (Guidelines suggested by the authors.)

	DURATION IN DAYS		
Job Classification	Minimum	Optimum	Maximum
Sedentary	1	5	14
Light	1	5	14
Medium	7	10	21
Heavy	7	14	28
Very Heavy	7	14	28

Chapter 19

bleeding is lower. For small resections where no catheter is left in place, patients may be able to return to work the following day. Larger resections will require longer recovery times.

Intravesical Immunotherapy

Intravesical chemotherapy is given to reduce the risk of recurrence or progression of non-muscle invasive bladder cancer. The most common form of intravesical chemotherapy used is actually immunotherapy with Bacillus Clamette-Guerin (BCG) instillation. The usual administration schedule course for BCG involves weekly instillations in the office for a total of 6 weeks. Each instillation involves a 1–2 hour office visit during which a catheter is placed for instillation. Some patients may receive additional maintenance BCG instillations every 3–6 months after the 6-week induction course. BCG is hypothesized to work by enhancing the patient's immune response to the cancer. Accordingly, the most common side effects are secondary to a brisk immune response in the bladder and include dysuria, urinary frequency, low-grade fever, and fatigue. These side effects can worsen with repeated treatments and sometimes require that the treatment be held.[35] The fatigue can be profound by the end of treatment and greatly limit work tolerance. Symptoms almost always resolve after the course of therapy is complete. While accommodations at work, such as convenient bathroom access and part-time work, may allow patients to continue working during therapy, many will find work difficult until induction is complete.

Summary

In summary, urologic disease are quite common in the United States population. Most affect work tolerance, although work capacity can also be temporarily affected following surgery. Return to work for patients with urologic disease can often be facilitated through the use of simple measures, such as availability of bathroom facilities, frequent breaks, and decreased lifting requirements. Urologic procedures are constantly evolving in an effort to become less invasive and decrease recovery time.

References

1. Litwin MS, Saigal CS. Introduction. In: Litwin MS, Saigal CS, eds. *Urologic Diseases in America.* Washington, DC: US Government Printing Office; 2007:3–7.

2. Reed P. *The Medical Disability Advisor: Workplace Guidelines for Disability Duration.* 6th ed. Westminster, Colo: Reed Group Ltd; 2009.

3. Merrill RM, Weed DL, Feuer EJ. The lifetime risk of developing prostate cancer in white and black men. *Cancer Epidemiol Biomarkers Prev*. Oct 1997;6(10): 763–768.

4. Jemal A, Siegel R, Ward E, Hao Y, Xu J, Thun MJ. Cancer statistics, 2009. *CA Cancer J Clin*. Jul-Aug 2009;59(4):225–249.

5. Penson DF, Chen JM. Prostate Cancer. In: Litwin MS, Saigal CS, eds. *Urologic Diseases in America*. Washington, DC: US Government Printing Office; 2007: 73–113.

6. Bivalacqua TJ, Pierorazio PM, Su LM. Open, laparoscopic and robotic radical prostatectomy: optimizing the surgical approach. *Surg Oncol*. Sep 2009;18(3):233–241.

7. El-Hakim A, Leung RA, Tewari A. Robotic prostatectomy: a pooled analysis of published literature. *Expert Rev Anticancer Ther*. Jan 2006;6(1):11–20.

8. Sultan R, Slova D, Thiel B, Lepor H. Time to return to work and physical activity following open radical retropubic prostatectomy. *J Urol*. Oct 2006;176 (4 Pt 1):1420–1423.

9. Webster TM, Herrell SD, Chang SS, et al. Robotic assisted laparoscopic radical prostatectomy versus retropubic radical prostatectomy: a prospective assessment of postoperative pain. *J Urol*. Sep 2005;174(3):912–914; discussion 914.

10. McLellan RA, Bell DG, Rendon RA. Effective analgesia and decreased length of stay for patients undergoing radical prostatectomy: effectiveness of a clinical pathway. *Can J Urol*. Oct 2006;13(5):3244–3249.

11. Lepor H. Status of radical prostatectomy in 2009: is there medical evidence to justify the robotic approach? *Rev Urol*. Spring 2009;11(2):61–70.

12. Eastham JA, Kattan MW, Rogers E, et al. Risk factors for urinary incontinence after radical prostatectomy. *J Urol*. Nov 1996;156(5):1707–1713.

13. Marsh DW, Lepor H. Predicting continence following radical prostatectomy. *Curr Urol Rep*. Jun 2001;2(3):248–252.

14. Konety BR, Sadetsky N, Carroll PR. Recovery of urinary continence following radical prostatectomy: the impact of prostate volume—analysis of data from the CaPSURE Database. *J Urol*. Apr 2007;177(4):1423–1425; discussion 1425–1426.

15. Konety BR, Joyce GF, Wise M. Bladder and Upper Tract Urothelial Cancer. In: Litwin MS, Saigal CS, eds. *Urologic Diseases in America*. Washington, DC: US Government Printing Office; 2007:225–277.

16. Donat SM, Siegrist T, Cronin A, Savage C, Milowsky MI, Herr HW. Radical cystectomy in octogenarians—does morbidity outweigh the potential survival benefits? *J Urol*. Jun 2010;183(6):2171–2177.

17. Maklebust J. United Ostomy Association visits and adjustment following ostomy surgery. *J Enterostomal Ther*. May-Jun 1985;12(3):84–92.

18. Lee CT. Quality of life following incontinent cutaneous and orthotopic urinary diversions. *Curr Treat Options Oncol*. Aug 2009;10(3–4):275–286.

19. Wallen EM, Joyce GF, Wise M. Kidney Cancer. In: Litwin MS, Saigal CS, eds. *Urologic Diseases in America*. Washington, DC: US Government Printing Office; 2007:337–373.

Chapter 19

20. Burgess NA, Koo BC, Calvert RC, Hindmarsh A, Donaldson PJ, Rhodes M. Randomized trial of laparoscopic v open nephrectomy. *J Endourol.* Jun 2007;21(6):610–613.

21. Jiang J, Zheng X, Qin J, et al. Health-related quality of life after hand-assisted laparoscopic and open radical nephrectomies of renal cell carcinoma. *Int Urol Nephrol.* 2009;41(1):23–27.

22. Dols LF, Kok NF, Terkivatan T, et al. Hand-assisted retroperitoneoscopic versus standard laparoscopic donor nephrectomy: HARP-trial. *BMC Surg.* 2010;10:11.

23. Nelson CP, Wolf JS, Jr. Comparison of hand assisted versus standard laparoscopic radical nephrectomy for suspected renal cell carcinoma. *J Urol.* May 2002;167(5):1989–1994.

24. Al-Said S, Al-Naimi A, Al-Ansari A, et al. Varicocelectomy for male infertility: a comparative study of open, laparoscopic and microsurgical approaches. *J Urol.* Jul 2008;180(1):266–270.

25. Eisenberg ML, Henderson JT, Amory JK, Smith JF, Walsh TJ. Racial differences in vasectomy utilization in the United States: data from the national survey of family growth. *Urology.* Nov 2009;74(5):1020–1024.

26. Nygaard I, Thom DH, Calhoun EC. Urinary Incontinence in Women. In: Litwin MS, Saigal CS, eds. *Urologic Diseases in America.* Washington, DC: US Government Printing Office; 2007:159–186.

27. Nitti VW, Blaivas JG. Urinary Incontinence: Epidemiology, Pathophysiology, Evaluation, and Management Overview. In: Wein AJ, Kavoussi LR, Novick AC, Partin AW, Peters CA, eds. *Campbell-Walsh Urology.* Vol 3. 9th ed: Saunders-Elsevier; 2007:2046–2070.

28. Novara G, Artibani W, Barber MD, et al. Updated systematic review and meta-analysis of the comparative data on colposuspensions, pubovaginal slings, and midurethral tapes in the surgical treatment of female stress urinary incontinence. *Eur Urol.* Aug 2010;58(2):218–38.

29. Ulmsten U, Henriksson L, Johnson P, Varhos G. An ambulatory surgical procedure under local anesthesia for treatment of female urinary incontinence. *Int Urogynecol J Pelvic Floor Dysfunct.* 1996;7(2):81–85; discussion 85–86.

30. Pearle MS, Calhoun EC, Curhan GC. Prostate Cancer. In: Litwin MS, Saigal CS, eds. *Urologic Diseases in America.* Washington, DC: US Government Printing Office; 2007:283–318.

31. Hollingsworth JM, Rogers MA, Kaufman SR, et al. Medical therapy to facilitate urinary stone passage: a meta-analysis. *Lancet.* Sep 30 2006;368(9542):1171–1179.

32. Wei JT, Calhoun EC, Jacobsen SJ. Benign Prostatic Hyperplasia. In: Litwin MS, Saigal CS, eds. *Urologic Diseases in America.* Washington, DC: US Government Printing Office; 2007:45–66.

33. Wasson JH, Bubolz TA, Lu-Yao GL, Walker-Corkery E, Hammond CS, Barry MJ. Transurethral resection of the prostate among medicare beneficiaries: 1984 to 1997. For the Patient Outcomes Research Team for Prostatic Diseases. *J Urol.* Oct 2000;164(4):1212–1215.

34. Fitzpatrick JM. Minimally Invasive and Endoscopic Management of Benign Prostatic Hypertrophy. In: Wein AJ, Kavoussi LR, Novick AC, Partin AW, Peters CA, eds. *Campbell-Walsh Urology*. Vol 3. 9th ed: Saunders-Elsevier; 2007.

35. Lamm DL, Blumenstein BA, Crissman JD, et al. Maintenance bacillus Calmette-Guerin immunotherapy for recurrent TA, T1 and carcinoma in situ transitional cell carcinoma of the bladder: a randomized Southwest Oncology Group Study. *J Urol*. Apr 2000;163(4):1124–1129.

Chapter 20

Working During Pregnancy

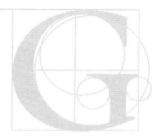

Anjel Vahratian, PhD, MPH

Pregnancy is a condition in which a woman is carrying a developing embryo or fetus. The length of pregnancy averages 40 weeks and is measured clinically from the day of a woman's last menstrual period and not conception. Data from 2008 show that approximately 4.2 million births were registered in the United States, a decline of 2% from 2007.[1] The majority of pregnancies occur to women 15 to 45 years of age, however their fertility window extends from the start of menstruation to the establishment of menopause. In 2008, the mean age for a woman at her first birth was 25.1 years.[1] Approximately 40% of live births were to unmarried mothers.[1]

Pregnancy is usually an uncomplicated experience for women, but it can be associated with an increased risk for complications, such as early pregnancy loss (miscarriage), gestational diabetes, pre-eclampsia, and preterm labor. This chapter will provide an overview of pregnancy, its potential complications, and its effect on a woman's risk, capacity, and tolerance for work. Current data on the average length of disability will be provided for different pregnancy outcomes, and a discussion of health policy regarding maternity leave will conclude this chapter.

Pregnancy: An Overview

Women often do not suspect that they are pregnant until they miss a menstrual period. Early and regular prenatal visits are encouraged to monitor the health and well-being of both the expectant mother and the developing fetus. These visits usually begin approximately 10 to 14 weeks gestation and, for an uncomplicated pregnancy, usually are scheduled every 4 weeks during the first and second trimesters and every 2 weeks during the third trimester. At 36 weeks gestation, women are asked to see their health provider on a weekly basis as delivery approaches. If a woman's pregnancy extends beyond her due date, she may be asked to see her provider 2 to 3 times a week to monitor the pregnancy more closely. Preconception care, or wellness visits prior to pregnancy, are also encouraged to promote a healthy pregnancy and for improving perinatal outcomes.[2]

Pregnancy: Prenatal Complications

During pregnancy, women may experience a broad range of complications. Fifteen percent of pregnancies result in an early pregnancy loss.[3] Gestational diabetes, or maternal glucose intolerance during pregnancy, occurs in 38.7 per 1,000 live births.[4] Gestational hypertension and pre-eclampsia, or maternal high blood pressure with or without protenuria during pregnancy, occurs in 38.0 per 1,000 live births.[4] Conditions such as these may impair the pregnancy from progressing to term safely.

Approximately 12% of births in the United States occur prematurely, or prior to 37 completed weeks of gestation.[1] Preterm birth may occur spontaneously (preterm labor) or arise due to a medical complication to the mother and/or fetus. While the exact cause of preterm labor is unknown, there are several conditions that are associated with an increased risk for preterm birth, such as hypertension, diabetes, pre-eclampsia, previous preterm labor, multiple pregnancies, cervical incompetence, substance abuse, and infection.[5] In evaluating a woman in preterm labor, the health care provider must consider the health of both the mother and fetus. The ability to prolong gestation to term is ideal, but not always possible. Careful monitoring may be necessary to ensure a healthy pregnancy outcome.

One of the most common interventions to prevent preterm birth is activity restriction or bed rest. The degree of restriction varies depending on the severity of symptoms.[6,7] For example, pregnant women may be advised to stay off their feet for extended periods, take naps during the day, or even remain confined to a bed for a portion of the remainder of their pregnancy. However, evidence to support the effectiveness of this intervention remains a source of debate.[7-9] For example, bed rest may have adverse health consequences on bone strength and muscle mass. Promislow et al. examined patterns of bone loss during pregnancy and showed that women who were prescribed bed rest had a mean bone loss of 4.6% compared to 1.5% among women who were not prescribed bed rest (p = 0.001).[10] Maloni et al. examined the effects of bed rest on maternal physical morbidity at 6 weeks postpartum and reported that at least 40% of the women sampled experienced fatigue, mood changes, tenseness, difficulty concentrating, back muscle soreness, and headache.[11] Activity restriction during pregnancy has also been associated with difficulty climbing up and down stairs, walking, and knee buckling.[12] In sum, this intervention has been widely used in pregnancy with little evidence to support that it reduces the risk for adverse pregnancy outcomes.

Pregnancy: Mode of Delivery

In addition to the timing of delivery, the mode of delivery is associated with some risk to the health of the expectant mother. While, the majority of women experience a vaginal birth, the rate of cesarean delivery in the United States is on the rise. In 2008, 32.3% of all births were delivered by cesarean section, an increase by more than 50% in the past decade.[1] Women often remain in the hospital for up to 48 hours following an uncomplicated normal delivery and up to 96 hours for an uncomplicated cesarean delivery. There are no Social Security Administration (SSA) listings for pregnancy.

Risk Assessment
Generally not considered an acute or a chronic condition, pregnancy presents a unique situation for the workplace. It is a dynamic condition. Thus, complications may arise suddenly and could have both short- and long-term effects on capacity and tolerance for work (see Chapter 2). Limited observational research on the effect of pregnancy complications, such as gestational diabetes, gestational hypertension, and/or pre-eclampsia, on the ability to work hinders our knowledge in this area and warrants further study.

Capacity
This term also assumes a degree of experience performing the activity in question prior to becoming pregnant. Most women can continue to work while pregnant, but as the pregnancy progresses their strength, flexibility, and endurance may diminish as they gain weight and their center of gravity shifts to accommodate the pregnancy.

Tolerance
During pregnancy, a woman's tolerance will vary depending on her health status and the stage of her pregnancy. As the pregnancy approaches term, her ability to maintain long working hours, standing, lifting, and/or shift work might lessen. A recent meta-analysis examined whether these occupational exposures are associated with low birth weight, preterm delivery, or pre-eclampsia/hypertension. While the authors note that the evidence

Chapter 20

may not be compelling to justify mandatory restrictions for common occupational exposures, such as prolonged working hours, shift work, lifting,
standing, and heavy physical workload, it is within reason and current
societal expectations to advise expectant mothers against working long
hours (more than 40 hours a week), prolonged standing, and heavy physical
work, especially in the third trimester.[13]

Table 20-1 lists the MDA consensus criteria for selected pregnancy
outcomes.

Family and Medical Leave Act

The Family and Medical Leave Act (FMLA) of 1993 "requires covered
employers to provide up to 12 weeks of unpaid, job-protected leave to "eligible" employees for certain family and medical reasons. Employees are
eligible if they have worked for their employer for at least one year, and
for 1,250 hours over the previous 12 months, and if there are at least 50
employees within 75 miles.[14]

Current data from the 2002 National Survey of Family Growth (NSFG)
shows that 70.2% of mothers who were employed at the time of their last
pregnancy took maternity leave after birth.[15]Advanced maternal age was
associated with taking maternity leave after childbirth, while a household
income less than 100% of the Federal Poverty Level or Hispanic origin were
characteristics of women who were less likely to take maternity leave after

Table 20-1 Length of Disability: Normal Vaginal and Cesarean Delivery

	DURATION, DAYS		
Job Classification	**Minimum**	**Optimum**	**Maximum**
Normal Vaginal Delivery			
Any Work	28	42	42
Cesarean Delivery			
Sedentary	28	42	42
Light	28	42	42
Medium	28	42	56
Heavy	42	49	84
Very Heavy	42	56	91

Reproduced with permission from Reed. www.mdguidelines.com.

childbirth. Eighty percent of women who took maternity leave during their last pregnancy indicated taking 12 weeks or less. Moreover, nearly 30% reported that their full leave was unpaid.

With the enactment of the FMLA, several studies have been conducted to assess the effect of maternity leave on maternal and child health outcomes. McGovern et al. analyzed data from a sample of women who delivered in Minnesota during 1991–1992 to assess the effect of time off work on the postpartum health of employed women.[16] The authors found that time off work had a positive effect on vitality for women taking more than 12 weeks leave, maternal mental health for women taking more than 15 weeks leave, and role function for women taking more than 20 weeks leave. However, most of these women didn't experience these positive effects because 75% of those studied returned to work by 12 weeks, 85% by 15 weeks, and 91% by 20 weeks after childbirth. The average duration of time off work postpartum in this study population was 10 weeks. Moreover, seventy percent of women reported limitations to daily role function. Limitations to this study included the time in which it was administered (early 1990's, prior to FMLA) and characteristics of the study population (91% white, 3% uninsured).

Chatterji and Markowitz, on behalf of the National Bureau of Economic Research, examined whether the length of maternity leave affected maternal health using data collected during the 1988 National Maternal and Infant Health Survey, a national sample of women between 15 and 49 years of age who had a pregnancy in 1988.[17] Their sample was limited to women who worked during their pregnancy and returned to work within 6 months of childbirth. The average duration of leave was 9 weeks, with more than 75% of women returning to work within 12 weeks. Using two measures of depression and a measure of overall health as an assessment of maternal health, the authors showed that returning to work later may reduce the number or frequency of depressive symptoms in postpartum women. The authors' state that "increasing maternal leave from 6 or fewer weeks to 8 weeks or 12 weeks is associated with an appreciable decline in depressive symptoms of approximately 11 percent and 15 percent respectively" (p 27).

Longer maternity leave has been associated with a reduction in infant mortality[18,19] and morbidity.[20] Moreover, in an analysis of data from the National Longitudinal Survey of Youth, Baum found that returning to work within the first three months of life was associated with lower cognitive scores during childhood.[21]

The duration of maternity leave has also been studied in regard to the effect of maternal employment on breastfeeding duration, which is shown to be associated with enhanced cognitive development among infants.[20] The American Academy of Pediatrics recommends women breastfeed exclusively for the first 6 months of life with continued breastfeeding for at least one year.[22] In addition to its beneficial effect on cognition, breast milk affords protection against certain illnesses.[23] Roe et al. showed in a survey of women who planned to return to work within 12 months of childbirth that the greatest decrease in breastfeeding duration occurred when employment was resumed in the first 12 weeks after birth.[24] Each additional week of leave from work increased breastfeeding duration by almost a half week. Moreover, a woman's time out of work was associated with an increase in breastfeeding frequency, which has broader implications for the practice of exclusive breastfeeding.

Guendelman et al. examined the implications of juggling work and breastfeeding on maternal health among a sample of 770 full-time working mothers in California.[25] The authors showed that a limited maternity leave (less than 12 weeks postpartum) was associated with a higher risk for early breastfeeding cessation. In particular, this relationship was strongest for women working in inflexible or nonmanagerial positions, where the psychosocial stress associated with negotiating life, work, and breastfeeding was more difficult. Pediatricians were advised to encourage their patients' mothers to take maternity leave and to support increased flexibility in working conditions for breastfeeding mothers.

However, a recent analysis suggests that even among those with paid antenatal and postpartum leave, most are hesitant to take full advantage of the entitlement. Guendelman et al. recently examined the utilization of California's legislation to provide paid pregnancy leave up to 4 weeks antenatally and 6 to 8 weeks postnatally for women working for public or private employers with five or more employees.[26] In an analysis of data based on postpartum interviews, the authors found that 52% of women worked until the time of delivery, 32% took antenatal leave with the expectation to return to their job after delivery, 9% quit their jobs, 5% cut back their hours, and 2% were fired during pregnancy. Sixty-three percent of women and 69% of those who took antenatal leave were offered leave by their employer. Moreover, 50% of leave takers, 51% of nonleave takers, and 15% of quitters returned to work by 3 months postpartum. The authors assert that antenatal leave is used in this population as a coping response to stress and tiredness versus as a health-promoting behavior. It is also used as a protective measure against occupational stressors such as night work and when a woman has limited control over the demands of her job. Overall, women seemed cautious in utilizing antenatal and/or postnatal leave.

Although barriers remain in accessing leave benefits, recent efforts at the state levels have sought to diminish their efforts. Since the enactment of the Act in 1993, six states and US territories (California, Hawaii, New Jersey, New York, Rhode Island, and Puerto Rico) have passed legislation to provide their residents with paid family and medical leave through short-term disability programs.[27] For example, in California more than 13 million workers have been offered partial wage replacement for family leave, and legislators have expanded eligibility in the state to all workers who pay into the system.

Summary

Most expectant mothers are able to work throughout their pregnancy. However, it is a dynamic condition. As women transition into the third trimester, the rapid weight gain may put a strain on their bodies, requiring more rest. A return to work postpartum will be dependent in part on the course of pregnancy and the delivery. Complications during the antenatal and postnatal periods may alter this timeline.

References

1. Martin J, Hamilton B, Sutton P, Ventura S, Mathews T, Osterman M. *Births: Final Data for 2008.* Hyattsville, MD: National Center for Health Statistics; Cited December 2010; Available from: http://www.cdc.gov/nchs/data/nvsr/nvsr59/nvsr59_01.pdf. Accessed February 16, 2011.

2. Atrash H, Johnson K, Adams M, Cordero J, Howse J. Preconception care for improving perinatal outcomes: the time to act. *Maternal and Child Health Journal.* 2006;10:S3–S11.

3. Wilcox A, Weinberg C, O'Connor J, et al. Incidence of early loss of pregnancy. *New England Journal of Medicine.* 1988;319:189–194.

4. Osterman M, Martin J, Menacker F. *Expanded health data from the new birth certificate, 2006.* Hyattsville, MD: National Center for Health Statistics; October 28, 2009. Available from: http://www.cdc.gov/nchs/data/nvsr/nvsr58/nvsr58_05.pdf. Accessed February 16, 2011.

5. Institute of Medicine, Committee on Understanding Premature Birth and Assuring Healthy Outcomes, Board on Health Sciences Policy. *Preterm Birth: Causes, Consequences, and Prevention.* Washington, D.C.: National Academies Press; 2007.

6. ACOG Committee on Obstetric Practice. ACOG Committee Opinion: Exercise during pregnancy and the postpartum period. *Obstetrics and Gynecology.* 2002;99:171–173.

Chapter 20

7. Sciscione A. Maternal activity restriction and the prevention of preterm birth. *American Journal of Obstetrics and Gynecology.* 2010;202:232.e231–232.e235.

8. Mozurkewich E, Luke B, Avni M, Wolf F. Working conditions and adverse pregnancy outcome: a meta-analysis. *Obstetrics and Gynecology.* 2000;95:623–635.

9. Pompeii L, Savitz D, Evenson K, Rogers B, McMahon M. Physical exertion at work and the risk of preterm delivery and small-for-gestational-age birth. *Obstetrics and Gynecology.* 2005;106:1279–1288.

10. Promislow J, Hertz-Picciotto I, Schramm M, Watt-Morse M, Anderson J. Bed rest and other determinants of bone loss during pregnancy. *American Journal of Obstetrics and Gynecology.* 2004;191:1077–1083.

11. Maloni J, Park S. Postpartum symptoms after antepartum bed rest. *JOGNN.* 2005;34:163–171.

12. Maloni J, Chance B, Zhang C, Cohen A, Betts D, Gange S. Physical and psychosocial side effects of antepartum hospital bed rest. *Nursing Research.* 1993;42:197–203.

13. Bonzini M, Coggon D, Palmer K. Risk of prematurity, low birthweight and pre-eclampsia in relation to working hours and physical activities: a systematic review. *Occup Environ Med.* 2007;64:228–243.

14. U.S. Department of Labor. *Employee Rights and Responsibilities Under the Family and Medical Leave Act.* Cited on August 2001. Available from: http://www.dol.gov/whd/regs/compliance/posters/fmlaen.pdf. Accessed on February 16, 2011.

15. U.S. Department of Health and Human Services, Health Resources and Services Administration. *Women's Health USA 2005.* Rockville, MD: U.S. Department of Health and Human Services;2005.

16. McGovern P, Dowd B, Gjerdingen D, Moscovice I, Kochevar L, Lohman W. Time off work and the postpartum health of employed women. *Medical Care.* May 1997;35(5):507–521.

17. Chatterji P, Markowitz S. *Working Paper 10206: Does the length of maternity leave affect maternal health?* Cambridge, MA: National Bureau of Economic Research; January 2004. Available from: http://www.nber.org/papers/w10206.pdf?new_window=1. Accessed on February 16, 2011.

18. Ruhm CJ. Parental leave and child health. *Journal of Health Economics.* Nov 2000;19(6):931–960.

19. Winegarden CR, Bracy PM. Demographic consequences of maternal-leave programs in industrial countries: evidence from fixed-effects models. *Southern Economic Journal.* Apr 1995;61(4):1,020–035.

20. Baker M, Milligan K. The early development and health benefits of maternity leave mandates. University of British Columbia and NBER. Cited on October 2006. Available from: http://www.aeaweb.org/annual_mtg_papers/2007/0107_1015_1702.pdf. Accessed on February 16, 2011.

21. Baum 2nd C. Does early maternal employment harm child development? An analysis of the potential benefits of leave-taking. *Journal of Labor Economics.* 2003;21:409–448.

22. American Academy of Pediatrics. Breastfeeding and the use of human milk. *Pediatrics*. 1997;99:e5.

23. Scariati PD, Grummer-Strawn LM, Fein SB. A longitudinal analysis of infant morbidity and the extent of breastfeeding in the United States. *Pediatrics*. Jun 1997;99(6):E5.

24. Roe B, Whittington LA, Fein SB, Teisl MF. Is there competition between breast-feeding and maternal employment? *Demography*. May 1999;36(2):157–171.

25. Guendelman S, Kosa J, Pearl M, Graham S, Goodman J, Kharrazi M. Juggling work and breastfeeding: effects of maternity leave and occupational characteristics. *Pediatrics*. 2009;123:e38–e46.

26. Guendelman S, Pearl M, Graham S, Angulo V, Kharrazi M. Utilization of pay-in antenatal leave among working women in Southern California. *Matern Child Health J*. Jan 2006;10(1):63–73.

27. National Partnership for Women and Families. Written testimony of Debra Ness for the Committee on Health, Education, Labor, and Pensions Subcommittee on Children and Families. Writing the Next Chapter of the Family and Medical Leave Act – Building on a Fifteen Year History of Support for Workers. February 13, 2008; Available from: http://www.nationalpartnership.org/site/DocServer/DebraNess_WrittenTestimony_2-13-08.pdf?docID=2941. Accessed February 16, 2011.

Chapter 20

Chapter 21

Hematology/Oncology

Michael Feuerstein, PhD and Gina L. Bruns, MA

The opinions and assertions contained herein are the private views of the authors and are not to be construed as being official or as reflecting the views of the Uniformed Services University of the Health Sciences or the Department of Defense.

More so than ever, because of earlier detection and more targeted treatments, cancer patients are able to work during or soon after their primary treatment. While cancer remains a life-threatening diagnosis, more patients are living longer and fuller lives than in the past. This fuller life means that work remains a goal for some patients and requires direct attention by providers. Work is often viewed as an important component of one's self-esteem.[1] Work is often a source of social support and for most provides necessary income. Work is also viewed by many as a useful distraction from the concerns that cancer survivors can experience and a place for accomplishment and self-worth.[2]

Given the importance of work in those with cancer, a recent meta-analysis of a heterogeneous group of patients who were employed at the time of diagnosis indicated that the pooled relative risk of unemployment for this group was 1.37 (95% CI = 1.21 – 1.55).[3] The percentage of unemployment for the cancer survivors was 33.8% while it was only 15.2% in the healthy controls. While not all cancer survivors can or choose to return to work posttreatment, we see from this large-scale analysis that a substantial difference in unemployment exists.

Many factors enter into a decision to *continue* to work following a diagnosis of cancer and may include the need to maintain health insurance, replace the income lost during the treatment for cancer, or cover both medical and nonmedical expenses related to diagnosis and treatment.[4] Similarly, myriad factors enter into a decision to *stop* working, including union membership, attaching less value to work, having children under the age of 18 in the household, being employed part-time, and earning a low income.[5] *Return to work* as an outcome has received the most attention in the cancer and work literature. A review of this literature indicates that a nonsupportive work environment and a job that involves manual labor are consistently associated with lower return-to-work rates.[6] However, return to work is not the only outcome the physician needs to consider. Other work-related problems such as the survivor's confidence in his or her ability to work, changes in work performance, and the likelihood of remaining at work (work retention) can also be affected by immediate, longer term, and late effects of cancer and its treatment.[7,8]

Factors that Influence Return-to-Work Decisions

At this stage of knowledge related to work and cancer, the prognostic factors identified do not represent traditional causal or risk factors and red flags. However, they are associated with various work outcomes, and providers should be aware of this in follow-up visits when talking with patients who indicate they are experiencing some type of challenge related to work. While there are many matters to cover in follow-up visits, a quick question about work can reveal problems that are often not considered. In a rare prospective study, Verbeek et al. identified independent risk factors for failure to return to work, including: blood, lymph, lung, CNS, or head-neck cancer; chemotherapy and/or radiotherapy exposure; severe fatigue; distress; age (more than 50 years of age); demanding physical work; low self-assessed work ability; leave or benefits lasting less than 12 weeks; little attachment to work; belief that employment does not provide a sense of normalcy; and the absence of frequent communication with one's supervisor.[9]

The only published review of multiple work outcomes (return to work, physical requirements of work, work dysfunction, job characteristics, and hours worked per week) in cancer survivors[10] found that working was influenced by self-perceived overall health, diagnosis, treatment type (toxicity, time from treatment termination), lifestyle habits, and the use of complementary and alternative medicine.

In a recent systematic review, our research group identified a set of variables in the broad areas of health and well-being, symptoms, function, work demands, work environment, policies, procedures, and economic factors that were associated with various work outcomes.[11] The work outcomes included return to work, work ability, work performance, and work retention. A literature search of PubMed and EMBASE included publications from January 2000 to March 2010, English language, studies on humans, and studies on adults. Three sets of terms used in the literature search included: (1) *cancer,*

cancer patient, cancer survivor, or *neoplasm*; (2) *employment, work, work-place, work environment, unemployment, return-to-work, work ability, work performance, work retention*, or *work demands*; and (3) *model, health, function, symptoms, policy, terms, conditions*, or *procedure*. Articles were removed if they were not original articles, lacked a control group or were not quantitative, did not investigate adult cancer patients and/or survivors, and were not related to at least one of the cancer and work topics in the conceptual framework.

This literature search yielded the following results. Lower levels of perceived ability to perform work tasks in cancer survivors is related to high levels of anxiety, the presence of comorbid diagnoses, and exposure to chemotherapy.[12,13] In contrast, greater perceived ability to work was related to maintaining the same job as prior to cancer diagnosis, a strong commitment to the work organization, and a good social climate at work.[12,13] Work performance (eg, varied working hours, sick leave due to cancer) is lower in cancer survivors than healthy controls,[14–18] especially among survivors who are older, experience fatigue, or report hot flashes.[7,17,19] Despite the reported work performance deficits, there is no evidence that existing work demands are met by survivors at a lesser rate than in noncancer controls. As would be expected, the presence of employer-sponsored health insurance is related to work retention postdiagnosis.[20] Cancer is also related to increased likelihood of retirement (especially among CNS, leukemia, and uterine cancer survivors) when compared to noncancer control groups.[21,22] Table 21-1 provides a convenient summary of factors to keep in mind based on our literature search.

Most broadly, a cancer survivor more than 50 years old is at increased risk of unemployment, working less hours, and reporting higher job demands.[5,17,20,23,24] As time from treatment increases, cancer survivors are more likely to maintain employment.[25,26] Health status is also important in that those with comorbid conditions are more likely to experience a change in work[12] and a higher level of impaired work ability.[13] A negative general health perception is related to unemployment.[26–28] Cognitive impairment, depression, pain, and physical functioning are all related to unemployment.[22,23,26,27,29] It is important to note that in the literature, distress, depression, and anxiety are typically indicated as being at a sub-threshold level, so sub-threshold levels of depression are related to heightened rates of unemployment. Fatigue and hot flashes are negatively related to work performance.[14,30] Additionally, several studies have demonstrated that poor mental health,[27,31,32] poor social functioning,[26,27] and decreased vitality[26,27,32] are all associated with higher rates of unemployment. The directionality of all these associations is currently unknown. However, mitigation of either end of this relationship should improve employment, vitality, mental health, and social functioning.

Chapter 21

Table 21-1 Literature Summary of "Red Flags" and Work Outcomes

Indicators of Work Outcome	Outcomes
Demographics	
Older cancer survivors (50–60) at time of diagnosis	↑ Unemployment[23]
Older cancer survivors (≥50)	↑ Job demands[43]
Older cancer survivors (50–59)	↑ Stopped working/changed jobs due to sequelae[19]
	↑ Unemployment[5]
Older cancer survivors (55–65) with new cancers	↓ Hours worked[17]
	↓ Full-time employment[17]
Older cancer survivors (55–64) with no job-related health insurance	↑ Unemployment[20]
	↑ Change jobs[20]
	↑ Move from full-time to part-time status[20]
Older cancer survivors (55–64)	↑ Managerial/professional/technical jobs[20]
Younger cancer survivors (<60 years old)	↑ Sick leave[19]
Older cancer survivors (≥60 years old)	↓ Daily activities limited due to sequelae[19]
Females (55–65) with new cancers	↓ Employment[17]
Older female survivors (≥55)	↑ Self-employed[44]
	↓ Confidence in finding new job[44]
Females	↓ Job control[43]
	↑ Job strain[43]
Older male survivors (≥50)	↑ Job demands[43]
Single marital status	↑ Disability[19]
Married	↑ Unemployment[45]
Treatment and Health	
3–4 years postdiagnosis	↑ Unemployment[45]
↑ Time from treatment (from 6 months to 18 months posttreatment)	↓ Job loss[25]
5–10 years posttreatment (vs >10 years)	↑ Daily activities limited due to sequelae[19]
Stages I & II (vs III)	↑ Work limitations[7]
↑ Comorbidity	↑ Work changes[12]
	↑ Impaired work ability[12,13]
Radiotherapy or endocrine therapy	↑ Stopped working/changed jobs due to sequelae[19]
Chemotherapy	↑ Work capacity (vs. surgery)[25]
	↑ Impaired work ability[13]
↓ General health perception	↑ Unemployment[26–28]
New cancer event	↑ Work cessation[5]

(Continued)

Table 21-1 *(Continued)*

Symptom Burden	
↑ Cognitive impairment (objective)	↑ Unemployment[29]
↑ Cognitive complaints (subjective)	↑ Unemployment[29]
↑ Self-reported memory problems	↑ Unemployment[29]
↑ Depression	↑ Unemployment[22,23]
↑ Fatigue	↑ Work limitations[8] ↓ Work performance[7]
↑ Pain	↑ Unemployment[26,27]
↓ Physical functioning	↑ Unemployment[26,27]
↑ Physical role limitations	↑ Unemployment[26,27]
↑ Hot Flashes	↓ Work performance[7]
Psychological Functioning and Well-Being	
↓ Emotional well-being	↑ Unemployment[14] ↑ Missing days of work[14]
↓ Existential well-being	↑ Unemployment[30]
↓ Functional well-being	↑ Unemployment[14]
↓ Physical well-being	↑ Unemployment[14] ↑ Missing days of work[14]
↓ Social well-being	↑ Missing days of work[14]
↑ Commitment to the work organization	↓ Impaired work ability[13]
↑ Good social climate at work	↓ Impaired work ability[13]
↓ Mental health	↑ Unemployment[27,31,32]
↑ Neuroticism	↓ Working capacity[25] ↓ Work ability[12]
↑ Quality of life	↑ Skill level of occupation[46] ↓ Disability[22] ↓ Work changes[12]
↑ Health-related quality of life	↑ Employment[26]
↑ Optimisism	↑ Work engagement[47]
↑ Role functioning due to emotional limitations	↑ Employment[26]
↑ Self-role	↑ Employment[25]
↓ Social functioning	↑ Unemployment[26,27]
↓ Vitality	↑ Unemployment[26,27,32]

↑ = increase
↓ = decrease

Intervention Options

Both a consideration of the influence of symptom burden and an appreciation of the workplace challenges the patient experiences as a result of cancer and its treatment can be helpful in forming an accurate picture of the individual's work situation. With this information, the physician can take necessary steps toward helping the survivor achieve a positive work experience.

At present, there is insufficient knowledge to develop evidence-based guidelines that facilitate improvements in work outcomes such as return to work, work ability, performance, or retention. A systematic review of return-to-work interventions in breast cancer survivors indicates that the literature is sparse.[33] In a review of 100 potential articles, only four studies met the inclusion criteria, and only one of these four used a control group. Return-to-work rates were quite high following interventions (75%–85%); however, the lack of control groups makes it difficult to conclude it was the intervention that led to the effect. The rehabilitation approaches highlighted in the review included group counseling, training of physical capacity, and encouragement to regain social activities. The one study that did use a control group[34] demonstrated that simple counseling, with a focus on the importance of engaging in work, along with social activities and advice on exercise significantly improved return-to-work rates 12 to 18 months post-surgery (counseling group 76%, control group 54%).

A Practical Approach

Because an active work life can be an important aspect of surviving cancer, the approach depicted in Figure 21-1 was generated to aid the physician in responding to this concern.

The approach includes three broad areas. The first is sufficient for most patients and includes identification of the red flags that can indicate problems either returning to work or maintaining an optimum level of productivity at work. Consistent with the review conducted for this chapter, the areas listed in Figure 21-1 represent areas that have consistently appeared in the literature. When the patient exhibits any of these red flags, the next step in Figure 21-1 is to ask a few more detailed questions as you would for any potential problem area. These questions should include an examination of the desire to work, expectations regarding work, possible barriers, and the person's ability to cope with a potentially stressful work situation. As with any assessment, feedback to the cancer patient and/or survivor is imperative. Each of the "yes" or "no" questions answered at this stage can guide a physician into one of the options for the third step.

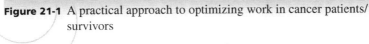

Figure 21-1 A practical approach to optimizing work in cancer patients/survivors

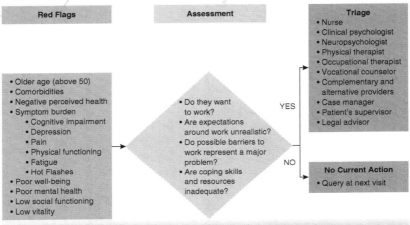

Step 3 in Figure 21-1 demonstrates that either consultation is deemed necessary or there does not appear to be a need for triage at the current time. However, in the case of no intervention necessary, follow-up on work concerns may need to be explored on future patient visits. Some work-related problems may be managed simply by discussion and some joint problem solving. One specific area in which the provider can initiate assistance to the survivor is in providing simple information regarding when and how to return to work. Previous research has shown that the provision of a simple informational pamphlet led to higher return-to-work rates in contrast to other samples that did not provide such information.[35] In a qualitative study of employed cancer survivors, they reported that a good relationship with their employer or manager was a major influence on return to work.[36] A brief discussion (with patient's consent) with a patient's employer or manager may also be helpful.

If a referral is necessary, there are many health care providers in the community who can offer problem specific care. For example, if there is a discrepancy between the patient's current level of physical capacity in relation to the work demands of the job and this mismatch seems modifiable, a physical therapist with workplace experience should be able to assist this patient. In the case of memory, organizational, or attention problems in relation to the type of work required, a clinical psychologist or neuropsychologist with experience in work-related rehabilitation can help the cancer survivor improve work outcomes.

Vocational counseling (state funded or private) represents another potential option, particularly when the patient cannot return to his or her former job. In two cross-sectional retrospective studies using administrative data from the national Rehabilitation Services Administration database, vocational services provided at no cost to the qualified applicant by the state (eg, counseling, miscellaneous training, rehabilitation technology services, job placement services, job search assistance, on-the-job support, maintenance services) were associated with improved work outcomes for young adult and adult cancer survivors.[37,38]

Although often not a simple process, employment laws such as those associated with the Americans With Disabilities Act (ADA)[39] can help the cancer survivor with the process of initiating and complying with reasonable accommodations that can reduce barriers to return to work or increase work ability and performance. However, it needs to be realized that despite this law, there is a higher level of perceived discrimination on the part of cancer survivors related to job loss, insurance, raises, and promotions when compared to other chronic illness groups.[40] Focus group studies indicate employers need more accurate information to dispel preconceptions about hiring and retaining people with a number of medical illnesses.[41] There are specific resources that provide information to cancer survivors at no cost, which can help cancer survivors either experiencing or attempting to prevent legal problems in the workplace (eg, Cancer Legal Resource Center: https://www.disabilityrightslegalcenter.org/about/cancerlegalresource.cfm). Being aware of these resources is important because workplace accommodations and disclosure of cancer survivorship in the workplace is related to maintaining employment.[42]

Risk

Risk in cancer survivors may be due to chemotherapy. If there is physical exam or electrodiagnostic test evidence of chemotherapy associated peripheral neuropathy, balance may be impaired, and restrictions that would prevent climbing to heights may be indicated. If corticosteroids or chemotherapy have resulted in osteoporosis, restrictions to prevent pathologic fracture may be indicated (limited climbing to heights, limited heavy lifting, etc). As long as immune system suppression exists after treatment, patients should be restricted from working with sick animals or humans and from fungal exposure (eg, gardening).

Capacity

Patients may have residual myopathy after chemotherapy, and functional testing may be indicated to quantitate residual functional capacity. Some chemotherapy agents have cardiac and pulmonary toxicity, and treadmill testing of exercise ability may be helpful to establish current ability. Similarly, some cancer surgery (eg, pneumonectomy) will decrease cardio-pulmonary function (capacity for work or exercise). Similarly, anemia may be significant during and after chemotherapy, and treadmill exercise testing can give both the physician and the patient an idea about exercise or work capacity.

Tolerance

Patients undergoing chemotherapy and/or radiation therapy typically have symptoms like nausea, diarrhea, and fatigue that are clearly due to their treatment, and in Western society these symptoms are traditionally judged to be severe enough to justify certification of work absence during the active phase of cancer treatment. Despite these symptoms, many of the self-employed and uninsured return to work.

Summary

While the evidence base for improving work outcomes in cancer survivors is limited at present, there is a body of literature that can guide efforts to assist those cancer survivors in need of some attention related to work out-comes. Cancer care and overall medical management of cancer survivors should at least consider the work-related concerns of patients. This can be done in a reasonable time frame during follow-up visits and thoughtful tri-age. The present chapter provides an approach that should help optimize work outcomes in cancer survivors.

References

1. Peteet JR. Cancer and the meaning of work. *Gen Hosp Psychiatry*. 2000;22: 200–205.

2. Main DS, Nowels CT, Cavender TA, Etschmaier M, Steiner JF. A qualitative study of work and work return in cancer survivors. *Psycho-Oncology*. 2005; 14:992–1004.

3. de Boer AGEM, Taskila T, Ojajarvi A, van Dijk FJH, Verbeek JHAM. Cancer survivors and unemployment: a meta-analysis and meta-regression. *JAMA*. 2009;301(7):753–762.

4. Short PF, Vasey JJ, Tunceli K. Employment pathways in a large cohort of adult cancer survivors. *Cancer*. 2005;103(6):1292–1301.

5. Drolet M, Maunsell E, Brisson J, Brisson C, Masse B, Deschenes L. Not work-ing 3 years after breast cancer: predictors in a population-based study. *J Clin Oncol*. 2005;23(33):8305–8312.

Chapter 21

6. Spelten ER, Sprangers MAG, Verbeek JHAM. Factors reported to influence the return to work of cancer survivors: a literature review. *Psycho-Oncology.* 2002;11:124–131.

7. Lavigne JE, Griggs JJ, Tu XM, Lerner DJ. Hot flashes, fatigue, treatment exposures and work productivity in breast cancer survivors. *J Cancer Survivorship.* 2008;2(4):296–302.

8. Hansen JA, Feuerstein M, Calvio LC, Olsen CH. Breast cancer survivors at work. *J Occup Environ Med.* 2008;50(7):777–784.

9. Verbeek J, de Boer A, Taskila T. Primary and occupational health care providers. In: Feuerstein M, ed. *Work and Cancer Survivors.* New York, NY: Springer; 2009.

10. Steiner JF, Cavender TA, Main DS, Bradley CJ. Assessing the impact of cancer on work outcomes: what are the research needs? *CANCER.* 2004;101(8): 1703–1711.

11. Feuerstein M, Todd BL, Moskowitz M, et al. Work and cancer survivors: a conceptual framework. *J Cancer Surviv.* 2010;4(4):415–437.

12. Gudbergsson SB, Fossa SD, Dahl AA. A study of work changes due to cancer in tumor-free primary-treated cancer patients. A NOCWO Study. *Supportive Care in Cancer.* 2008;16(10):1163–1171.

13. Taskila T, Martikainen R, Hietanen P, Lindbohm ML. Comparative study of work ability between cancer survivors and their referents. *Eur J Cancer.* 2007;43:914–920.

14. Avis NE, Crawford S, Manuel J. Quality of life among younger women with breast cancer. *J Clin Oncol.* 2005;23(15):3322–3330.

15. Chirikos TN, Russell-Jacobs A, Cantor AB. Indirect economic effects of long-term breast cancer survival. *Cancer Practice.* 2002;10(5):248–255.

16. Feuerstein M, Hansen JA, Calvio LC, Johnson L, Ronquillo LG. Work productivity in brain tumor survivors. *J Occup Environ Med.* 2007;49(7):803–811.

17. Short PF, Vasey JJ, Moran JR. Long-term effects of cancer survivorship on the employment of older workers. *Health Serv Res.* 2008;43(1):193–210.

18. Yabroff KR, Lawrence WF, Clauser S, Davis WW, Brown ML. Burden of illness in cancer survivors: findings from a population-based national sample. *J Natl Cancer Inst.* 2004;96(17):1322–1330.

19. Peuckmann V, Ekholm O, Sjogren P, et al. Health care utilisation and characteristics of long-term breast cancer survivors: nationwide survey in Denmark. *Eur J Cancer.* 2009;45:625–633.

20. Tunceli K, Short PF, Moran JR, Tunceli O. Cancer survivorship, health insurance, and employment transitions among older workers. *Inquiry.* 2009;46(1):17–32.

21. Taskila-Abrandt T, Pukkala E, Martikainen R, Karjalainen A, Hietanen P. Employment status of Finnish cancer patients in 1997. *Psycho-Oncology.* 2005;14(3):221–226.

22. Bradley S, Rose S, Lutgendorf S, Costanzo E, Anderson B. Quality of life and mental health in cervical and endometrial cancer survivors. *Gynecol Oncol.* 2006;100:479–486.

23. Carlsen K, Dalton SO, Diderichsen F, Johansen C. Risk for unemployment of cancer survivors: a Danish cohort study. *Eur J Cancer.* 2008;44:2866–1874.

24. Gudbergsson SB, Fossa SD, Sanne B, Dahl AA. A controlled study of job strain in primary-treated cancer patients without metastases. *Acta Oncologica.* 2007;46(4):534–544.

25. Chan YM, Ngan HY, Yip PS, Li BY, Lau OW, Tang GW. Psychosocial adjustment in gynecologic cancer survivors: a longitudinal study on risk factors for maladjustment. *Gynecol Oncol.* 2001;80(3):387–394.

26. Fang FM, Chiu HC, Kuo WR, et al. Health-related quality of life for nasopharyngeal carcinoma patients with cancer-free survival after treatment. *Int J Radiat Oncol Biol Phys.* 2002;53(4):959–968.

27. Fleer J, Hoekstra HJ, Sleijfer DT, Tuinman MA, Klip EC, Hoekstra-Weebers JEHM. Quality of life of testicular cancer survivors and the relationship with sociodemographics, cancer-related variables, and life events. *Supportive Care in Cancer.* 2006;14:251–259.

28. Hewitt M, Roland JH, Yancik R. Cancer survivors in the United States: age, health, and disability. *J Gerontol.* 2003;58(1):82–91.

29. Harder H, Cornelissen JJ, vVan Gool AR, Duivenvoorden HJ, Eijkenboom WMH, van den Bent MJ. Cognitive functioning and quality of life in long-term adult survivors of bone marrow transplantation. *Cancer.* 2002;95:183–192.

30. Shin HW, Noh DY, Lee ES, et al. Correlates of existential well-being and their association with health-related quality of life in breast cancer survivors compared with the general population. *Breast Cancer Res Treatment.* 2009;118:139–150.

31. Fang FM, Tsai WL, Chien CY, Chiu HC, Wang CJ. Health-related quality of life outcome for oral cancer survivors after surgery and postoperative radiotherapy. *Jpn J Clin Oncol.* 2004;34(11):641–646.

32. Mols F, Aaronson NK, Vingerhoets AJJM, et al. Quality of life among long-term non-Hodgkin lymphoma survivors. *Cancer.* 2007;109:1659–1667.

33. Hoving JL, Broekhuizen MLA, Frings-Dresen MHW. Return to work of breast cancer survivors: a systematic review of intervention studies. *BMC Cancer.* 2009;9:117–126.

34. Maguire P, Brooke M, Tait C, Sellwood RR. The effect of counseling on physical and social recovery after mastectomy. *Clin Oncol.* 1983;9:319–324.

35. Nieuwenhuijsen K, Bos-Ransdorp B, Uitterhoeve LLJ, Sprangers MAG, Verbeek JHAM. Enhanced provider communication and patient education regarding return to work in cancer survivors following curative treatment: a pilot study. *J Occup Rehabil.* 2006;16:647–657.

36. Amir Z, Neary D, Luker K. Cancer survivors' view of work 3 years post diagnosis: a UK perspective. *Eur Jour Oncol Nurs.* 2008;12:190–197.

37. Chan F, Strauser D, Cardoso EdS, Zheng LX, Chan JYC, Feuerstein M. State vocational services and employment in cancer survivors. *Journal of Cancer Survivorship.* 2008;2:169–178.

38. Strauser D, Feuerstein M, Chan F, Arango J, Cardoso EdS, Chiu C-Y. Vocational services associated with competitive employment in 18–25 year old cancer survivors. *J Cancer Survivorship.* in press.

39. ADA. American Disability Act. Job Accommodation Network: Report to Congress on the Job Accommodation 1990.

40. Feuerstein M, Luff GM, Harrington CB, Olsen CH. Pattern of workplace disputes in cancer survivors: a population study of ADA claims. *J Cancer Survivorship.* 2007;1:185–192.

41. Grizzard WR. Meeting demand-side expectations and needs. Paper presented at: APA 15th Anniversary Seminar 2005; Washington, DC.

42. Pryce J, Munir F, Haslam C. Cancer survivorship and work: symptoms, supervisor response, co-worker disclosure and work adjustment. *J Occup Rehabil.* 2007;17(1):83–92.

43. Gudbergsson SB FS, Sanne B, Dahl AA. A controlled study of job strain in primary-treated cancer patients without metastases. *Acta Oncologica.* 2007.46(4):534–44.

44. Norredam M, Meara E, Landrum MB, Huskamp HA, Keating NL. Financial status, employment, and insurance among older cancer survivors. *J Gen Intern Med.* 2009;24(Suppl 2):438–445.

45. Syse A, Tretli S, Kravdal O. Cancer's impact on employment and earnings - a population-based study from Norway. *J Cancer Survivorship.* 2008;2:149–158.

46. Awadalla AW, Ohaeri JU, Gholoum A, Khalid AOA, Hamad HMA, Jacob A. Factors associated with quality of life of outpatients with breast cancer and gynecologic cancers and their family caregivers: a controlled study. *BMC Cancer.* 2007;7:102–116.

47. Hakanen JJ, Lindbohm ML. Work engagement among breast cancer survivors and the referents: the importance of optimism and social resources at work. *J Cancer Survivorship.* 2008;2(4):283–295.

Chapter 22

Working With Common Psychiatric Problems

Joel Steinberg, MD

This chapter, like most other chapters in this book, will focus on risk assessment, capacity, and tolerance. First, however, there are two other important considerations.

1. Analogous to what is describes in Chapter 23, Working with Common Functional Syndromes: Fibromyalgia and Chronic Fatigue Syndrome, mental health problems and conditions are collections of symptoms. The diagnostic system used by mental health professionals in the United States is the *Diagnostic and Statistical Manual*, fourth edition, text revision (DSM IV-TR).[1] Like fibromyalgia and chronic fatigue syndrome, mental health diagnoses are also based on collections of symptoms and are not based on objectively establishing the presence of an underlying etiology or pathophysiologic disorder. Diagnoses made by reviewing a group of symptoms are called *syndromic diagnoses*. Most other medical specialties deal with well-defined and measurable pathophysiologic conditions and/or conditions with a definite etiology and/or a measurable difference or distinction from the normal. Diseases diagnosed on the basis of specific pathophysiology, laboratory abnormalities, and results of objective testing frequently have more predictable levels of expected symptom severity and disease trajectory. Symptom severity of non-syndromic medical conditions frequently is proportional to the known underlying pathophysiology.

2. Generally speaking, as stated, there is no currently proven underlying pathophysiology for most conditions that we call mental illnesses (Introduction, pp xxx-xxxi).[1] Correspondingly, there are no objective findings on physical examination or routine laboratory studies to document the presence of any given condition and/or its severity. Cause is often not something that can be established with any reasonable

degree of certainty in most categories of mental illness because mental illnesses are syndromic diagnoses, not diagnoses that deal with causation. (Exceptions include some neurologic conditions listed in DSM IV-TR—conditions designated as "due to a general medical condition," heritable conditions, and probably some of the dementing disorders, to name a few.)

Psychological testing is as close as we can currently come to getting objective data in the mental health field, although promising technology in the form of advanced neuroimaging is in various stages of development and may prove helpful in the future. Further discussion on this topic is beyond the scope of this text. Furthermore, the American Psychiatric Association is in the process of revising the *Diagnostic and Statistical Manual*, so much of the current terminology may be modified, at least to some extent, in the near future. As understanding increases, some conditions that were once defined as mental illness (eg, homosexuality, which in the earliest editions of the DSM was considered a mental disorder) no longer are. New conditions may be described. Conditions may be refined, combined, or divided into more than one diagnostic entity.

Regardless, in the mental health field a diagnosis reveals very little about the degree of impairment. The determination about whether a person with a given diagnosis can work or not has to do in large part with the level of severity of the existing impairment (symptoms) and the risks and remaining capacities associated with the diagnosed condition. When mental problems are not associated with substantial impairment in activities of daily living (ADLs), typically the mental health problem(s) is/are not work prohibitive. Clearly, even patients who have significant psychotic disorders can stabilize with medication and be gainfully employed over many years.

Beginning with DSM-III (1980), a multiaxial diagnostic system has been used with a descriptive approach. The descriptive approach attempted to be neutral with respect to theories of etiology (Introduction, p xxxvi).[1] DSM-IV-TR offers that "a compelling literature documents that there is much 'physical' in 'mental' and much 'mental' in 'physical' disorders," (Introduction, p xxx). It also instructs, "All medical conditions are defined on various levels of abstraction—for example, structural pathology (eg, ulcerative colitis), symptom presentation (eg, migraine), deviance from a physiological norm (eg, hypertension), and etiology (eg, pneumococcal pneumonia). Disorders have also been defined by a variety of concepts (eg, inflexibility, irrationality, distress, dysfunction, dyscontrol, disadvantage, disability, syndromal pattern, etiology, and statistical deviation).

Confounding Factors

The DSM-IV offers the following comment (Introduction, p xxxi): "Neither deviant behavior (eg, political, religious, or sexual) nor conflicts that are primarily between the individual and society are mental disorders unless the deviance or conflict is a symptom or a dysfunction in the individual . . ." and finally, importantly, it states, "[i]n DSM-IV, there is no assumption that each category of the mental disorder is a complete entity with absolute boundaries dividing it from other mental disorders or from another mental disorder. There is also no assumption that all individuals described as having the same mental disorder are alike in important ways."

Severity

The DSM-IV[1] clarifies (Introduction, p xxxiii): ". . . assignment of a particular diagnosis does not imply a specific level of impairment or disability . . . a diagnosis does not carry any necessary implications regarding the causes of disorder or its associated impairments. Inclusion of a disorder classification (as in medicine generally) does not require that there be knowledge about its etiology." Lastly, it cautions on that page that the "use of DSM-IV in forensic settings should be informed by an awareness of the risks and limitations discussed above."

Exaggeration

Importantly, because there are no objective correlates for most mental health disorders, issues of symptom exaggeration are potentially ubiquitous. The degree of exaggeration can range from mild all the way to frank malingering, and can be produced by conscious intent or via unconscious processes. Some mental health professionals and other scholars even have declared that mental illness itself as a category of illness, is a myth.[2] Estimates vary as to how frequently exaggeration/malingering is an issue, but particularly in circumstances where workers' compensation, disability, and personal injury are concerned, estimates range to as high as 30% to 50% of all cases.[3] Clues about exaggeration/malingering can be obtained from data reported in the physical exam (eg, presence of Waddell's signs, a positive Hoover's test, etc) and variations in histories recorded by various prior interviewers. More definitive data regarding mental health issues and these potential exaggeration/malingering problems can often be determined with the benefit of results from psychological testing, and, in particular, symptom validity testing.[4]

Individuals often provide less accurate histories than their records, possibly owing to poor recall at times, but sometimes the inaccuracies occur purposely.[5,6] Discrepancies between various renditions of the history should be addressed. Hints of a longstanding mental disorder(s) (that may very well be manifestations of an underlying personality disorder) include a failure to complete high school, a general discharge or worse from the military, a discontinuous work history, antisocial behavior with or without a history of criminal justice involvement, lengthy periods of unemployment, and/or lack of social support.*

Exaggerated behavior may stem from either conscious or unconscious psychiatric pathology. Signs on physical exam that may suggest an underlying psychosocial issue include multiple and/or florid signs of exaggerated or magnified illness behavior; discrepancies such as a difference between supine and seated straight leg raising; bizarre responses and complaints; inexplicable findings (Waddell's signs and a positive Hoover test are mentioned above), etc. Psychiatric disorders are not likely to occur for the first time in the time period shortly after an injury, although a person may attempt to link the two—more plausible alternatives may be that there was a pre-existing mental condition. "Desperation surgery" and even "minimally invasive surgery" typically lead to poor results in people with longstanding or even just recently developed illness behavior.

Risk

In terms of risk, the major risks of returning someone to work who has a mental illness involve issues of potential violent or aggressive behaviors and also issues of possible injury due to inattention and/or poor judgment. Aggressive behaviors can potentially be directed against persons, meaning assaultive, suicidal, or homicidal behaviors, or directed against property. Statistics show that in the absence of paranoia and substance abuse, even profound mental illnesses like schizophrenia do not show any meaningful increase over the general population in the incidence of violence toward other persons.[7] The presence of paranoid ideation does increase the risk of violence, however. So do certain agents used by drug abusers, especially methamphetamine. The available information also shows that most if not all mental illnesses are attenuated or ameliorated by work. That is to say that work has a salutary effect on people with mental illnesses.[8–10]

Hence the risk of worsening the mental illness by returning a given person to work is usually not serious, and it is generally outweighed by the potential benefits of being back in the workplace. Clearly, there are benefits with respect to socialization and being part of a peer group, but beyond that,

---

* Wiley, Susan, MD. Deception and Detection in Psychiatric Diagnosis. Psychiatric Clinics of North America, Vol 21, #4, Dec. 1998.

epidemiologic data indicate that physical health status—including longevity—is improved in members of the workforce when compared to their nonworking counterparts.[11]

One of the best ways to assess risk of violence is the personal history of the person being evaluated. A history of violence, and particularly repeated violence, establishes a higher risk for repeat violent behaviors. In this situation, the past is one of the best ways to predict the future. Of course, that does not mean that any current threats of violence from persons without a history of violence should be disregarded. Threats of violence cannot be disregarded, and assessment may be beyond the level of expertise of the nonmental health care provider. Generally, as might be expected, patients who have no history of violence are much less likely to manifest violent behavior in the present, while those with a history of violence are more likely to repeat this pattern. Paranoia and the use of certain kinds of drug, especially if specific persons are identified as part of the menacing scheme(s), should raise red flags, as mentioned above. Another risk factor that must be considered is that problems with attention, concentration, and judgment may lead to injuries to the person or to co-workers, or to property damage.

Specific Risk Issues:

- Paranoid schizophrenia and delusional disorders would be rational reasons for permanent disqualification from safety-sensitive jobs like police officer or any job that provides access to weapons or classified information. Similarly, commercial driving and airplane piloting would be precluded by the Department of Transportation regulations. Other jobs in which other people depend on the performance of the patient (physician, nurse, explosive material manager, and so-called safety-sensitive jobs) would also be prohibited with these disorders.

- Individuals expressing homicidal ideation, if directed toward coworkers, should not return to that workplace. These situations may require consideration of psychiatric hospitalization and warning of intended victims. The "Tarasoff duty to warn" preempts patient consent to release medical information. Most states provide for this as an exception to physician-patient and psychiatrist-patient confidentiality.

- Pedophilia and antisocial behavior would usually preclude return to work for teachers, guidance counselors, or coaches. Individuals with these disorders can work, but they require supervised structured jobs and ongoing treatment.

Capacity

Safety (risk) is an overriding consideration, and these risk factors must be taken into account when determining a patient's status. After risk has been considered, capacity issues or work limitations are then considerations. Capacity issues include difficulties with attention, concentration, judgment, etc, that stem from the underlying mental condition and the additional effects on these functions from medications used to treat the condition or other health conditions. Problems in these areas of functioning may impair work attendance, work performance, and work safety (risk). Jobs that are familiar, simple, and/or jobs that do not require sustained or high levels of attention or multitasking are less difficult to adapt to when these problems are present.

Tolerance

Looking at the issue of tolerance, motivation is one of the chief factors determining who tolerates (chooses to) work and who does not tolerate (chooses not to) work. As indicated above, work has a beneficial effect on most mental illnesses: improvement in the mental health condition is to be expected with work. Interpersonal conflict with supervisors or coworkers can masquerade as depression or anxiety, but are not in themselves reasons to certify work absence for a mental disorder.

Assessment

In many chapters of this book, it is clear that symptoms without objective findings generally should be thought of as properly being assessed in the category of tolerance—whether or not a patient will (choose to) tolerate symptoms that are generated or exacerbated by work. It is to be hoped that the reader will ask him- or herself, "Is there any reason that mental health symptomatology should be thought of differently?" In the previous edition of this book, it may have been suggested that symptoms associated with psychiatric syndromes should be given high weight and credibility. Yet it is well known, as is pointed out above, that exaggeration is a crucial problem in mental health assessments, and in fact even well-trained mental health professionals are not particularly reliable at discerning the difference between true symptoms versus exaggerated symptoms or malingering.[12]

Prognosis

Statistics demonstrate that approximately 50% of people out of work for 8 weeks or more will not return to work, and more than 85% of persons off work for 6 months or more will never return to work on a sustained basis.[13–14]

Work Cessation

Disability can be thought of as a disease in and of itself. Disabled workers do not enjoy life, and they die earlier than their working counterparts. Disability can place a substantial burden on society, both financially and in terms of overutilization of medical and mental health services. Generally, returning to work is beneficial and can be thought of as a rehabilitation procedure in and of itself.[9,15] For these reasons alone, every reasonable effort should be devoted to a prompt return to work, even if it is to modified duty status, and to avoid approval of unnecessary time away from work.

Because of the risks and the momentous effects on a given person's life (and the lives of other family members), the decision to place and/or continue a person on out-of-work status because of mental symptoms, for the most part, should be made by mental health professionals who can/should/will pay close attention to issues described in the preceding paragraphs.[13]

Return to Work

Return-to-work decisions can often be made by primary care professionals just as well or better than by mental health professionals because of their familiarity with the overall situation, including personal and family dynamics, and because of the issue of tolerance. As has been emphasized throughout this book, work is beneficial to health and to survival; therefore, any physician or other care provider who can help his or her patient make a decision to return to work is probably acting in the patient's best interest. Analogous to comments made in this book about working after sustaining brain trauma, there is no serious evidence to suggest that working has an adverse effect on the underlying mental health problem(s) in the overwhelming majority of cases.

Help With Assessment of Severity

The physician or other health or mental health care provider has to assess to what degree the currently reported symptomatology impairs the worker. More severe psychiatric symptoms such as homicidal or suicidal thoughts with intent or plan, psychotic or manic symptoms, and profound lethargy or morbid guilt are more reliably associated with significant psychiatric impairment. Often at that level of severity, hospitalization, either voluntary or involuntary, or other forms of intensive treatment are warranted. Usually in these severe cases, there are serious abnormalities of the mental status examination, such as marked disturbance of organization of thought, perception of reality, cognitive functioning, behavior, speech or communication, and/or poor hygiene. More severe impairments of the performance of daily activities such as performing household tasks, driving, reading, shopping, interacting with others, or managing finances are expected accompaniments when there are claims of a disabling level of psychiatric symptomatology.

The description of symptoms should be detailed, including their intensity, frequency, and duration, and specifically how they affect/limit the person's ability to function. For example, if someone reports panic attacks, ideally the symptoms associated with these attacks would be described; how severe they are; how long they last; how frequently they occur; what methods the person has used to try to control them; how successful he or she has been in this endeavor; and how do these attacks affect the person's ability to function. It would be expected that a mental disorder severe enough to prevent performance of all work duties would also cause a notable impairment in most or all other life activities. It would be highly, highly unlikely that a mental disorder would be severe enough to preclude work and yet have little or no impact on activities of daily living and social functioning. Work is typically one of the last areas of functioning to be affected by most mental disorders.

Results of Surveys

Mental health problems are nearly ubiquitous. Large population studies have shown that as many as 30% of any given group of urban dwellers report severe mental illness symptomatology. Milder symptomatology affects far more people than severe illnesses do.[16]

Forty percent of males receiving Social Security disability benefits and 30% of females receiving disability benefits received them because of psychiatric illnesses.[17]

The annual incidence of mental illness in the US is about 22.1 percent of American adults annually or 44.3 million people.[18] In addition, the fourth of the ten leading causes of disability in the United States and other western countries is mental disorders. These include major depression, bipolar disorder, schizophrenia, and obsessive-compulsive disorder.

Confounding Issues

Complaints that derive from issues like conflicts with a supervisor, other types of job dissatisfaction, a wish to take time off work for various personal reasons, etc, must be separated from symptoms due to mental illness. These problems are often referred to as psychosocial problems. Many readers will be familiar with the Boeing aircraft study that showed that in terms of back pain, other than a history of prior episodes of back pain, the greatest risk factor for a future complaint of back pain was dissatisfaction with the job, regardless of whether the job was heavy or light in terms of physical requirements.[19] There is no reason to believe that mental health complaints are dissimilar in this respect.

A noncausal relationship—or correlation—exists when a circumstance other than the event in question is responsible for a medical outcome. For example, gray hair and cerebrovascular accidents tend to occur in the same population (because of aging), but they are not connected causally. A large percentage of asymptomatic individuals has significantly abnormal spinal imaging—disc protrusions, facet degeneration, disc degeneration and dehydration, annular tears, spondylosis, spinal stenosis, foraminal stenosis, and congenital deformities. One must be aware of the possibility of unrelated conditions that predated or postdated the alleged causal event(s). The fallacy of post hoc, ergo propter hoc ("after this, therefore because of this") must always be considered. That is to say that an event taking place subsequent to another event is not necessarily a consequence of the preceding event. The temporal relationship of events does not necessarily confirm a causal relationship.

Pain and Mental Issues

Functional somatic syndromes is a term that applies to conditions such as multiple chemical sensitivity, sick building syndrome, repetitive stress injury, side effects of silicone breast implants, chronic whiplash, chronic fatigue syndrome, irritable bowel syndrome, fibromyalgia, and probably to at least some cases of Gulf War Syndrome. Not surprisingly, these syndromes have similar epidemiologic characteristics and are associated with a higher prevalence of psychiatric comorbid conditions.[15]

Commonly people who complain of chronic pain also complain of psychiatric problems, particularly depressive disorders.[20–22] Often these complaints become much more prominent when financial support for physical disability comes to an end ("maximum medical improvement" in workers compensation.) The role of medications, particularly strong opioids and other medications that affect alertness and cognition in their presentation, must also be considered.

Primary care physicians evaluating and treating mental illnesses may want to utilize screening and surveillance instruments for mental illnesses, like the PHQ-9[23] for depression, for example. Such instruments can be useful, but because the meaning of the questions are transparent and because there are no internal validity measures, they may be susceptible to deliberate over-reporting or manipulation by some patients.

Mental Illness and Work

Most mental illnesses do not have an identifiable cause.[24] Criterion 3 of the NIOSH criteria[25] asks: "What evidence, particularly objective, is there that the level of exposure is of the frequency, intensity, and duration to rise to the level that would support a work relatedness determination?" For mental illness, there simply is no objective method for establishing that such a level of exposure actually occurred. Findings from scientific studies have actually made it even more difficult to assert with credibility that adult life experience is a cause of mental illness, by indicating a lack of relationship or an inverse relationship (eg, work seems to be a protective factor against psychological dysfunction rather than a cause of it; psychopathology can be a cause of adult life events rather than vice versa). The burden of proof is on the claimant's or plaintiff's side of the argument. There is a lack of definitive causation science for mental illness as related to the workplace. Involvement in workers' compensation and tort systems leads to worse clinical outcomes (worse than the outcomes obtained with the same health or mental health problems in persons who do not become involved in workers compensation or litigation).[26-28] If work is not the cause of mental illness, then return to that work is usually not a risk to the patient.

It is an ethical violation under both the American Psychiatric Association and the American Psychological Association standards for a treating clinician to offer conclusions about causation (or any other forensic issues).[29-31] Thus, if a treating general medical or mental health professional is tempted to certify a patient with a mental disorder absent from the workplace because of the risk of work making the mental disorder worse (causation) ethical guidelines would require the patient be referred for a forensic evaluation by a nontreating professional for this assessment.

Research findings have indicated that reliance on an examinee's self-reported history is always a less than credible practice because of a tendency for examinees to underreport pre-existing symptoms and because of the tendency for reported histories to be influenced by an examinee's belief about the cause of his or her current problem.[25] Research findings show that these natural human tendencies are compounded by an additional tendency among claimants to endorse an artificially low level of general difficulties for the period of their life that preceded a medico-legal claim (abnormally low compared with nonclaimants).[32] Given such scientific findings, a claimant's self-reported history of preclaim versus postclaim differences in his or her health cannot credibly be used for attempting to establish occupational or tort relevant causation.

In the American Psychiatric Association's guidelines for the assessment of malingering,[1] the guidelines call for consideration of the examinee's level of cooperation with the examination, and psychological testing is one of the objective, standardized, and reliable means of assessing cooperation. In addition, the malingering guidelines call for examiners to consider any discrepancies between subjective complaints and objective findings, and psychological testing can be an important source of objective findings.

Many examining mental health professionals performing evaluations fail to offer an Axis II diagnosis. Personality disorders by definition are relatively fixed ways of behaving that arise in childhood or adolescence and thus long before an adult workplace event. The identification of a personality disorder creates an obstacle to credibly claiming that work and/or experiences at work are the relevant causative factors for any manifestation of distress or impairment. The critical importance of this standard part of the diagnostic process is illustrated by scientific findings that 70% of workers compensation claimants with claims of low back pain were found to have a personality disorder (when the possibility was actually assessed).[33,34] This finding is consistent with a long history of research findings that have revealed a high percentage of personality disorders among patients with chronic pain. The rationale behind such claims of mood disorders secondary to chronic pain involves a belief that injury caused the chronic pain, and chronic pain subsequently caused a mood disorder, thereby establishing occupational or tort relevant causation for the mood disorder. Mood disorders are predictive of a lack of general medical findings for pain complaints, therefore a major shortcoming of such claims is the scientific evidence that the presence of a mood disorder increases the likelihood that there will be no findings to account for the reported pain.[35] Thus, the development of a mood disorder tends to militate against the injury (or any general medical condition) being the cause of the pain complaints. A simultaneous manifestation of chronic pain and a mood disorder tends to move the entire clinical picture away from injury relatedness, rather than justifying a claim of occupational causation for relevant mental illness.

In addition, many nonmental health professionals fail to distinguish between patients being unhappy with life circumstances when they sustain an injury in a job they dislike and the patient actually having a mental illness. Unhappiness with life circumstances is not a major depressive disorder. Clinicians tend to assume that the information provided by the claimant is accurate and free from bias. Usually clinicians do not routinely evaluate for symptom exaggeration or malingering. The health care professional often fails to differentiate between a psychosocial issue and a genuine psychological concern. Psychosocial issues can include workplace interpersonal differences, motivational issues such as job dissatisfaction, inappropriate employee workplace behavior, perceived discrimination, concern about job security, etc.

Mental health concerns represent the fifth leading reason for short-term disability and the third leading cause of long-term disability.[36] By the year 2020, the World Health Organization reported that major depressive disorder will be the number one cause of disability for all ages, globally. Currently major depressive disorder is the second cause of disability for ages 15 to 44 (WHO, 2004). At least 64% of individuals with physical concerns (such as musculoskeletal, cardiac, cancer, stroke, etc) are likely to experience a concurrent mental health concern.[37,38]

Mental Illness and Disability

The US Social Security Disability criteria have been the standard way to evaluate mental illnesses for several editions of the AMA *Guides to the Evaluation of Permanent Impairment* (from the third through the fifth editions). The Sixth Edition of the *Guides*[15] uses different standards. Under the Social Security Administration (SSA) and the former editions of the *Guides* cited, individuals are evaluated along four functional axes:

- Activities of daily living (ADLs);

- The quality of social relationships;

- The ability to maintain pace, persistence, and concentration (ie, work);

- The ability to tolerate stress as measured by the absence of multiple and lengthy episodes of decompensation under stress.

For most mental health conditions, when two or more of these four functional areas are evaluated as markedly impaired, the individual is usually found to be disabled on a categorical basis. The same system was used for impairment rating in the third, fourth, and fifth editions of the *Guides*.

In the sixth edition of the *Guides,* the four functional axis scales are broken down into six scales by dividing social relationships into two different scales and by adding a scale having to do with the ability to travel. Those six areas make up the rating system called the Psychiatric Impairment Rating Scale (PIRS). Other rating system scales include the Global Assessment of Function (GAF) and the Brief Psychiatric Rating System (BPRS). Each of the three scales leads to an impairment value. The criteria for assessing the effect of mental illness (impairment) may help physicians and mental health professionals evaluate claims of work disability due to mental illness.

Bottom Line

Mental health diagnoses are syndromic for the most part. The diagnosis tells very little or nothing about causation, the degree of impairment, or the level of severity of the underlying condition. Basically the risks of working with a mental health diagnosis have to do with the potential for out-of-control aggressive behavior and the results of lapses of attention, concentration, and judgment. When concentration, attention, and judgment are impaired, tasks that can most easily be accomplished are those that are familiar to a given individual and those that are relatively simple. These latter factors of concentration, attention, and judgment also affect capacity. Tolerance and motivation are viewed as two sides of the same coin.

- Work is beneficial to the health and mental health of an individual and to society.

- The longer a given individual is absent from work, the less likely that person is to return to work.

- Reported mental health problems are quite common, yet the vast majority of those with mental health symptoms work every day. Under some conditions nearly 100% of the population may report mental health symptomatology.

- Many reported mental health problems are misrepresented for a variety of reasons, both conscious and unconscious. Evaluation for potential exaggeration issues must be considered in any complete evaluation. Symptom validity testing, especially by use of the forced choice technique and personality tests that contain internal validity scales, are among the best ways to accomplish assessment of these issues.

- The concomitant existence or presence of mental health problems and physical problems and/or work-related problems does not prove cause and effect. Just because one event follows another or occurs simultaneously does not necessarily establish a causal link.

- A suggested set of manifestations of limitations and dysfunctions likely to accompany more severe mental health impairments has been provided in this chapter. Mental illnesses without accompanying major impairment in ADLs are rarely incapacitating in terms of work.

- Continuing to work, even if modifications are necessary, and/or early return to work are desirable for the reasons described above.

- Primary care providers are often the decision makers about both return-to-work issues and disability issues. Such decisions are potentially life-changing events. An appropriate level of concern and consideration is called for. Requests to be placed on disability should be as carefully evaluated as requests for narcotic prescriptions. Staying at work and/or early return to work is critically important to the health and well-being of your patients, whenever it can be accomplished.

- Mental health professionals are available for consultative assistance when these areas are unclear to the primary provider.

Questions to ask if a patient is out of work with a mental disorder:

- What is the DSM diagnosis?

- What symptoms support this diagnosis?

- How does the individual spend his or her time away from work? What activities does the individual still participate in? (Impairment should be in all aspects of life, and not just at work.)

- Is there conflict at work with a supervisor or coworker?

- Could the individual return to work in the same job if work at a different work site or with a different supervisor were available? (If "yes," a mental disorder is not preventing return to work; a personality conflict is the issue.)

- Could the individual return to work in a different job? If "yes," what job?

- Has a psychiatrist been consulted? If not, why not?

References

1. American Psychiatric Association. *Diagnostic and Statistical Manual of Mental Disorders,* 4th ed., text revision. Washington, DC: American Psychiatric Association; 2000.

2. Szaz T. *The Myth of Mental Illness.* New York: Harper & Row; 1961.

3. Sall, Richard E., *Strategies in Workers Compensation.* Lanham, Maryland, 2004.

4. Richmond J., Green P, Gervais R, et al. Objective tests of symptom exaggeration in independent medical examinations. *J Occup Environ Med.* 2006;48:303–311.

5. Don AS, Carragee EJ. Is the self-reported history accurate in patients with persistent axial pain after a motor vehicle accident? *Spine J.* 2009;9:4–12.

6. Barsky AJ. Forgetting, fabricating, and telescoping: the instability of the medical history. *Arch Intern Med.* 2002;162:981–984.

7. Friedman RA. Violence and mental illness—how strong is the link? *NEJM.* 2006;355:2064–2066.

8. Partnership for Workplace Mental Health, a Program of the American Psychiatric Foundation: *Assessing and Treating Psychiatric Occupational Disability.* http://www.workplacementalhealth.org/APDisabilityProjectExecSumm.pdf. Accessed 06/12/2010.

9. Waddell G, Burton AK. Is Work Good for Your Health and Well-being? London: The Stationery Office. 2006. http://www.workingforhealth.gov.uk/documents/is-work-good-for-you.pdf Accessed 06/12/2010.

10. Blustein DL. The Role of Work in Psychological Health and Well-Being: A Conceptual, Historical, and Public Policy Perspective. *Amer Psychologist.* 2008;63(4):228–240.

11. Haralson RH. Forward. In: Melhorn JM, Ackerman WE. *Guides to the Evaluation of Disease and Injury Causation.* Chicago, IL: American Medical Association; 2008.

12. Larrabee, GJ., 2007. *Assessment of Malingered Neuropsychological Deficits.* Oxford Press, New York.

13. *Assessing and Treating Psychiatric Occupational Disability: New Behavioral Health Functional Assessment Tools Facilitate Return to Work* A Report from the Partnership for Workplace Mental Health. Taskforce on Disability and Return to Work. American Psychiatric Foundation. www.workplacementalhealth.org. Assessed 09/10/2010.

14. Pilley MD. How the Primary Care Physician Can Help Negotiate the Return-to-Work Disability Dilemma. In: *A Physician's Guide to Return to Work.* Chicago, IL: American Medical Association; 2005.

15. Melhorn JM, Ackerman WE. *Guides to the Evaluation of Disease and Injury Causation,* Chicago, IL: American Medical Association; 2008.

16. Langner, T. S., and Michael, S.: Life stress and mental health: the Midtown Manhattan Study. Free Press, New York, 1963.

17. Thorlacius, Sigurdur, et al., 2003., Prevalence of disability in Iceland 2001 and comparison with other Nordic countries. *Disability Medicine.* Vol 3, No. 2, April–June 2003.

18. The Numbers Count: NIMH http://www.nimh.nih.gov/health/publications/the-numbers-count-mental-disorders-in-america/index.shtml. Accessed 06/12/2010.

19. Bigos SJ, Battié MC, Spengler DM, et al. A prospective study of work perceptions and psychosocial factors affecting the report of back injury. *Spine.* 1991;16:1–6.

20. Ohayon MM, Schatzberg AF. Chronic pain and major depressive disorder in the general population. *J of Psychiatric Res.* 2010:8; 44(7):454–61.

21. Beesdi K, Jacobi F, Hoyer J, et al. Pain associated with specific anxiety and depressive disorders in a nationally representative population sample. *Soc Psychiat Epidemiol.* 2010; 45:89–104.

Chapter 22

22. Dersh J, Gatchel RJ, Polatin P, et al. Prevalence of psychiatric disorders in patients with chronic disabling occupational spinal disorders. *Spine.* 2006;31:1156–1162.

23. Patient Health Questionnaire-9. http://muskie.usm.maine.edu/clinicalfusion/DHHS/phq9.pdf. Accessed 06/12/2010.

24. Barth RJ. Chapter 16, Mental Illness. In: Melhorn JM, Ackerman WE. *Guides to the Evaluation of Disease and Injury Causation.* Chicago, IL: American Medical Association; 2008.

25. NIOSH publication 79–116. A Guide to the Work-Relatedness of Disease. http://www.cdc.gov/niosh/pdfs/79–116.pdf. Accessed 06/12/2010.

26. Dommerholt J. Persistent myalgia following whiplash. *Curr Pain Headache Rep.* 2005;9(5):326–330.

27. Downs DG. Nonspecific work-related upper extremity disorders. *American Family Physician.* 1997;55:1296–1302.

28. Harris I, Multford J, Solomon M, et al. Association between compensation status and outcome after surgery. *JAMA.* 2005;293:1644–1652.

29. Greenberg SA, Shuman DW. Irreconcilable conflict between therapeutic and forensic rules. *Prof Psychol Res Pr.* 1997:28:50–57.

30. Hales RE, Yudofsky SC. *The American Psychiatric Publishing Textbook of Clinical Psychiatry, Fourth Edition.* Washington, DC: American Psychiatric Publishing; 2002.

31. Barth RJ, Brigham CR. Who is in the better position to evaluate, the treating physician or an independent evaluator? *The Guides Newsletter* 2005 (Sep/Oct):8–11.

32. Lee's-Haley PR, Williams CW, English LT. Response bias in self-reported history of plaintiffs compared with nonlitigating patients. *Psychology Reports.* 1996;79:811–18.

33. Gatchel RJ, Weisberg JN. *Personality Characteristics of Patients with Pain.* Washington, DC: American Psychological Association; 2000.

34. Dersh J, Gatchel RJ, Mayer T, et al. Prevalence of psychiatric disorders in patients with chronic disabling occupational spinal disorders. *Spine.* 2006;31(10):1156–1162.

35. Magni G. On the relationship between chronic pain and depression when there is no organic lesion. *Pain.* 1987;31:1–21.

36. Department of Mental Health and Substance Dependence, Noncommunicable Diseases and Mental Health. *Investing in Mental Health.* World Health Organization, Geneva, Switzerland, 2003.

37. Buist-Bowman MA, deGraff R, Vollebergh WAM, Ormel J. Comorbidity of physical and mental disorders and the effect on work-loss days. *Acta Psychiatica Scandanavia.* 2005;111;6:436–443.

38. Dersh J, Gatchel RJ, Polatin P, Mayer T. Prevalence of psychiatric disorders in patients with chronic work-related musculoskeletal pain disability. *J Occup Environ Med.* 2002 May;44(5):459–68.

Chapter 23

Working With Common Functional Syndromes: Fibromyalgia and Chronic Fatigue Syndrome

James B. Talmage, MD

Fibromyalgia and chronic fatigue syndrome are syndromes. As syndromes, they are labels for collections of symptoms. There is no currently proven pathophysiology for these syndromes.[1,2] The diagnosis of many clinical conditions is similarly based on subjective criteria established by consensus of experienced physicians. Migraine headache, irritable bowel syndrome, and major depression are examples.

Fibromyalgia is a syndrome of widespread chronic pain (above and below the diaphragm, and on the left and right sides of the body), usually accompanied by some combination of stiffness, fatigue, headaches, bowel and/or bladder complaints, sleep disturbance, paresthesias, and cognitive difficulties. This diagnosis is generally verified by determining the presence of tender points.[2,3]

Fibromyalgia may be a disorder of the central nervous system.[4] Fibromyalgia patients report pain at low levels of cutaneous pressure and display increased CNS activation on functional MRI[5] with increased connectivity between central neurons.[6]

Fibromyalgia has genetic underpinnings with immediate relatives of individuals having an eight times increased risk of the disorder,[7] most likely due to genetic mutations in neurotransmitters such as catechol O methyl transferase, and serotonin receptor and transporter.

Chronic fatigue syndrome is characterized by new-onset significant fatigue that does not resolve with rest, that reduces the premorbid activity level, and that persists without obvious explanation by systemic disease for at least six months.[8,9]

While these syndromes are discussed separately in many texts and articles, this chapter follows the example of other authors and discusses them as a single entity. The overlap in symptoms between these conditions is extensive, and the label given to a particular patient may depend more on the specialty of the physician making the diagnosis than on the features of the disease.[3,10] This chapter discusses these conditions when they are present in isolation and not when they accompany other conditions like rheumatoid arthritis and systemic lupus erythematosus. For those more complex cases with comorbidity, primary care physicians should consult with appropriate specialists (rheumatologists). In cases in which fibromyalgia is a comorbidity to a primary rheumatologic disorder like rheumatoid arthritis, the primary disorder will determine the individual's work ability and work restrictions.

Social Security Administration's Criteria for Total Disability

Fibromyalgia syndrome and chronic fatigue syndrome are not discussed in the Social Security Administration's (SSA's) guide for physicians.[11] Because the US Social Security system is based on the biomedical model, in which severe objective impairment is the criterion for disability, and because these syndromes have no objective findings on physical examination, laboratory tests, electromyography, muscle biopsy, and routine imaging studies, these conditions are not mentioned in the text for physician evaluators of disability for the SSA.

Countries differ in their approach to disability for functional syndromes. In Norway, for example, 11% of the female population met the criteria for a diagnosis of fibromyalgia, and it became the single most frequent diagnosis for disability.[12] In Iceland, when claims for government-funded disability began to be filed for patients with fibromyalgia, these claims were rejected by the system. In many cases the patients' physicians filed amended applications for disability, listing a secondary psychiatric diagnosis.[13] In Iceland the psychiatric comorbidity may be a basis for state-funded disability.

While most patients with fibromyalgia do not have a current psychiatric illness, patients with fibromyalgia have a higher rate of current or past psychiatric illness than normal controls. In addition, the presence of a comorbid psychiatric illness makes fibromyalgia patients more likely to seek health care and to seek disability certification.[3]

Risk

Risk is not an issue. These conditions are not associated with the criteria of the Americans With Disabilities Act of 1990 (ADA) of "significant risk" of "substantial harm" that is "imminent" (see Chapter 8). These patients experience symptoms, like pain and fatigue, with activity; however, the increase in subjective symptoms without any detectable objective correlate is not significant harm. If these patients are willing job applicants, there is no basis for a preplacement examining physician to recommend against the hiring and placement of these individuals into jobs of any degree of difficulty, despite the fact that these syndromes have been diagnosed and are still symptomatic. Fibromyalgia has been shown to improve with aerobic exercise,[2,14,15] and progressive exercise is recommended as treatment. Work may involve exercise, and thus be therapeutic, in addition to its psychosocial benefits, as discussed in Chapter 1.

Some medications used to treat fibromyalgia syndrome may have sedation and/or cognitive impairment as side effects, and these medications may prevent an individual from working in a few careers due to regulation (pilots, commercial drivers, nuclear power plant operators, etc), or due to company policy on safety sensitive jobs.

Capacity

Capacity in fibromyalgia is not usually an issue. Patients dislike doing what they can do because it hurts. Both fibromyalgia and chronic fatigue syndrome patients complain of fatigue. Both groups may have a decreased exercise capacity from deconditioning documented on treadmill testing. Both conditions frequently result in patients adopting a sedentary lifestyle, so cardiovascular deconditioning is to be expected. For heavy and very heavy jobs, aerobic exercise capacity may be an issue and may be a basis for physician-described work limitations. However, the result of treadmill exercise testing in chronic fatigue syndrome may change on a day-to-day basis, so the result of a single test may not be a valid test of disability.[16] This is especially true if the test is stopped by "fatigue" (tolerance) long before the predicted maximal heart rate is reached (exercise testing) or the anaerobic threshold is crossed (cardiopulmonary exercise testing).

If cognitive complaints affect job performance in intellectually demanding jobs, formal neuropsychological testing by a neuropsychologist may document a problem with intellectual capacity that would be a basis for physician-described work limitations. If psychiatric comorbidity is suspected, psychiatric referral is indicated for diagnosis and treatment. Psychiatric comorbidity may be a basis for work limitations. Some medications used to treat fibromyalgia syndrome have sedation and cognitive impairment as side effects, and these may hinder work performance.

Because these are chronic conditions that do not generally respond dramatically to treatment, there is no logical basis for temporary work modification. Physicians would not be able to state that temporary work modifications would permit time for effective treatment that would result in expected prompt return to full duty.

Tolerance

Tolerance for subjective symptoms is generally the issue in these conditions. As long as Western society is using a biomedical model for disability, in which severe impairment is expected to be present to justify physician certification of disability, these functional syndromes with no objective findings would not qualify for work restrictions (risk) or work limitations (capacity). The fibromyalgia syndrome patient's inability to tolerate symptoms (especially pain) may well be due to "central sensitization" or enhanced symptom perception.[3] The pain and fatigue may be real, but physicians have yet to discover a way to measure either pain or fatigue. These patients' plight is similar to that of the patients with nonspecific regional arm pain (Chapter 13) or mechanical low back pain (Chapter 12), in which significant symptoms exist without confirmatory objective findings.

Chapter 2 stated that when tolerance in the Western biomedical model is believable on the basis of the presence of severe objective pathology, physicians will probably agree on supporting a patient's disability application. In these cases there is no basis for physician-imposed work restrictions or physician-described work limitations. Thus a disability application for a patient with fibromyalgia syndrome can only be supported by a physician notation on a disability certification form under "comments" that the patient has symptoms with activity and that it is medically safe for him or her to work.

Because work tolerance is not an area of medical science, physicians will disagree according to their perspectives and biases. It is sobering to remember that in a study to determine whether experienced pain clinic physicians could correctly distinguish individuals with fibromyalgia from paid volunteers simulating fibromyalgia, simulators were misidentified as fibromyalgia patients in one-third of the judgments, and fibromyalgia patients were misidentified as simulators in one-fifth of the judgments.[17] Thus, the best course for physicians is to agree that there is no contraindication to work activity (no need for physician-imposed restrictions and no basis for physician-described activity limitations), and the decision of whether or not the rewards of work outweigh the symptoms experienced is the patient's choice. It is not the physician's decision to certify or not certify disability. It is the patient's decision to work or not to work.

Summary

Fibromyalgia and chronic fatigue syndrome are syndromes, with symptoms but no objective findings. In the Western biomedical model of disability, there is usually no basis for physician-imposed work restrictions (risk) or physician-described work limitations (capacity). The issue is tolerance for the symptoms experienced during activity that the patient can do. Whether or not the rewards of work outweigh the symptoms is the patient's choice, and physicians should not certify disability in patients with these syndromes based only on tolerance.

References

1. Abeles AM, Pillinger MH, Solitar BM, et al. Narrative Review: The Pathophysiology of Fibromyalgia. *Ann Intern Med.* 2007;146:726–734.

2. Simms RW. Fibromyalgia syndrome: current concepts in pathophysiology, clinical features, and management. *Arthritis Care Res.* 1996;9:315–328.

3. Goldenberg DL. Fibromyalgia syndrome a decade later: what have we learned? *Arch Intern Med.* 1999;159:777–785.

4. Arnold LM, Clauw DJ. Fibromyalgia syndrome: practical strategies for improving diagnosis and patient outcomes. *Am J Med.* 2010;123(6):S2.

5. Gracely RH, Petzke F, Wolf JM, et. al. Functional magnetic resonance imaging evidence of augmented pain processing in fibromyalgia. *Arthritis Rheum.* 2002;46(5):1333–1343.

6. Napadow V, LaCount L, Park K, et al. Intrinsic brain connectivity in fibromyalgia is associated with chronic pain intensity. *Arthritis Rheum.* 2010;62(8):2545–2555.

7. Arnold LM, Clauw DJ. Fibromyalgia syndrome: practical strategies for improving diagnosis and patient outcomes. *Am J Med.* 2010;123(6):S2.

8. Holmes GP, Kaplan JE, Gantz NM. Chronic fatigue syndrome: a working case definition. *Ann Intern Med.* 1988;108:387–389.

9. Komaroff AL, Buchwald D. Symptoms and signs in chronic fatigue syndrome. *Rev Infect Dis.* 1991;13(suppl):S12–S18.

10. Buchwald D, Garrity D. Comparison of patients with chronic fatigue syndrome, fibromyalgia, and multiple chemical sensitivities. *Arch Intern Med.* 1994;154:2049–2053.

11. *Disability Under Social Security*. Baltimore, MD: Social Security Administration; January 2003. SSA publication 64–039.

12. Brusgaard D, Evensen AR, Bjerkedal T. Fibromyalgia: a new cause for disability pension. *Scand J Soc Med*. 1993;21:116.

13. Thoriacius S. Fibromyalgia and chronic fatigue syndrome. *Disability Med*. 2001;1:14–15.

14. Fontaine KR, Lora Conn L, Clauw DJ. Effects of Effects of lifestyle physical activity on perceived symptoms and physical function in adults with fibromyalgia: results of a randomized trial. *Arthritis Research & Therapy*. 2010;12:R55.

15. Wang C, Schmid CH, Rones R, et al. A randomized trial of tai chi for fibromyalgia. *NEJM*. 2010;363:743–54.

16. Alpern HL, Ranavaya MI, Govindan S. *Chronic Fatigue Syndrome: Impairment and Disability Issues*. Chicago, IL: American Academy of Disability Evaluating Physicians; 1999.

17. Khostanteen I, Tunks ER, Goldsmith GH. Fibromyalgia: can one distinguish it from simulation? *J Rheumatol*. 2000;27:2671–2676.

Chapter 24

International Perspectives
on Return to Work

Editor's Note: This chapter is new to the second edition of this book.
Countries around the world are confronting disability and return-to-work
issues. They also face the tasks of evaluation as well as the need for legal
interfaces for handling these claims. To elucidate these issues, we have
solicited brief overviews from experts in five countries. The authors were
given great latitude in content, allowing them to reflect on their specific
experiences and emphasize what they see as the most important issues.
The reader should take away a sense of the growing global challenges in
the disability field.

International Perspectives on Return to Work: Introduction

David Linklater, MD, MBA

Disability benefits are growing considerably across a number of international jurisdictions, and the range of disability benefits offered vary widely. The main types of disability insurance are social security benefits, workers' compensation, private illness insurance (short-term and long-term disability), and social pension insurance.

Comparisons Across Jurisdictions

The table below provides information about Disability Benefit Recipients (% of population) ages 20 to 64.[1]

The source of funds to finance disability insurance is either the individual or a combination of public and private means including employers. The situation in most OECD nations is a combination of public, private, and employer contributions and disability insurance systems.[2]

Disability Benefit Recipients of Population (%): 20–64 Years of Age

Country	Mid-1990s	2007*	Annual Change
Sweden	8.2	10.8	2.32
Norway	7.7	10.3	2.48
Finland	10.0	8.5	−1.35
Netherlands	9.4	8.3	−1.52
Denmark	7.4	7.2	−0.26
Great Britain	7.0	7.0	0.06
USA	4.7	5.9	2.04
Australia	4.2	5.4	2.14
France	4.0	4.9	2.34
Germany	4.2	4.4	0.51
Canada	4.3	4.3	0.02
Spain	3.1	3.8	1.66
Mexico	0.7	0.7	−0.43
OECD average	5.5	5.8	0.47

* or last available year

References

1. Sickness, Disability and Work: Keeping on Track in the Economic Downturn. Organisation for Economic Co-operation and Development (OECD). 2009.

2. Assessing disability: an international comparison of workers' compensation systems. Munchener Ruckversicherungs-Gesellschaft, 2004.

International Perspectives on Return to Work: Australia

Dwight Dowda, MB, BS, MPH

Australia, with a population of approximately 22 000 000, consists of the states of New South Wales, Victoria, Western Australia, South Australia, Queensland, and Tasmania, as well as the Northern Territory and Australian Capital Territory.

Historically, workers compensation legislation in Australia first existed in the Australian colonies between 1882 and 1895 in the Employer Liability Act of 1880 (enacted in Britain). The Commonwealth of Australia was inaugurated in 1901 (Federation), and new workers' compensation legislation that incorporated no-fault principles came about after that.

Within Australia, there are now 11 workers' compensation systems. Eight of these systems have idiosyncratic laws specific to their respective state or territory. There are also three Commonwealth workers compensation systems. One is for Australian government employees, Australian Defence Force personnel who had service prior to July 1, 2004, and the employees of licensed self-insurers under the Safety Rehabilitation Compensation Act of 1998. The second is for certain seafarers under the Seafarers Rehabilitation Compensation Act of 1992, and the third is for Australian Defence Force personnel with service on or after July 1, 2004, covered by the Military Rehabilitation Compensation Act of 2004.

Accordingly, despite the relatively small population of Australia, history has seen the evolution of significant inconsistencies in the operation and application of its various workers' compensation laws. Largely, these inconsistencies have been driven by varying industrial profiles and economic environments of each jurisdiction and specific judicial decisions that have led to legislative amendments.

Currently in Australia there is a very strong drive toward harmonizing the various jurisdictions, not only with respect to workers' compensation legislation but in other legislations as well. The focus is on the states and territories adopting harmonized occupational health and safety legislation. The difficulties inherent in administering across state and territory boundaries create an administrative and financial burden on companies that operate nationally.

Each of the states and territories has progressively amended or even dramatically altered its respective workers' compensation legislation, and such change is ongoing.

In the early 1900s, the focus was on defining work-related injury and improving benefits for injured workers. In the latter part of the 20th century, the emphasis shifted to the role of occupational health and safety, in particular focusing on the need for injured workers to undergo rehabilitation.

Many jurisdictions in Australia highlighted this change of focus by adding the word "rehabilitation" to the names of their laws. For example, in 1991 in Western Australia, the Workers' Compensation Act of 1902, amended in 1981, was renamed the Workers' Compensation & Rehabilitation Act of 1981. In South Australia, the Workman's Compensation Act of 1900 was amended in 1986 and renamed the Workers' Rehabilitation & Compensation Act 1986; and in Tasmania, the Workers' Compensation Act of 1927 was changed dramatically under the Tasmanian Law Reform Commission in 1986 and was renamed the Workers' Rehabilitation & Compensation Act in 1988. Clearly, the focus has shifted to early rehabilitation, along with return to safe and durable work for injured workers.

Nearly all the jurisdictions for workers' compensation in Australia have a requirement that employers define and provide suitable duties that accommodate an individual who has sustained a work-related injury. These duties can be the same as the ones the individual had previously or an equivalent position. The specific preinjury position provisions depend on the jurisdiction. There remains within each workers' compensation program throughout Australia a common general intention that the injured worker is returned in a timely, safe, and durable manner to his or her work environment. Details of this extend beyond the limits of this publication but may be found in the publication by Safe Work Australia, which contains an extensive contemporary comparison of workers' compensation in Australia and New Zealand.[1]

Workers' compensation legislation that exists throughout Australia has the intent of creating a balance between early return to work and ensuring that a worker has had all reasonable and necessary treatment to allow recovery to maximum medical improvement.

Mechanisms of dispute resolution are as varied as the different jurisdictions in which they are found. In some jurisdictions (for example, New South Wales) disputes are lodged with the Workers' Compensation Commission, which is an independent statutory tribunal. An exception to dispute resolution occurring within the structure of the Workers' Compensation Commission is for matters relating to coal miners, which are heard and determined in the District Court. Within the Victorian system, dispute resolution can start at the level of conciliation. This can be escalated in the case of medical questions to a medical panel and further escalation of the claim can be taken to the level of the Magistrate's Court (for claims up to $100 000.00) or the County Court for claims of greater amounts. In Western Australia, dispute resolution can occur at the level of conciliation by tele-conference, direct face-to-face conciliation, arbitration, review, appeal to the Commissioner (who is a District Court judge), District Court hearings, or by a constituted medical assessment panel in cases in which the dispute is on medical issues.

Chapter 24

Reference

1. Safe Work Australia: Comparison of Workers Compensation Arrangements in Australia and New Zealand, Commonwealth of Australia 2010.

International Perspectives on Return to Work: Canada

David Linklater, MD, MBA

Canada (like the United States and Australia) has no federal level workers' compensation. In these jurisdictions, each state or province has its own workers' compensation insurance system.[1]

Canadian workers' compensation originated in the province of Ontario, which charged Sir William Meredith with reviewing the program in 1912. Following visits to key European nations (Belgium, England, France, and Germany) and reviewing acts of 39 countries,[2] Meredith proposed a new workers' compensation statute for the province. The statute was based on a historic trade-off in which workers gave up the right to sue for work-related injuries (regardless of fault) in return for guaranteed compensation for accepted claims. This trade-off remains the cornerstone of workers' compensation in Canada.[3]

Ontario adopted workers' compensation legislation in 1914, and this was soon followed in other provinces: Nova Scotia (1915), Manitoba (1916), British Columbia (1917), and Alberta (1918). The Canadian workers' compensation system, provincially organized and administered, has common components:

1. **Financing.** The premiums are paid fully by employers.

2. **Eligibility for Coverage.** Each province has its own legislation outlining which workers are eligible; in most provinces, traditional "heavy" industries are covered; there is variation on the eligibility of certain types of office workers (eg, bank workers). The military and the national police force (The Royal Canadian Mounted Police) are excluded.

3. **Diseases and Injuries Covered.** The injuries are covered if they are "work related." In general, the condition must arise out of employment and in the course of employment. Certain provincial jurisdictions have specific legislation including or excluding certain diagnoses or conditions, but this is the exception rather than the rule.

4. **Benefits Provided.** All provinces provide wage replacement for time lost from work and pay the medical costs for work-related injuries (diagnostic, examination, rehabilitation, drugs, and devices). For more serious injuries, supported care may be provided, as are medically required devices (eg, beds, wheelchairs). Finally, if a fatality is work related, benefits are provided to survivors, though these benefits vary amongst the provinces.

Canadian Interprovincial Comparison of Benefits and Workers' Compensation Board Responsibility for Prevention[4]

Jurisdiction	Maximum Compensable Earnings (CDN)	% of Earnings Benefits is Based on	WCB Responsible for Prevention
Alberta	$77,000	90% net	No
British Columbia	$71,200	90% net	Yes
Manitoba	No maximum	90% net	Partial
New Brunswick	$56,300	85% loss of earnings	Yes
Newfoundland	$51,235	80% net	Yes
Northwest Territories/Nunavut	$75,200	90% net	Yes
Nova Scotia	$50,800	75% net 1st 26 wks, then 85% net	Yes
Ontario	$77,600	85% net	No
Prince Edward Island	$47,500	80% net 1st 38 wks, then 85% net	Yes
Quebec	$62,500	90% net	Yes
Saskatchewan	$55,000	90% net	No
Yukon Territories	$77,610	75% gross	Yes

Chapter 24

Challenges

There are a number of challenges that face all disability systems regardless of location.[5–8] These challenges are as follows:

- an increase in the absolute number of disability benefit recipients,
- a low number of recipients who return to work,
- the younger average age of recipients,
- a longer period during which recipients receive benefits,
- the shift from musculoskeletal to mental illness claims,
- the inclusion of symptom-based diagnoses for physical claims,
- the disability and delayed recovery caused by obesity,
- the use and abuse of prescription drugs,
- the migration of workers and recipients across borders,
- an aging population.

Physicians who are aware of these important challenges will recognize the important role that they play in helping reduce the human and financial costs through accurate return-to-work assessments.

References

1. Williams CAJ. *An International Comparison of Workers' Compensation.* Norwell, Kluwer Academic Publishers. 1991, pp. 2–3.

2. Meredith WR. Final Report on Laws Relating to the Liability of Employers to Make Compensation to Their Employees for Injuries Received in the Course of their Employment Which are in Force in Other Countries, and as to How Far Such Laws Are Found to Work Satisfactorily. *Workers' Compensation in Saskatchewan.* S. W. C. Board. Regina, Saskatchewan Workers' Compensation Board. 1913.

3. Hick S (2004). *Social Welfare in Canada: Understanding Income Security.* Toronto: Thompson Educational Publishing; 2004, pp. 158–159.

4. Comparison of Workers' Compensation Legislation 2009. Association of Workers' Compensation Boards of Canada, 2009.

5. Disability benefits: Turning back the rising tide. International Social Security Association, 2006.

Chapter 24

6. Tompson W. The Netherlands: Reform of disability insurance, 2002–06. Chapter 13 in *The Political Economy of Reform*, OECD, 2009.

7. Sengupta I, Reno V, Burton JF. *Workers' Compensation: Benefits, Coverage, and Costs, 2007.* Washington, DC: National Academy of Social Insurance. 2009.

8. James E, Iglesias A. *Integrated Disability and Retirement Systems in Chile.* Washington, DC: National Center for Policy Analysis; 2007.

International Perspectives on Return to Work: Ireland

Clement Leech, MD

In Ireland, particularly in the past two decades, there has been a marked increase in chronic disability resulting from common health problems (musculoskeletal disorders, mental health problems and cardio-pulmonary diseases). This is in spite of the introduction of health and safety legislation, improved ergonomic practice, automation, and advances in technology and medical science. There is no evidence of an increase in the actual prevalence

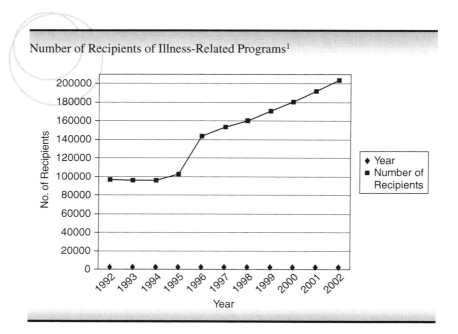

Number of Recipients of Illness-Related Programs[1]

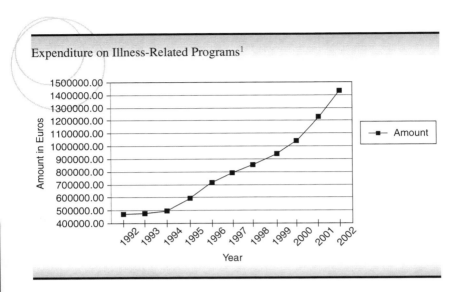

Expenditure on Illness-Related Programs[1]

of these common health problems. The difference is in the progression to a state of chronic pain and disability.

This problem had continued in Ireland during a period of virtual full employment, but it is expected to deteriorate further in these times of economic difficulties in which the unemployment rate is reaching 13.5%.

In facing its challenge, the Irish Department of Social and Family Affairs (recently renamed the Department of Social Protection [DSP]) decided to analyze the problem. There is strong evidence showing that work is generally good for physical and mental health and well-being. Unemployment is associated with poorer physical and mental health and well-being. Work can be therapeutic and can reverse the adverse health effects of unemployment. This is true for healthy people of working age, for disabled people, for most people with common heath problems, and for social security beneficiaries, as long as account is taken of the nature and quality of work and its social context: jobs should be safe and accommodating.

The DSP decided to address the problem by intervening in the acute stage using international evidence-based guidelines in a social security setting.[2]

First, the DSP addressed the problem of low back pain by designing and implementing the Renaissance Project, the aim of which was to determine if using these guidelines in this setting would decrease the incidence of progression to chronic disability.

The outcomes of the Renaissance Project resulted in a significant reduction in the progression to chronic disability from simple low back pain.[3] The effect of this early intervention in the acute stage should result not only in the improved health of sufferers of low back pain in the long term but also in decreased healthcare costs, reduced absenteeism, increased production, and significant savings in long-term benefit programs.

The Renaissance Project has now been extended nationwide in Ireland and also extended to another major common health problem, mental health, with significant positive outcomes.

To support and to robustly justify these changes in assessment practice, it was deemed necessary to modernize our disability assessment system.

Project Background and Objectives

Chapter 24

The Medical Review and Assessment Service (MRAS) of the DSP assesses the medical eligibility of claimants for all illness, disability, and carer payment programs. The 27 Medical Assessors (MAs) assess more than 113 000 claims and reviews per year.

Claimant's medical eligibility is assessed by means of either an in-person assessment at one of the 50 review centers across the country or through reports provided by their medical practitioner.

In 2005, an independent review of the operation of MRAS identified opportunities for modernization, including:

- introduction of evidence-based medical protocols to support medical decision making,
- use of information technology (IT) in performing medical assessments,
- use of IT to support the prioritization and management of referrals for medical assessment, and
- improved reporting of illnesses, outcomes, and trends.

In 2009, the DSP initiated an 18-month project to modernize both the administrative and medical streams of MRAS. This project represented a major progression of the department's overall Service Delivery Modernization program to introduce new ways of working supported by technology improvements.

The project has developed in four key phases:

- Management of Certificate Stock and Payments to Medical Certifiers (Registered Medical Practitioners contracted to the department for initial certification of people unfit for work): introducing new administrative processes to support the reconciliation of payments due to Medical Certifiers for certificates and medical reports furnished. This involved the automated scanning and processing of the 70 000 medical certificates issued per week.

- Desk Assessment and Scheduling: introducing facilities for MAs to view medical reports online and record the outcome of their assessment. New electronic scheduling tools were developed to support the management of claimants who are required to be seen at an in-person assessment.

- Activation: introducing facilities for MAs to refer claimants who would benefit from early intervention.

- Medical Protocols and In-Person Assessment: introducing mechanisms for MAs to perform in-person assessments online with the support of evidence-based medical protocols.

Approach

The new ways of working were developed in a collaborative manner involving the medical and administrative areas of MRAS working with the department's project team.

The Chief Medical Advisor established a core working group of MAs who played a leading role in representing the needs of the medical cadre. This core group provided crucial input on the opportunities for improvement and feedback on the feasibility of potential solutions.

A key aspect of the collaborative approach to developing the new MRAS system were the "Agile Methodology Planning Game" workshops. These planning games provided the MA core group with the opportunity to use a prototype (ie, mock-up) of the new system and provide direct feedback to the development team. This prototype enabled changes to be rapidly incorporated and re-assessed prior to development of the final system.

A collaborative approach helped ensure that the system met the needs of the MA group, in particular by being clear, intuitive, and easy to use.

Key Benefits of the Modernization

The modernization project has introduced transformational changes in the ways of working in both the medical and administrative streams of MRAS. Key benefits of this modernization include:

- Early intervention for priority referrals,

- Introduction of evidence-based medical protocols to support medical decision making,

- Increased transparency and flexibility by moving from paper-based assessments to on-line and in-person assessments, and

- Development of a comprehensive database of illness and outcomes via the capture of ICD-10 codes.

Early Intervention

Since its introduction in 2004, the Renaissance Project of early intervention for low back pain has delivered significant benefits for the DPS, providing consistent and robust results while reducing the time claimants are awaiting assessment.

Previously, a manual administrative process was required to identify these early intervention and other priority referrals. Indeed, a paper case file was created for each referral. The new IT system replaces this paper file with an online electronic referral containing details of the claimant's illness or disability and all relevant medical reports. The system automatically routes each referral for either desk or in-person assessment based on predefined profiling criteria. This automatic profiling supports early intervention by automatically routing Renaissance and common mental heath cases for an in-person medical assessment as a matter of priority.

A technological approach provides flexibility for the future introduction of further early intervention programmes.

Evidence-Based Medical Protocols

Evidence-based medical protocols were developed following a review of accepted standard medical references and research of current literature. These protocols form a comprehensive knowledge base of up-to-date evidence-based research. The protocol documents are structured in the following manner:

- Overview and definition
- Epidemiology
- Etiology
- Diagnosis
- Differential diagnosis and comorbidity
- Treatment
- Prognosis
- Guidelines for information gathering at the in-person assessment
- Analysis of effect on functional ability.

The protocol documents were subject to a rigorous internal review led by the CMA and an external review panel. A comprehensive set of 27 protocols were developed to cover the most common illnesses and disabilities, namely:

Mental Health:

- Depression, anxiety, stress, PTSD
- Intellectual disabilities
- Substance and drug dependency
- Alcohol dependency
- Eating disorders
- Nervous System:
  - Epilepsy
  - Headache, migraine
  - Stroke
- Respiratory System:
  - Asthma
  - COPD
- Circulatory System:
  - Ischemic heart disease, cardiac failure
  - Hypertension

- General Alimentary System
- Musculoskeletal System:
  - Renaissance – Back
  - Renaissance – Neck and shoulder
  - Rheumatoid Arthritis
  - Osteoarthritis – Upper limbs
  - Osteoarthritis – Lower limbs
- Endocrine System:
  - Thyroid
  - Diabetes
- General genitourinary system
- General obstetrics and gynecology
- General ENT system
- Dermatological:
  - Eczema, psoriasis
  - Dermatitis
- Miscellaneous:
  - Chronic Fatigue
  - Chronic pain, fibromyalgia

In addition to forming evidence-based reference documents, key aspects of the protocols have been integrated into the design of the electronic in-person assessment form (MR1). Scheme eligibility is determined primarily by the degree of disability and its expected duration. To support MAs in their decision making, key indicators of severity of disability from the medical protocols have been incorporated into the electronic MR1 form completed by the MA.

Electronic MR1 Form

One of the most fundamental changes to be introduced by the MRAS modernization project is the move to paperless in-person medical assessments. Currently MAs complete an MR1, a paper form, during the in-person assessment while referring to paper copies of any relevant medical reports supplied by the claimant.

The 12-page paper MR1 form, successfully operated for many years, captures the key information required to perform the in-person assessment, in a structured manner, including:

- History taking
- Claimant's account of the affect of the illness or disability
- Medical evidence furnished
- Examination and clinical findings
- Disability assessment
- Work capacity assessment
- Program eligibility.

While the introduction of technology to the assessment process provides many benefits, the design of the new "electronic MR1" posed a number of key challenges, including:

- Maintaining the structure and integrity of the assessment process,
- Ensuring there was no increase in the time required to complete the assessment process,
- Maintaining the personal nature of the assessment process (ie, the technology should not overly distract the MA from engaging with the claimant), and
- The need to support MAs with a range of IT literacy levels.

Over a number of months, these challenges were addressed through the joint working of the MA core and the project team. Consequently, the following key features were incorporated into the design of the electronic MR1:

- Claimant Questionnaire – All claimants attending an in-person assessment will be sent a questionnaire requesting details of their medical history and details of how their illness or disability affects their activities of daily living. The MA will have online access to this information during the in-person assessment, thereby significantly reducing the need for the MA to record background information on the system.

- Minimal Typing – Wherever possible, the electronic form has been designed to allow for the clicking of boxes and items on menus. For example, where the claimant's questionnaire contains all relevant information regarding their medical history, the MA can simply click on a box to refer to the questionnaire. However, the ability to capture typed notes and comments is available should there be the need to capture additional information.

- System review and medical examination – In performing a review of the claimant's system, the MA indicates which, if any, systems are abnormal. Where a system is indicated as abnormal, the MA is provided with the opportunity of selecting a relevant protocol (eg, asthma or COPD for the respiratory system). By selecting a protocol, the MA is provided with a set of questions relating to indicators of the severity of Ability/Disability.

Chapter 24

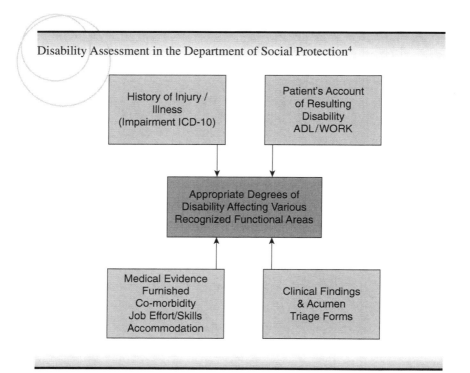

Disability Assessment in the Department of Social Protection[4]

Claimants' Questionnaire or Statement

Claimants Questionnaire

Please complete questionnaire below in full

Telephone Number:_____	**Mobile Number:**_____
Occupation:	
Date last worked: **"Working Y/N: "** Text for Disablement only:	

Work History – Type of Work	<u>From</u>	<u>To</u>
1.		
2.		
3.		

Level of Education:					
Primary ☐		Secondary ☐		Third Level ☐	

Training Courses Completed:

1.

2.

Past Serious Illnesses / Operations:

1.

2.

Attending GP
No ☐   Yes ☐

If yes, specify

Specialist Referral
No ☐   Yes ☐

If yes, specify

Investigations
No ☐   Yes ☐

If yes, specify

(Continued)

Claimants' Questionnaire or Statement *(Continued)*

Medication No ☐ Yes ☐ If yes, specify	

Does your Condition affect the activities of your Typical Day under the following headings?

Bathing No ☐ Yes ☐ Describe how	
Dressing No ☐ Yes ☐ Describe how	
Grooming No ☐ Yes ☐ Describe how	
Toileting No ☐ Yes ☐ Describe how	
Care of Family No ☐ Yes ☐ Describe how	
Driving No ☐ Yes ☐ Describe how	
Doing Housework No ☐ Yes ☐ Describe how	
Shopping No ☐ Yes ☐ Describe how	
Cooking No ☐ Yes ☐ Describe how	
Walking No ☐ Yes ☐ Describe how	
Climbing Stairs No ☐ Yes ☐ Describe how	
Sitting No ☐ Yes ☐ Describe how	

Chapter 24

(Continued)

Claimants' Questionnaire or Statement *(Continued)*

Watching TV No ☐ Yes ☐ Describe how	
Reading No ☐ Yes ☐ Describe how	
Sleeping No ☐ Yes ☐ Describe how	
Hobbies/Leisure Activities No ☐ Yes ☐ Describe how	

The following figure demonstrates the selection of a protocol based on clicking on boxes for the systems review within the MR1 form.

- Electronic capture of ability-disability profile – The assessment culminates in the MA completing an ability-disability profile for the claimant based on his or her examination and clinical findings. The ability-disability profile, together with all the supporting information captured in the electronic MR1, will be maintained on the MRAS system for future reference.

Systems Review and Protocol

General state of health: Good ▾ **Height:** ____ **Weight:** ____

BP: 000/000 **Urine:** ____

	NORMAL	ABNORMAL
Mental Health	●	○
Nervous System	●	○
Respiratory System	○	●
Circulatory System	●	○
Alimentary System	●	○
Musculo-skeletal System	●	○
Endocrine	●	○
Genitourinary System	●	○
Obs and Gyne	●	○
ENT	●	○
Dermatological System	●	○
Other (Please Specify)	●	○

Asthma ▾
Select...
Asthma
COPD

(Continued)

Systems Review and Protocol *(Continued)*

Asthma

Normal	Yes / No
Does not complain of restriction in Activities of Daily Living, especially walking, running or climbing stairs	○ ○
Exhibits no evidence of breathlessness during interview or examination	○ ○
Mild	**Yes / No**
Taking regular preventative treatment, i.e. steroid inhalers	○ ○
Intermittent oral steroids	○ ○

Chapter 24

The following figure demonstrates the ability-disability profile completed online by an MA.

For example, if a claimant's cause of incapacity is COPD, the electronic MR1 form will prompt the MA to complete the following questionnaire.

The completion of this questionnaire, together with the relevant clinical findings, will support the MA in his or her assessment of the claimant's functional ability and disability. This assessment is summarized in the profile shown on page 459.

Normal to Profound Scale Form

Normal	Yes / No
Capable of usual Activities of Daily Living	☐ ☐
Mild	**Yes / No**
Breathless on moderate exertion	☐ ☐
Occasional use of short acting bronchodilators	☐ ☐
Exhibits no evidence of breathlessness during interview or examination	☐ ☐

(Continued)

Normal to Profound Scale Form *(Continued)*

Moderate	Yes / No	
Breathless on walking 100m, or climbing one flight of stairs at a normal pace	☐	☐
Attends chest clinic – no hospital admissions in the last 12 months	☐	☐
FEV1/FVC < 70%, FEV1 50–80% (if available)	☐	☐
On short and long acting bronchodilators	☐	☐
On home nebulisers	☐	☐
Exhibits some evidence of breathlessness during examination process	☐	☐
Severe	**Yes / No**	
Stops for breath after a few minutes on level ground	☐	☐
FEV1/FVC < 70%, FEV1 30–50% (if available)	☐	☐
Has required treatment with courses of oral steroids and antibiotics every two months in the last 12 months during acute exacerbations	☐	☐
Barrel shaped chest	☐	☐
Tachypnoea	☐	☐
Breath sounds reduced with a prolonged expiratory phase and/or rhonchi	☐	☐
Profound	**Yes / No**	
Incapable of independent living	☐	☐
Virtually bed, or wheelchair, bound and dependant on carers for bodily care	☐	☐
On maximum medication and domiciliary oxygen	☐	☐
History of multiple admissions during acute exacerbations	☐	☐
FEV1/FVC < 70%, FEV1 < 30% (if available)	☐	☐
Central cyanosis	☐	☐
Signs of right ventricular failure	☐	☐

Chapter 24

ICD-10 Coding

The new MRAS system will enable the capture of ICD-10 codes for desk and in-person assessments performed. MAs will have the flexibility to either directly enter the relevant code(s) or search the WHO ICD Web site to obtain the relevant code.

Over time this ICD coding information will provide an extensive database of illness and disabilities. Combined with data analysis tools, this database will be an invaluable tool for trend analysis and outcome reporting.

Ability-Disability Profile

Clinical description of effects of claimant's Illness/Accident/Disablement

Indicate, if any, the degree to which the claimant's condition has affected his/her ability in the following areas:

	Normal	Mild	Moderate	Severe	Profound
Mental Health	◉	○	○	○	○
Learning/Intelligence	◉	○	○	○	○
Consciousness/Seizures	◉	○	○	○	○
Balance/Co-ordination	◉	○	○	○	○
Vision	◉	○	○	○	○
Hearing	◉	○	○	○	○
Speech	◉	○	○	○	○
Continence	◉	○	○	○	○
Reaching	◉	○	○	○	○
Manual Dexterity	◉	○	○	○	○
Lifting/Carrying	◉	○	○	○	○
Bending/Kneeling/Squatting	◉	○	○	○	○
Sitting	◉	○	○	○	○
Standing	◉	○	○	○	○
Climbing Stairs	○	◉	○	○	○
Walking	○	○	◉	○	○

Chapter 24

References

1. Leech C. Presentation to 2nd Annual Conference of Pain Society of Ireland, Tallaght Hospital, Dublin Nov 2002.

2. Renaissance Project Leech C. The Stationary Office, Government Publications Sales Office, Sun Alliance House, Molesworth Street Dublin 2. Government of Ireland 2004.

3. http://www.welfare.ie/EN/Policy/ResearchSurveysAndStatistics/Pages/renaissance.aspx.

4. Leech C. Presentation to 1st International Disability Evaluating Medicine Conference, Royal College of Physicians of Ireland 1996.

International Perspectives on Return to Work: Korea

Jong Uk Won, MD, Dr. PH

The workers' compensation insurance system in Korea was first legislated as a national social security program in 1963. The Korea Workers' Compensation & Welfare Service, which is an affiliated corporation of the Ministry of Employment and Labor established by the Industrial Accident Compensation Act, oversees the program. In 1964, the year in which the workers' compensation insurance system first went into effect, it was applied to companies in the mining and manufacturing industries that hired more than 500 workers. The range of application was gradually expanded into most companies except the worksites of some excluded industries such as domestic, farming, and fishing industries. Workers' compensation insurance is mandatory in Korea.

The workers' compensation benefits consist of medical care, temporary disability, matching to 70% of average wages, permanent disability, nursing care, and survivors' and funeral expenses. Vocational rehabilitation, which was newly legislated in 2008, is now an additional benefit.[1]

Recent Return-to-Work Status in Korea

Rehabilitation of injured workers is being provided by the Korea Workers' Compensation and Welfare Service Corporation under workers' compensation insurance in Korea. The rate of return to work increased from 40.0% in 2002 to 57.2% in 2009, showing an upward trend. According to a recent survey, 35.2% of workers among 35 569 of newly injured workers returned to their previous companies, and more than 20% of workers found other work, including being self-employed[2,3] (see table).

Chapter 24

Annual Return-to-Work Rates of Injured Workers in Korea

Year	Number of Injured Workers	Types of Return to Work				Not Returned	Unable to Survey
		Subtotal	Previous Worksite	Another Worksite	Own Business		
2009	35,569	20,334 (57.2%)	12,511 (35.2%)	6,684 (18.8%)	1,139 (3.2%)	12,330 (34.7%)	2,905 (8.2%)
2008	37,178	19,950 (53.7%)	12,962 (34.9%)	6,031 (16.2%)	957 (2.6%)	13,905 (37.4%)	3,323 (8.9%)
2007	36,553	18,220 (49.8%)	12,216 (33.4%)	5,223 (14.3%)	781 (2.1%)	13,459 (36.8%)	4,874 (13.3%)
2006	38,872	17,681 (45.5%)	11,794 (30.3%)	45,472 (14.1%)	415 (1.1%)	15,095 (38.8%)	6,096 (15.7%)
2005	37,119	15,680 (42.2%)	10,144 (27.3%)	4,958 (13.4%)	578 (1.6%)	13,225 (35.6%)	8,214 (22.1%)
2004	34,320	14,420 (42.0%)	9,829 (28.6%)	4,060 (11.8%)	531 (1.5%)	11,576 (33.7%)	8,324 (24.3%)
2003	30,363	12,192 (40.2%)	8,663 (28.5%)	3,302 (10.9%)	227 (0.7%)	10,448 (34.4%)	7,723 (25.4%)
2002	26,546	10,627 (40.0%)	7,421 (28.0%)	3,017 (11.4%)	189 (0.7%)	5,666 (21.3%)	10,253 (38.6%)

Institutional Supports for Occupational Rehabilitation and Return to Work

The return to work of disabled workers was lacking in the early years of workers' compensation. The return-to-work system had been inadequate in facilitating timely professional therapy and rehabilitation because the compensation system had focused on acute medical care and cash benefits. However, the importance of rehabilitation that facilitates return to work began to be realized in the late 1990s. The concepts of promoting rehabilitation and return to society for workers were specified in the provision of workers' compensation insurance by the amendment of 2000. A 5-year project (from 2001 to 2005) was planned and implemented with the purpose of consolidating return to society with medical, vocational, and social rehabilitation.[4] The rehabilitation project was converted from a budget project to a legal vocational rehabilitation benefit by a 2008 amendment, allowing rehabilitation services to support workers and return them to workplace and society.

Support for occupational training includes allowances to promote programs needed to return to work. The expenses for occupational training courses at the public or private occupational training agencies are paid to the institutes, and training allowances that meet the daily minimum wage are paid to the injured workers.

Return-to-work subsidies are paid to the employers or companies that help the occupationally injured and permanently impaired workers return to and maintain their jobs. These subsidies consist of return-to-work subsidies, adaptation training expenses, and/or rehabilitation exercises expenses.

Present Issues of Return to Work in Korea

It is well known that the return to work rate decreases with increasing disability duration. As previously stated, many efforts are being made to help injured workers return to their work in Korea. However, the rate of return to work is still low, partly due to the long duration of treatment.

Chapter 24

According to the studies investigating the treatment duration of injured workers, treatment duration is longer in the workers' compensation insurance than in the National Health Insurance, and the portion of long-term care patients is increasing.[5] This is partly due to the severity of the illnesses and injuries of injured workers, but lack of control on the medical care of the workers' compensation patients could be the more important cause. The duration of treatment may be longer due to insufficient management and control of the health care providers as well as workers' preference for longer care to get more temporary disability benefits. So a vicious cycle is created because a prolonged disability period makes return to work more difficult, and workers try to extend treatment duration due to the difficult return-to-work situation.

However, despite a prolonged medical care period, workers' satisfaction with the medical care they receive is low. In recognition of these problems, efforts are being made to increase the quality of medical care provided under workers' compensation. In addition, case management for individual workers will soon be implemented.

Meanwhile, a few large enterprises have been operating return-to-work programs for their injured workers. These programs consist of work hardening, job modification, and return-to-work planning. Although these programs ought to be provided to every injured worker, they are currently limited to the workers of a few large enterprises in Korea.

Conclusion

Vocational rehabilitation and return to work are new issues in Korea. Only recently, specific policies and plans for implementation to facilitate return to work have been set up, even though the importance of return to work had been recognized earlier. However, focus remains on workers who have significant impairments and return to work of workers with minimal disability is not a subject of much interest. Although return to work has to be the main goal during care of injured workers, it has not received much attention until recently. The way to facilitate return to work has to be a team approach with cooperation by doctors, social workers, and specialists in vocational rehabilitations, as well as employers, employees, and the government. Return to work in Korea can be improved by systemic cooperation between the government and employers.

References

1. http://www.kcomwel.or.kr.

2. Internal statistics materials from the Korea Workers' Compensation & Welfare Service 2009.

3. Kim YB. A thesis about standard of injured workers' return to work: a literature review. *J Vocational Rehabil.* 2009;19(1):203–224.

4. Choi YY. A study on the funding for return to work and policy for injured workers. *J Vocational Rehabil.* 2009;19(2):71–90.

5. Park SK. A study on the rehabilitation of long-term patients in industrial accidents hospital. *Disability & Employment.* 2003;50:5–20.

Chapter 24

Return to Work: Scandinavia, with a Focus on Sweden

Karen Belkić, MD, PhD

Legislative Framework and Actual Developments

In all Nordic countries, legislation has been passed explicitly stating that working conditions must respect the physical and mental health of the workforce.[1] This includes the Amended Swedish Work Environment Act (Act No. 677, 1991), which states that working conditions shall be adapted to people's differing physical and psychological circumstances.[1] Therein, it is mandated that employers are responsible for organized work rehabilitation and must make a rehabilitation investigation when an employee has been sick-listed for more than 4 weeks. The interventions should aim at improving the employee's functional capacity, health, and well-being.[2] In Sweden prior to 1991, vocational rehabilitation was unusual in private companies, and persons with functional impairment generally were employed in semi-public organizations or they became disability pensioners.[3] General sickness insurance began in 1955.[4]

According to the Swedish Work Environment Act, together with the National Insurance and Security of Employment and Trade Union Representation Acts, a Disability Ombudsman monitors issues relating to the rights and interests of people with disabilities. Shop stewards have special responsibilities for enforcing safety regulations to prevent accidents. Union representatives have strong legal rights and by law cannot be fired for complaining or enforcing legal action. The employee can request union support when discussing rehabilitation alternatives.[5] Since 1999, according to Swedish law, employers of all sizes are responsible for the rehabilitation of their employees. The government is responsible for covering the costs of rehabilitation of the unemployed.[3]

In practice, however, the provision of rehabilitation services in Sweden has been inconsistent.[3] Four different organizations are involved: health services, social services, the employer, and the insurance authorities. Differences in work capacity assessment have been observed among the various agencies, with lack of scientific knowledge by these professionals noted.[6] Poor cooperation has been reported between the social security and employment agencies vis-à-vis unemployed persons on sick leave.[7]

As unemployment has increased, there has been greater difficulty with a negative effect on selection and hiring of persons at risk. Employers are more likely to fire a less productive worker rather than to get involved with rehabilitation.[5] In the nineties, there were major reductions in the public service sector, resulting in an increased workload for those who stayed in the workforce.[8] Persons exposed to work-related strain frequently became long-term sick listed.[8]

As stated by Millet and Sandberg:[9] "Sweden has had the long-standing aim to create a modern healthy working environment that improves quality of living. Nevertheless a crisis exists today." Since 1997 there has been a notable increase in the number of persons and length of time on sick leave, with a heavy burden on governmental social insurance agencies and upon vocational rehabilitation services. Costs for sickness absence and disability pension in Sweden have equaled the costs of health care. This does not include the costs to employers, to the persons who are on sick leave, and to private insurance companies.[10] A key problem is that longer-term sick leave diminishes chances of return to work.[9]

The Role of the Physician

In Sweden a physician's certificate is required after 7 days of absence due to sickness. The first 14 days of sick leave are paid by the employer. Subsequently, the government insurance system pays for the sick leave. The insurance authorities can change sick leave to temporary or permanent disability pension.[11] Physicians frequently fail to provide needed information on functional capacity and other data concerning sickness certification, leading to delays in receipt of benefits and initiation of return-to-work activities.[12] According to the late Professor Gösta Tibblin, "Sickness certification may be regarded as a drug with effects and side-effects. It should be used in proper doses and thus should be handled in the same way as a medical prescription."[13] Experienced Swedish physicians have been found to certify patients as sick more often than their less experienced colleagues.[13]

Comparison of Sweden and the United States Regarding Vocational Rehabilitation

Stubbs and Deaner[3] note that there are "fundamentally different strategies" for Sweden and the United States. The Swedish system is seen to be medically oriented and usually engages a multi-disciplinary team, whereas in the United States one individual generally handles vocational rehabilitation. These authors point to particular problems for small Swedish companies vis-à-vis vocational rehabilitation. This is especially important because this sector has been growing substantially for the last two decades, and as mentioned, since 1999, small enterprises are responsible for the rehabilitation of their employees.

Recent Initiatives to Improve Vocational Rehabilitation

There have been a number of intervention programs aimed at improving the cooperation among the providers of vocational rehabilitation services. This includes a "multi-professional, cooperative approach."[14] At 6-month follow-up, participation in such programs has shown 5 times higher likelihood of being employed compared to the period prior to rehabilitation. At 24 month follow-up, the probability of being employed rose even further, to 7 times that prior to rehabilitation.[15] A rehabilitation model that included promotion of a healthy psychosocial work environment together with productivity considerations was found to be feasible, yielding a reduction in sick leave from 12% to 3% and diminished costs (lowered per employee from 1860 Euros per month to 440 Euros per month) as applied to a middle-sized Swedish engineering company.[16] Promoting pride and empowerment according to "theories of social emotions" are also emphasized as important components of the return-to-work process.[17] It has been noted that in countries such as Finland, with high coverage of occupational health services, occupational health professionals could play a key role as return-to-work coordinators.[18]

Partial return to work has been identified as a useful strategy for helping maintain occupational activity. Jobs with relatively low demands and high control have been found to promote full as well as partial return to work among Swedish public sector employees who were out sick 28 days or more.[19] In Sweden it is possible to prescribe 25%, 50%, or 75% of full working hours. This part-time sick leave was found to be a potential solution for persons who had been on long-term sick leave.[11] Long waiting times before the employee met with the company physician motivated a change mandating more rapid completion of the administrative aspects and rehabilitation plan.[20] New rules have recently been established to simplify the rehabilitation process in Sweden, with a focus on return to work for those on long-term sick leave.[21] Another initiative has been the newer Swedish law termed "resting disability pension" which permits those out on disability to go back to work without jeopardizing their benefits.[22]

Experience in Various Areas of Medicine Regarding Return to Work

Musculoskeletal Disorders Including Early Rheumatoid Arthritis

Musculoskeletal disorders are the major cause of sickness absence in Sweden.[8] Physicians trained in social insurance medicine give sickness certification more often to patients with musculoskeletal disorders compared to physicians without such training.[13] Emphasis has been placed upon early rehabilitation, which increases the likelihood of return to work.[23] Six-year follow-up has been performed on a multi-professional 8-week rehabilitation program among 122 participants with musculoskeletal disorders.[24] Fifty-two percent had returned to work compared to 13% of the referents. Relative to the period prior to rehabilitation, there was a significantly higher level of activity, as well as reduction in pain and analgesic consumption among the participants.[24] A 2-year prospective Swedish study of 110 patients with early rheumatoid arthritis examined an active team support program, including rehabilitation meetings with the employer, together with disease-modifying medications. This program was found to effectively prevent or delay work disability.[25]

Mental Health Disorders and Stroke

Since 1990, burnout and other stress-related psychiatric disorders have greatly increased as a cause of sick leave and disability in Sweden.[26] Persons with mentally or socially restricted work capacity were found to be nearly twice as likely not to be employed after rehabilitation compared to those with somatic work restriction.[14] Initiatives to promote return to work among persons with mental health disorders include the so-called "clubhouse model."[27] Therein, the persons organized themselves with work as the main rehabilitation tool. The goal was to create links of mutual trust, co-operation, solidarity, and voluntary responsibilities. In a qualitative evaluation, the work-ordered day successfully functioned as a framework. In a small qualitative study of patients who had suffered a cerebrovascular accident, return to work was found to be facilitated by "understanding and positive attitude of co-workers."[28] Will and self-efficacy were also found to be important factors contributing to return to work.[28]

Oncology

Considerable attention has been paid to promoting return to work after cancer treatment in Scandinavia. A series of studies from Oslo, Norway was devoted to rehabilitation to working life among patients with breast, prostate, and testicular cancer without early relapse after primary treatment.[29] It was confirmed that holding a job was a key prerequisite for maintaining healthy living conditions.[29,30] In Stockholm, a team rehabilitation program was developed for women with lymphedema after breast cancer surgery. The team consisted of a physiotherapist, social worker, oncologist, occupational therapist, and nurse. A large number of the participants increased the percentage of working time after participating in the program. Several participants considered that this special rehabilitation program played a critical role in their ability to return to work.[31]

The Occupational Stress Index (OSI)

As noted, persons exposed to work-related strain frequently become long-term disabled.[8] A critical factor can be the possibility of returning to modified, *healthier* work conditions.[2,32,33] Our initial experience in Sweden and elsewhere within the clinical setting of burnout, depression, cancer, and cardiovascular disease is that a strategy based upon the OSI is effective in helping identify and ameliorate occupational stressors during return to work.[32–35] The OSI is an additive-burden model, which incorporates key aspects of the leading sociological work-stressor models but was developed from a cognitive ergonomics perspective.[35] The OSI is of clinical utility, helping physicians incorporate the workplace into diagnostic and management strategies. We are currently using the OSI to help develop evidence-based return-to-work guidelines for patients with cancer, neuropsychiatric, and cardiovascular disorders.

Summary

Sweden and other Scandinavian countries have aimed at providing a healthy work environment with ample measures for effective return to work in the face of illness. However, the magnitude and costs of sickness absence have become unwieldy. Numerous innovations to promote early and effective return to work have been introduced. These have met with noteworthy success, including within the clinical setting of musculoskeletal and mental health disorders, as well as oncology.

The author thanks the Signe and Olof Wallenius Stiftelse, Cancerfonden, and King Gustav the Fifth's Jubilee Foundation for support.

References

1. Levi L. Legal and legislative issues: legislation to protect work CV health in Europe. *Occup Med.* 2000;15:269–273.

2. Söderberg S, Jumisko E, Gard G. Clients' experiences of a work rehabilitation process. *Disab Rehab.* 2004;26:419–424.

3. Stubbs J, Deaner G. When considering vocational rehabilitation: describing and comparing the Swedish and American systems and professions. *Work.* 2005;24:239–249.

4. Järvholm B, Karlsson B, Mannelqvist R. [Work capacity and sickness insurance as described in concept and law] [Swedish] *Läkartidningen.* 2009;106: 1178–1181.

5. Trygged S. Making work work. Vocational rehabilitation in Sweden. The Sköndal Institute, 1998, Working Paper #7.

6. Söderberg E, Vimarlund V, Alexanderson K. Experiences of professionals participating in inter-organisational cooperation aimed at promoting clients' return to work. *Work.* 2010;35:143–151.

7. Eriksson UB. Engström LG. Starrin B. Janson S. Falling between two stools; how a weak co-operation between the social security and the unemployment agencies obstructs rehabilitation of unemployed sick-listed persons. *Disab Rehab.* 2008;30:569–576.

8. Holmgren K, Dahlin Ivanoff S. Women on sickness absence—views of possibilities and obstacles for returning to work. *Disab Rehab.* 2004;26:213–222.

9. Millet P, Sandberg KW. Sweden. *Work.* 2005;24:213–214.

10. Alexanderson K, Hensing G. More and better research needed on sickness absence. *Scand J Public Health.* 2004;32:321–323.

11. Sieurin L, Josephson M, Vingård E. Positive and negative consequences of sick leave for the individual, with special focus on part-time sick leave. *Scand J Public Health.* 2009;37:50–56.

12. Söderberg E, Alexanderson K. Sickness certificates as a basis for decisions on entitlement to sickness insurance benefits. *Scand J Public Health.* 2005;33: 314–320.

13. Norrmén G, Svärdsudd K, Andersson D. Impact of physician-related factors on sickness certification in 1° health care. *Scand J Primary Health Care.* 2006;24:104–109.

14. Jakobsson B, Ekholm J, Bergroth A, Schüldt Ekholm K. Improved employment rates after multiprofessional cross-sector cooperation in vocational rehabilitation: a 6-year follow-up with comparison groups. *Int J Rehab Res.* 2010;33: 72–80.

15. Jakobsson B, Bergroth A, Schüldt K, Ekholm J. Do systematic multiprofessional rehabilitation group meetings improve efficiency in vocational rehabilitation? *Work.* 2005;4:79–90.

16. Sjöbom V, Marnetoft SU. A new model for vocational rehabilitation at an organizational level—a pilot study with promising results. *Work.* 2008;30:99–105.

17. Svensson T, Müssener U, Alexanderson K. Pride, empowerment, and return to work: on the significance of promoting positive social emotions among sickness absentees. *Work*. 2006;27:57–65.

18. Martino P-K. Reducing sickness absenteeism at the workplace—what to do and how? *Scand J Work Environ Health*. 2006;32:253–255.

19. Josephson M, Heijbel B, Voss M, Alfredsson L, Vingård E. Influence of self-reported work conditions and health on full, partial and no return to work after long-term sickness absence. *Scand J Work Environ Health*. 2008;34:430–437.

20. Sedvall M, Gunnarsson LG. [Unnecessarily long sick leave caused by the Social Insurance Office and the employers]. [Swedish] *Lakartidningen*. 2006;103: 2570–2571.

21. Närlid M. [The rehabilitation chain]. [Swedish] *Läkartidningen*. 2008;105: 1997–1998.

22. Edén L, Andersson IH, Ejlertsson G, et al. Return to work still possible after several years as a disability pensioner due to musculoskeletal disorders: a population-based study after new legislation in Sweden permitting 'resting disability pension.' *Work*. 2006;26:147–155.

23. Lydell M, Grahn B, Månsson J, Baigi A, Marklund B. Predictive factors of sustained return to work for persons with musculoskeletal disorders who participated in rehabilitation. *Work*. 2009;33:317–328.

24. Norrefalk JR, Linder J, Ekholm J, Borg K. A 6-year follow-up study of 122 patients attending a multiprofessional rehabilitation programme for persistent musculoskeletal-related pain. *Int J Rehab Res*. 2007;30:9–18.

25. Nordmark B, Blomqvist P, Andersson B, et al. A two-year follow-up of work capacity in early rheumatoid arthritis: a study of multidisciplinary team care with emphasis on vocational support. *Scand J Rheumatol*. 2006;35:7–14.

26. Engström LG, Janson S. Stress-related sickness absence and return to labour market in Sweden. *Disab Rehab*. 2007;29:411–416.

27. Norman C. The Fountain House movement, an alternative rehabilitation model for people with mental health problems. *Scand J Caring Sci*. 2006;20:184–192.

28. Medin J, Barajas J, Ekberg K. Stroke patients' experiences of return to work. *Disab Rehab*. 2006;28:1051–1060.

29. Gudbergsson SB. Life after cancer: work experiences, living conditions and impact of cancer in tumour-free cancer survivors. Doctoral Dissertation, University of Oslo, Faculty of Medicine, 2007.

30. Gudbergsson SB, Fosså SD, Borgeraas E, Dahl AA. A comparative study of living conditions in cancer patients who have returned to work after curative treatment. *Support Care Cancer*. 2006;14:1020–1029.

31. Johnsson A. [Rehabilitation from breast cancer—women who have undergone surgery and were afflicted by lymphedema—development of multidisciplinary care]. [Swedish] *Report to Cancerfonden* 2001–2003, Stockholm.

32. Belkić K. Return to healthy work for patients who have been treated for cancer: a proactive clinical perspective informed by occupational health psychology. In: Giga S, Plaxman P, Houdmont J, Ertel M, *European Academy of Occupational*

Chapter 24

Health Psychology Conference Proceedings, Series, I-WHO Publications, Nottingham, England, 2003:25.

33. Belkić K, Savić Č. The occupational stress index: an approach derived from cognitive ergonomics applicable to clinical practice. *Scand J Work Environ Health.* 2008;(Suppl 6):169–175.

34. Belkić K, Savić Č, Theorell T, Cizinsky S. *Work stressors and cardiovascular risk: Assessment for Clinical Practice* (Stress Research Report No. 256) Stockholm: Section for Stress Research Karolinska Institute and World Health Organization Psychosocial Center, 1995.

35. Belkić K. *The Occupational Stress Index: An Approach Derived from Cognitive Ergonomics and Brain Research for Clinical Practice*, Cambridge International Science Publishing, Cambridge, 2003.

Index

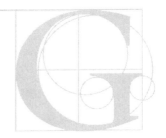

Index

Index

Index

Index

Index

Index

Index

Index

Index

Index

Index

Index

Index

Index

Index

Index

Index

Index

Index

Index

Index

S

Index

Index

Index

Index

Index